WEIGHT IN AMERICA

OBESITY, EATING DISORDERS, AND OTHER HEALTH RISKS

D1377577

ISSN 1551-2118

WEIGHT IN AMERICA
OBESITY, EATING DISORDERS, AND OTHER HEALTH RISKS

Barbara Wexler

INFORMATION PLUS® REFERENCE SERIES
Formerly Published by Information Plus, Wylie, Texas

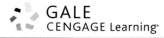

GALE
CENGAGE Learning·

Detroit • New York • San Francisco • New Haven, Conn • Waterville, Maine • London

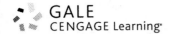

Weight in America: Obesity, Eating Disorders, and Other Health Risks

Barbara Wexler

Kepos Media, Inc.: Paula Kepos and Janice Jorgensen, Series Editors

Project Editors: Kimberley McGrath, Kathleen J. Edgar, Elizabeth Manar

Rights Acquisition and Management: Christine Myaskovsky, Kimberly Potvin

Composition: Evi Abou-El-Seoud, Mary Beth Trimper

Manufacturing: Cynde Lentz

Gale
27500 Drake Rd.
Farmington Hills, MI 48331-3535

ISBN-13: 978-0-7876-5103-9 (set)   ISBN-10: 0-7876-5103-6 (set)
ISBN-13: 978-1-4144-8150-0   ISBN-10: 1-4144-8150-0

ISSN 1551-2118

This title is also available as an e-book.
ISBN-13: 978-1-4144-9726-6 (set)
ISBN-10: 1-4144-9726-1 (set)
Contact your Gale sales representative for ordering information.

Printed in the United States of America
1 2 3 4 5   16 15 14 13 12

FD284

TABLE OF CONTENTS

PREFACE

Weight in America: Obesity, Eating Disorders, and Other Health Risks is part of the *Information Plus Reference Series*. The purpose of each volume of the series is to present the latest facts on a topic of pressing concern in modern American life. These topics include the most controversial and studied social issues of the 21st century: abortion, capital punishment, care for the elderly, crime, health care, the environment, immigration, minorities, social welfare, women, youth, and many more. Even though this series is written especially for high school and undergraduate students, it is an excellent resource for anyone in need of factual information on current affairs.

By presenting the facts, it is the intention of Gale, Cengage Learning to provide its readers with everything they need to reach an informed opinion on current issues. To that end, there is a particular emphasis in this series on the presentation of scientific studies, surveys, and statistics. These data are generally presented in the form of tables, charts, and other graphics placed within the text of each book. Every graphic is directly referred to and carefully explained in the text. The source of each graphic is presented within the graphic itself. The data used in these graphics are drawn from the most reputable and reliable sources such as from the various branches of the U.S. government and from private organizations and associations. Every effort has been made to secure the most recent information available. Readers should bear in mind that many major studies take years to conduct and that additional years often pass before the data from these studies are made available to the public. Therefore, in many cases the most recent information available in 2012 is from 2009 or 2010. Older statistics are sometimes presented as well, if they are landmark studies or of particular interest and no more-recent information exists.

Even though statistics are a major focus of the *Information Plus Reference Series*, they are by no means its only

content. Each book also presents the widely held positions and important ideas that shape how the book's subject is discussed in the United States. These positions are explained in detail and, where possible, in the words of their proponents. Some of the other material to be found in these books includes historical background, descriptions of major events related to the subject, relevant laws and court cases, and examples of how these issues play out in American life. Some books also feature primary documents or have pro and con debate sections that provide the words and opinions of prominent Americans on both sides of a controversial topic. All material is presented in an evenhanded and unbiased manner; readers will never be encouraged to accept one view of an issue over another.

HOW TO USE THIS BOOK

The United States has a serious weight problem. The majority of Americans weigh more than they should, and roughly one-third are considered obese. Overweight and obesity have serious health consequences, and their epidemic levels in the United States have had a major impact on society. Yet, overweight and obesity are not the only problems that Americans face when it comes to food. Some suffer from eating disorders, such as anorexia nervosa and bulimia nervosa, that can have a devastating effect on their health. This book brings together information from academic and governmental sources on every aspect of overweight, obesity, and eating disorders, including their prevalence in the United States, their consequences, public opinion about them, and methods to prevent them.

Weight in America: Obesity, Eating Disorders, and Other Health Risks consists of 11 chapters and three appendixes. Each chapter is devoted to a particular aspect of weight in the United States. For a summary of the information that is covered in each chapter, please see the synopses provided in the Table of Contents. Chapters generally begin with an overview of the basic facts and background information on the chapter's topic, then proceed to examine subtopics of particular interest. For example, Chapter 5: Dietary Treatment for Overweight and Obesity begins by considering the history of dieting and the changing norms for body weight over time. This is followed by a discussion of modern-day diets and products such as sugar substitutes. The next section describes the composition of Americans' diets and the development of the U.S. dietary guidelines. The chapter concludes with a section that examines how diets work and the ongoing debate about whether low-fat diets are superior to low-carbohydrate diets. Readers can find their way through a chapter by looking for the section and subsection headings, which are clearly set off from the text. They can also refer to the book's extensive Index if they already know what they are looking for.

Statistical Information

The tables and figures featured throughout *Weight in America: Obesity, Eating Disorders, and Other Health Risks* will be of particular use to readers in learning about this issue. These tables and figures represent an extensive collection of the most recent and important statistics on weight and related issues. For example, graphics cover the percentage of obese adults by state, race, and ethnicity; the prevalence of obesity among adults; the names found on ingredient labels for added sugars; dubious diet claims; and fruit and vegetable consumption rates of adults and teens. Gale, Cengage Learning believes that making this information available to readers is the most important way to fulfill the goal of this book: to help readers understand the issues and controversies surrounding overweight and obesity in the United States and reach their own conclusions about them.

Each table or figure has a unique identifier appearing above it, for ease of identification and reference. Titles for the tables and figures explain their purpose. At the end of each table or figure, the original source of the data is provided.

To help readers understand these often complicated statistics, all tables and figures are explained in the text. References in the text direct readers to the relevant statistics. Furthermore, the contents of all tables and figures are fully indexed. Please see the opening section of the Index at the back of this volume for a description of how to find tables and figures within it.

Appendixes

Besides the main body text and images, *Weight in America: Obesity, Eating Disorders, and Other Health Risks*

has three appendixes. The first is the Important Names and Addresses directory. Here, readers will find contact information for a number of government and private organizations that can provide further information on aspects of weight and eating disorders and their impact on health. The second appendix is the Resources section, which can also assist readers in conducting their own research. In this section, the author and editors of *Weight in America: Obesity, Eating Disorders, and Other Health Risks* describe some of the sources that were most useful during the compilation of this book. The final appendix is the detailed Index. It has been greatly expanded from previous editions and should make it even easier to find specific topics in this book.

ADVISORY BOARD CONTRIBUTIONS

The staff of Information Plus would like to extend its heartfelt appreciation to the Information Plus Advisory Board. This dedicated group of media professionals provides feedback on the series on an ongoing basis. Their comments allow the editorial staff who work on the project to continually make the series better and more user-friendly. The staff's top priority is to produce the highest-quality and most useful books possible, and the Information Plus Advisory Board's contributions to this process are invaluable.

The members of the Information Plus Advisory Board are:

- Kathleen R. Bonn, Librarian, Newbury Park High School, Newbury Park, California
- Madelyn Garner, Librarian, San Jacinto College, North Campus, Houston, Texas
- Anne Oxenrider, Media Specialist, Dundee High School, Dundee, Michigan
- Charles R. Rodgers, Director of Libraries, Pasco-Hernando Community College, Dade City, Florida
- James N. Zitzelsberger, Library Media Department Chairman, Oshkosh West High School, Oshkosh, Wisconsin

COMMENTS AND SUGGESTIONS

The editors of the *Information Plus Reference Series* welcome your feedback on *Weight in America: Obesity, Eating Disorders, and Other Health Risks*. Please direct all correspondence to:

Editors
Information Plus Reference Series
27500 Drake Rd.
Farmington Hills, MI 48331-3535

CHAPTER 1
AMERICANS WEIGH IN OVER TIME

More die in the United States of too much food than of too little.

—John Kenneth Galbraith, *The Affluent Society* (1998)

In 2011 more Americans were fatter than ever before—in fact, they remain the heaviest since the U.S. government started tracking patterns of body weight of the U.S. adult population during the first half of the 20th century. The Centers for Disease Control and Prevention (CDC) reports in "Obesity—Halting the Epidemic by Making Health Easier: At a Glance 2011" (May 26, 2011, http://www.cdc.gov/chronicdisease/resources/pub lications/AAG/obesity.htm) that over one-third of adults in the United States—more than 72 million—are considered obese. In "Prevalence of Overweight, Obesity, and Extreme Obesity among Adults: United States, Trends 1960–1962 through 2007–2008" (June 2010, http://www .cdc.gov/NCHS/data/hestat/obesity_adult_07_08/obesity _adult_07_08.pdf), Cynthia L. Ogden and Margaret D. Carroll discuss data from the CDC's 2007–2008 National Health and Nutrition Examination Survey. The researchers reveal that in 2007–08, 34.2% of American adults aged 20 years and older were overweight, 33.8% were obese, and 5.7% were extremely obese. Despite billions of dollars spent on diet programs, overweight and obesity are widespread and increasingly prevalent throughout the United States.

Even though Americans' body weight had been increasing incrementally during the last century, obesity skyrocketed between 1988 and 2008. Ogden and Carroll note that even though the prevalence of overweight was essentially stable during this period, obesity rose from 22.9% to 33.8%. Normal-weight adults are now a minority in the United States; nearly one-third of the adult population is obese, and childhood obesity is at an all-time high. According to the CDC, in *Obesity Trends among U.S. Adults between 1985 and 2010* (July 13, 2011, http://www.cdc.gov/obesity/downloads/obesity_trends

_2010.pdf), in 1990, 10 states had obesity prevalence rates of less than 10% and no states had rates at or above 15%. By 2010 no states had obesity prevalence rates of less than 20%, 36 states had rates of 25% or higher, and 12 of these states (Alabama, Arkansas, Kentucky, Louisiana, Michigan, Mississippi, Missouri, Oklahoma, South Carolina, Tennessee, Texas, and West Virginia) reported rates of 30% or greater. (The prevalence rate is the number of cases of a disease or condition present during a specified interval of time, usually a year, divided by the population.) Figure 1.1 maps the geographic distribution of obesity throughout the United States in 1990, 2000, and 2010.

The prevalence of obesity varies by state. According to the CDC, in 2010 Colorado reported the lowest percentage of obesity (21%), followed by Nevada (22.4%), Connecticut (22.5%), and Utah (22.5%). Mississippi reported the highest rate of obesity (34%), followed by West Virginia (32.5%), Alabama (32.2%), and Kentucky (31.3%).

An analysis of data from the CDC's 2010 Behavioral Risk Factor Surveillance System (BRFSS) and the 2007–2008 National Health and Nutrition Examination Survey reveals that the obesity epidemic affects men and women of all ages, races, ethnic origins, smoking status, and educational attainment. Even though the prevalence of obesity among U.S. adults disproportionately affects older age groups, African-Americans, and Hispanics, and declines with increasing educational attainment, no group remains untouched by this epidemic.

In "Surveillance of Health Status in Minority Communities—Racial and Ethnic Approaches to Community Health across the U.S. (REACH U.S.) Risk Factor Survey, United States, 2009" (*Morbidity and Mortality Weekly Report*, vol. 60, no. 6, May 20, 2011), Youlian Liao et al. of the CDC compare the prevalence of obesity in a representative sample of minority populations—

FIGURE 1.1

Obesity trends* among U.S. adults, 1990, 2000, and 2010

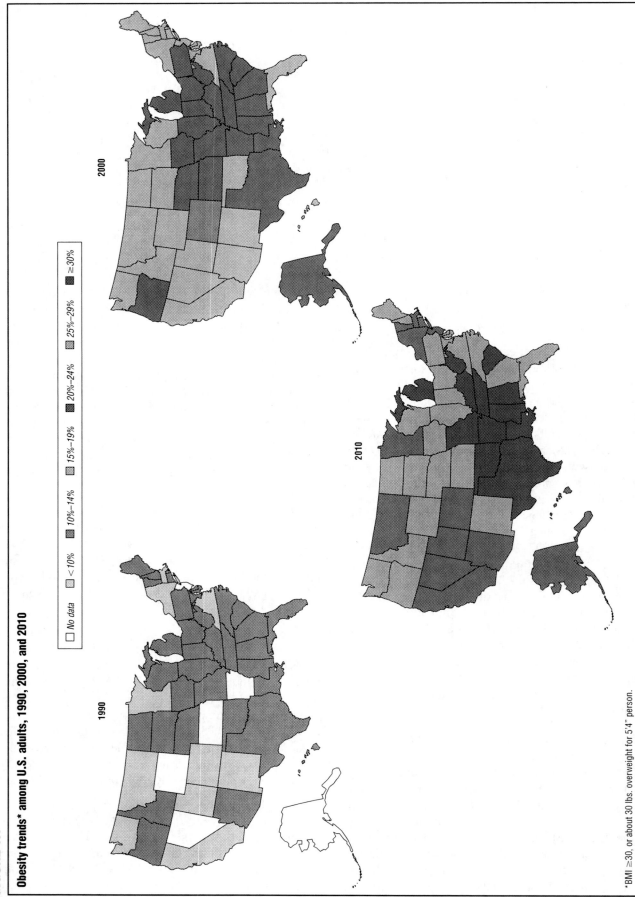

*BMI ≥30, or about 30 lbs. overweight for 5'4" person.

SOURCE: "Obesity Trends among U.S. Adults, BRFSS, 1990, 2000, 2010," in *Obesity Trends among U.S. Adults between 1985 and 2010*, Centers for Disease Control and Prevention, National Center for Chronic Disease Prevention and Health Promotion, Division of Nutrition, Physical Activity, and Obesity, July 21, 2011, http://www.cdc.gov/obesity/data/trends.html (accessed September 26, 2011)

African-American, Hispanic, Asian and Pacific Islander (A/PI), and Native American—in 28 communities located in 17 states with national prevalence data from the BRFSS. The researchers find that with the exception of the A/PI communities, the prevalence of obesity was higher in the minority populations than in the county or state in which the minority populations were located. For example, 45% of Native American men and women and African-American women were obese in the surveyed communities in 2009, compared with slightly more than a quarter of adults nationally. (See Table 1.1.) An exception were A/PIs, with an obesity prevalence of 45.3% in

TABLE 1.1

Percentage of adults who are obese in selected communities, by race/ethnicity and sex, compared with national rates, 2009

	REACH U.S. racial/ethnic populations				BRFSS
	Black	Hispanic	A/PI	AI	MMSA/county/state
Community	%	%	%	%	%
Men					
Richmond, Virginia	32.3	NA	—	—	28.6
West Philadelphia, Pennsylvania	29.2	—	—	—	29.4
Kanawha and McDowell Counties, West Virginia	41.6	—	—	—	31.8
Boston, Massachusetts	19.3	—	—	—	22.1
Charleston and Georgetown Counties, South Carolina	30.8	—	—	—	29.8
Fulton County, Georgia	21.9	—	—	—	25.4
YMCA of the Greater Cleveland, Ohio	28.9	—	—	—	28.4
Community Health Council of Los Angeles, California	31.7	—	—	—	24.1
City Neighborhoods of Chicago, Illinois	28.8	33.9	—	—	27.0
Southeast Chicago, Illinois	36.8	45.0	—	—	27.0
South Los Angeles, California	40.4	28.2	—	—	24.1
East Harlem, New York	24.9	32.0	—	—	21.8
Southwest Bronx, New York	27.1	25.9	—	—	21.8
Humboldt Park and West Town, Chicago, Illinois	32.4	35.1	—	—	27.0
YMCA of the Santa Clara Valley, California	—	28.4	—	—	17.7
Pima County, Arizona	—	36.9	—	—	28.0
Grant and Hidalgo Counties, New Mexico	—	30.6	—	—	25.7
Lawrence, Massachusetts	—	25.1	—	—	25.5
Seattle and King County, Washington	29.3	32.3	10.9	—	22.0
Los Angeles and Orange Counties, California	13.0	32.0	20.4	—	24.1
Special Service for Group, California	—	—	9.6	—	24.1
Waianae, Hawaii	—	—	45.3	—	24.5
New York City, New York	—	—	8.7	—	21.8
Orange County A/PI Community Alliance, California	—	—	4.8	—	24.1
Eastern Band of Cherokee Indians, North Carolina	—	—	—	53.6	29.9
Choctaw Nation of Oklahoma	—	—	—	39.4	32.5
Intertribal Council of Michigan	—	—	—	43.1	30.3
Oklahoma	—	—	—	49.3	32.5
Median	29.3	32.0	10.3	46.2	28.6*
Low	13.0	25.1	4.8	39.4	15.8*
High	41.6	45.0	45.3	53.6	35.0*
Women					
Richmond, Virginia	45.1	—	—	—	27.2
West Philadelphia, Pennsylvania	46.6	—	—	—	32.4
Kanawha and McDowell Counties, West Virginia	47.3	—	—	—	31.8
Boston, Massachusetts	32.5	—	—	—	17.9
Charleston and Georgetown Counties, South Carolina	48.9	—	—	—	30.9
Fulton County, Georgia	38.8	—	—	—	23.6
YMCA of the Greater Cleveland, Ohio	45.9	—	—	—	26.4
Community Health Council of Los Angeles, California	38.7	—	—	—	23.9
City Neighborhoods of Chicago, Illinois	52.1	42.3	—	—	26.6
Southeast Chicago, Illinois	48.8	51.2	—	—	26.6
South Los Angeles, California	46.3	33.7	—	—	23.9
East Harlem, New York	40.1	42.4	—	—	22.4
Southwest Bronx, New York	44.2	31.2	—	—	22.4
Humboldt Park and West Town, Chicago, Illinois	44.2	39.8	—	—	26.6
YMCA of the Santa Clara Valley, California	—	36.6	—	—	22.2
Pima County, Arizona	—	33.3	—	—	23.9
Grant and Hidalgo Counties, New Mexico	—	35.9	—	—	25.6
Lawrence, Massachusetts	—	36.9	—	—	18.7
Seattle and King County, Washington	25.4	36.2	5.8	—	20.3
Los Angeles and Orange Counties, California	39.3	41.9	8.6	—	23.9
Special Service for Group, California	—	—	6.7	—	23.9
Waianae, Hawaii	—	—	38.2	—	19.9
New York City, New York	—	—	6.6	—	22.4
Orange County A/PI Community Alliance, California	—	—	4.5	—	23.9
Eastern Band of Cherokee Indians, North Carolina	—	—	—	50.2	29.8
Choctaw Nation of Oklahoma	—	—	—	35.1	30.6
Intertribal Council of Michigan	—	—	—	55.1	29.5

TABLE 1.1

Community	REACH U.S. racial/ethnic populations				BRFSS
	Black	**Hispanic**	**A/PI**	**AI**	**MMSA/county/state**
	%	%	%	%	%
Oklahoma	—	—	—	40.7	30.6
Median	44.7	36.8	6.7	45.5	26.0*
Low	25.4	31.2	4.5	35.1	18.7*
High	52.1	51.2	38.2	55.1	36.0*

Abbreviations: AI = American Indian, A/PI = Asian/Pacific Islander, MMSA = metropolitan and micropolitan statistical area, NA = not applicable, REACH = Racial and Ethnic Approaches to Community Health, BRFSS = Behavioral Risk Factor Surveillance System.
*Data from 2009 the Behavioral Risk Factor Surveillance System (BRFSS) from the 50 states and the District of Columbia.
Note: Obesity is body mass index ≥30.0 kg/m² based on self-reported height and weight.

SOURCE: Adapted from Youlian Liao et al., "Table 7. Percentage of Adults Who are Obese, in 28 Racial and Ethnic Approaches to Community Health (REACH) U.S. Communities, 2009, and in the Comparison Populations from the Behavioral Risk Factor Surveillance System (BRFSS), 2007–2009, by Race/Ethnicity and Sex—United States," in "Surveillance of Health Status in Minority Communities—Racial and Ethnic Approaches to Community Health across the U.S. (REACH U.S.) Risk Factor Survey, United States, 2009," *Morbidity and Mortality Weekly Report*, vol. 60, no. 67, May 20, 2011, http://www.cdc.gov/mmwr/pdf/ss/ss6006.pdf (accessed September 26, 2011)

men and 38.2% in women, compared with the 24.5% of men and 19.9% of women in the general population in Waianae, Hawaii.

Obesity was not as prevalent in most A/PI communities. For example, in 2009 the median prevalence (median values are midpoints—half the population is above and half is below) of obesity among A/PI men and women was 10.3% and 6.7%, respectively, compared with a prevalence of 46.2% among Native American men and 45.5% among Native American women. (See Table 1.1.) In *F as in Fat: How Obesity Threatens America's Future, 2011* (July 2011, http://healthyamericans.org/assets/files/TFAH 2011FasInFat10.pdf), Jeffrey Levi et al. of the Trust for America's Health indicate that in 15 states more than 40% of African-Americans were obese and in four states over 35% of Latinos were obese. By contrast, whites in just four states (Kentucky, Mississippi, Tennessee, and West Virginia) had obesity rates of 30% or more.

In October 2011, amid reports of the rising tide of obesity in the United States, the Gallup-Healthways Well Being Index survey offered some of the first favorable news about Americans' weight in more than a decade. According to Roy Strom, in "Obesity Rate Declines Slightly, Study Finds" (Reuters, October 8, 2011), the survey indicates that the percentage of normal or healthy weight Americans increased slightly in 2011, rising from 35.6% in 2010 to 36.6% in 2011. However, the survey finds that overweight and obese Americans continue to constitute more than 60% of the U.S. population. Even though this survey suggests that obesity and overweight are declining, from 26.6% and 36%, respectively, in 2010 to 25.8% and 35.8%, respectively, in 2011, researchers have not pinpointed a reason for the decline. They speculate that it may be related to the economy, with more Americans choosing to eat at home rather than dining out.

In the United States many researchers believe that obesity is the second-leading cause of preventable death after smoking. There is conclusive scientific evidence that mortality (death) risk increases with increasing weight and that even slightly overweight adults—people of average height who are 10 to 20 pounds (4.5 to 9.1 kg) above their ideal weight—are at increased risk of premature death. The rising prevalence of overweight and obesity not only foretells increasing adverse effects on health and longevity but also guarantees increased costs for medical care. Overweight and obesity increase the risk of developing a range of ailments including heart disease, stroke, selected cancers, sleep apnea (interrupted breathing while sleeping), respiratory problems, osteoarthritis (loss of joint bone and cartilage), gallbladder disease, fatty liver disease (the deposition of fats, such as triglycerides in the liver, which may lead to an enlarged liver and elevated liver enzymes), and diabetes mellitus (abnormally high blood glucose resulting from the body's inability to use blood glucose for energy). Levi et al. observe that 10% of annual U.S. health care spending—an estimated $147 billion—is related to obesity and that people who are obese spend 42% more on health care than do healthy-weight people.

Overweight and obesity also exact a personal toll, with affected individuals at increased risk for emotional, psychological, and social problems. Overweight children, teens, and adults suffer from depression, low self-esteem, and other mental health and emotional problems more than their normal-weight counterparts. Along with a physical inability to participate in many activities, people who are overweight or obese may encounter weight-based stigmatization, bias, and discrimination in school and at the workplace and may be excluded from social opportunities.

TRENDS IN U.S. BIRTH WEIGHTS

Americans are not born overweight. In fact, Joyce A. Martin et al. of the CDC indicate in "Births: Final Data for 2008" (*National Vital Statistics Reports*, vol. 59, no. 1, December 8, 2010) that the mean (average) birth weight of infants born as singletons (births of one infant as opposed to twins or other multiple births) has steadily declined since 1990. (The reasons for this decline are not yet completely understood but may include changes in characteristics of mothers, such as an increase in older mothers and more preterm births and high-risk pregnancies.) In 2008 the mean birth weight for all singletons was approximately 7 pounds, 4 ounces (3,296 g). The mean birth weight for twins was 5 pounds, 2 ounces (2,330 g) and for triplets, 3 pounds, 10 ounces (1,666 g). (See Table 1.2.)

Even though the ideal birth weight varies based on the expectant mother's ethnicity, for women in the United States the average ideal birth weight is approximately 7 pounds, 8 ounces (3,402 g), close to the average weight of singletons born in 2008. In the United States the percentage of babies born with low birth weight (LBW)—less than 5 pounds, 8 ounces (2,500 g)—rose steadily between 1990 and 2006. (See Table 1.3.) According to Martin et al., the LBW rate rose from 5.9% in 1990 to 6.49% in 2006, the highest level reported in more than three decades, and then declined slightly to 6.4% in 2008. The percentage of infants with very low birth weight (VLBW)—less than 3 pounds, 4 ounces (1,500 g)—remained steady between 2000 (1.11%) and 2008 (1.11%). In 2008 more than twice as many non-Hispanic African-American mothers gave birth to LBW and VLBW infants, 11.6% and 2.49%, respectively, as did non-Hispanic white mothers (5.26% LBW and 0.82% VLBW).

LBW and VLBW are major predictors of infant morbidity (illness or disease) and mortality. For LBW infants, the risk of dying during the first year of life is more than five times that of infants born at normal weight; the risk for VLBW infants is nearly 100 times higher. The risk of delivering an LBW infant is greatest among the youngest and oldest mothers; however, many of the LBW births among older mothers are attributable to their higher rates of multiple births.

Birth Weight Influences Risk of Disease

Even though the relationship between birth weight and development of disease in adulthood is an emerging field of research, and scientists cannot yet fully explain how and why birth weight is a predictor of health and illness in later life, mounting evidence indicates that both LBW and higher-than-average birth weight are linked to future health problems. Research reveals that LBW infants are more likely than normal-weight infants to develop disease in later life. Male infants with LBW who gain weight rapidly before their first birthday appear to be at the highest risk. Researchers hypothesize that LBW infants have fewer muscle cells at birth and that rapid weight gain during the first year of life may lead to disproportionate amounts of fat to muscle and above-average body mass. Infants with LBW who later develop above-average body mass have an increased risk for developing diseases such as type 2 diabetes (an inability to produce sufficient insulin, the hormone that regulates blood glucose), hypertension (high blood pressure), and cardiovascular disease (heart disease and stroke).

Keith M. Godfrey, Hazel M. Inskip, and Mark A. Hanson find in "The Long-Term Effects of Prenatal Development on Growth and Metabolism" (*Seminars in*

TABLE 1.2

Birthweight characteristics, 2008

	Twins	Triplets	Quadruplets	Quintuplets and higher-order multiples[a]	Singletons
Number	138,660	5,877	345	46	4,102,766
Percentage very preterm[b]	11.6	38.5	56.5	89.1	1.6
Percentage preterm[c]	58.9	93.1	92.2	95.7	10.6
Mean gestational age in weeks (standard deviation)	35.3 (3.6)	32.0 (3.9)	30.7 (3.9)	28.5 (4.3)	38.7 (2.4)
Percentage very low birthweight[d]	10.1	36.1	59.9	82.2	1.1
Percentage low birthweight[e]	57.0	94.6	98.6	93.3	6.4
Mean birthweight in grams (standard deviation)	2,330 (628)	1,666 (567)	1,371 (489)	1,253 (806)	3,296 (561)

[a]Quintuplets, sextuplets, and higher-order multiple births are not differentiated in the national data set.
[b]Less than 32 completed weeks of gestation.
[c]Less than 37 completed weeks of gestation.
[d]Less than 1,500 grams.
[e]Less than 2,500 grams.

SOURCE: Joyce A. Martin et al., "Table H. Gestational Age and Birthweight Characteristics, by Plurality: United States, 2008," in "Births: Final Data for 2008," *National Vital Statistics Reports*, vol. 59, no.1, December 8, 2010, http://www.cdc.gov/nchs/data/nvsr/nvsr59/nvsr59_01.pdf (accessed September 26, 2011)

TABLE 1.3

Percentage of low birthweights and very low birthweights by race and Hispanic origin, selected years, 1990–2008

Year	Very low birthweight[a]	Low birthweight[b]
All races[c]		
2008	1.11	6.40
2007	1.14	6.45
2006	1.14	6.49
2005	1.14	6.41
2000	1 11	6.00
1995	1.08	6.05
1990	1.05	5.90
Non-Hispanic white[d]		
2008	0.82	5.26
2007	0.83	5.32
2006	0 85	5.37
2005	0.84	5.32
2000	0.80	4.88
1995	0.78	4.87
1990	0.73	4.56
Non-Hispanic black[d]		
2008	2.49	11.60
2007	2.65	11.78
2006	2.61	11.85
2005	2.71	11.90
2000	2.62	11.28
1995	2.55	11.66
1990	2.54	11.92
Hispanic[e]		
2008	0.96	5.74
2007	0.97	5.74
2006	0.98	5.79
2005	0.97	5.69
2000	0.94	5.36
1995	0.93	5.36
1990[f]	0.87	5.23

[a]Less than 1,500 grams (3 lb.4 oz.)
[b]Less than 2,500 grams (5 lb. 8 oz.)
[c]Includes races other than white and black and origin not stated.
[d]Race and Hispanic origin are reported separately on birth certificates. Persons of Hispanic origin may be of any race. Race categories are consistent with 1977 Office of Management and Budget standards. Thirty states reported multiple-race data for 2008 that were bridged to single-race categories for comparability with other states.
[e]Includes all persons of Hispanic origin of any race.
[f]Excludes NewHampshire and Oklahoma, which did not report Hispanic origin.

SOURCE: Joyce A. Martin et al., "Table F. Percentage of Singleton Births of Very Low and Low Birthweight, by Race and Hispanic Origin of Mother: United States, 1990, 1995, 2000, and 2005–2008," in "Births: Final Data for 2008," *National Vital Statistics Reports*, vol. 59, no.1, December 8, 2010, http://www.cdc.gov/nchs/data/nvsr/nvsr59/nvsr59_01.pdf (accessed September 26, 2011)

Reproductive Medicine, vol. 29, no. 3, May 2011) that LBW and poor rates of infant growth and development are associated with an increased risk for cardiovascular disease (diseases of the heart and blood vessels), type 2 diabetes, and osteoporosis (thinning of the bones that makes them more likely to fracture). The risk of developing these diseases increases when restricted early growth and development are followed by increased weight gain during childhood. The researchers also note that abnormally high birth weights are associated with an increased risk for obesity and type 2 diabetes.

LBW has also been linked to the development of asthma. In "Is the Association between Low Birth Weight and Asthma Independent of Genetic and Shared Environmental Factors?" (*American Journal of Epidemiology*, vol. 169, no. 11, June 1, 2009), a study of 21,588 twins, Eduardo Villamor, Anastasia Iliadou, and Sven Cnattingius find that LBW is associated with asthma during childhood and adult life.

Evidence also indicates that birth weight is related to a risk of developing breast cancer. Xiaohui Xu et al. consider 18 epidemiological (population) studies that detail 16,424 cases of breast cancer to determine whether birth weight influenced the risk of developing breast cancer in adulthood. The results of the study were published in "Birth Weight as a Risk Factor for Breast Cancer: A Meta-analysis of 18 Epidemiological Studies" (*Journal of Women's Health*, vol. 18, no. 8, August 2009). The researchers find that women who weighed more than 8 pounds, 13 ounces (4,000 g) when they were born were at greater risk for breast cancer than women who had birth weights of less than 5 pounds, 8 ounces to 6 pounds, 10 ounces (2,500 to 3,000 g) and that this risk followed a classic dose-response pattern—each incremental increase in birth weight increased the risk of developing the disease.

Athanasios Michos, Fei Xue, and Karin B. Michels indicate in "Birth Weight and the Risk of Testicular Cancer: A Meta-Analysis" (*International Journal of Cancer*, vol. 121, no. 5, September 1, 2007) that both LBW and high birth weight (HBW; greater than 8 pounds, 13 ounces) increase the risk of testicular cancer in men. Men with LBW were 18% more likely and men with HBW were 12% more likely to develop testicular cancer than men of average birth weight.

HBW is also associated with an increased risk for childhood cancer. Michael R. Sprehe et al. observe in "Comparison of Birth Weight Corrected for Gestational Age and Birth Weight Alone in Prediction of Development of Childhood Leukemia and Central Nervous System Tumors" (*Pediatric Blood Cancers*, vol. 54, no. 2, February 2010) that HBW is most closely linked to an increased risk of developing acute lymphoblastic leukemia (a cancer of the blood and bone marrow and one of the most common cancers in children).

In "Birth Size, Infant Weight Gain, and Motor Development Influence Adult Physical Performance" (*Medicine and Science in Sports and Exercise*, vol. 41, no. 6, June 2009), Charlotte L. Ridgway et al. look at birth weight as an influence on adult physical performance measures, including muscle strength, endurance, and aerobic fitness. The researchers find that LBW is associated with impaired aerobic fitness and a higher resting pulse rate in adulthood, independent of adult body size. Higher birth weight is associated with earlier motor development, as evidenced in standing unaided and walking at younger ages. It is also associated with increased handgrip strength in adolescents, young adults, and even in older adults, which suggests that the effects of birth weight on physical performance may be lifelong. Higher birth weight, greater infant weight gain, and earlier motor development were independently associated with muscle strength and endurance, whereas higher birth weight and lower infant weight gain were associated with higher levels of aerobic fitness. Ridgway et al. explain that the link between higher birth weight and greater muscle strength and endurance may in part reflect the relationship between birth weight and lean muscle in adults— people with higher birth weights are likely to have increased muscle mass. Similarly, the relationship between lower infant weight gain and improved aerobic fitness may be attributable to the fact that rapid weight gain during infancy may preferentially produce fat rather than lean muscle tissue.

The only action that can alter the birth weight of an infant is if the mother modifies her weight gain during the pregnancy. In 2011 most health professionals concurred that for normal-weight women the optimal weight gain during pregnancy ranged between 15 and 25 pounds (6.8 and 11.3 kg) of fat and lean mass. Furthermore, the landmark study "Composition of Gestational Weight Gain Impacts Maternal Fat Retention and Infant Birth Weight" (*American Journal of Obstetrics and Gynecology*, vol. 189, no. 5, November 2003) conducted by Nancy F. Butte et al. of the Children's Nutrition Research Center in Houston, Texas, reveals that a newborn's birth weight and the mother's postpregnancy weight are influenced not only by how much weight is gained during the pregnancy but also by the source of the excess weight. The researchers conducted body scans of 63 women before, during, and after their pregnancies and recorded changes in the women's weight from water, protein, fat, and potassium—a marker for changes in muscle tissue, which is one component of lean mass. Butte et al. find that increases in lean mass, and not fat mass, appeared to influence infant size. Independent of how much fat the women gained during pregnancy, only lean body mass increased the birth weight of the infant, with women who gained more lean body mass giving birth to larger infants.

In "The Effects of Maternal Weight Gain Patterns on Term Birth Weight in African-American Women" (*Journal of Maternal-Fetal and Neonatal Medicine*, vol. 23, no. 8, August 2010), Vinod K. Misra, Calvin J. Hobel, and Charles F. Sing examine the relationship between maternal weight gain at different times during pregnancy and infant birth weight in African-Americans and compare these findings to those of non-African-Americans. The researchers chose to focus on African-Americans because as a group they are at higher risk for preterm delivery, LBW, and higher rates of infant mortality than other Americans. Misra, Hobel, and Sing also wondered whether the timing of weight gain during pregnancy was related to birth weight. By measuring maternal weight gain at three time points during pregnancy, the researchers were able to distinguish how birth weight was influenced by the magnitude and rate of change of maternal weight during each trimester of pregnancy. Misra, Hobel, and Sing find that African-American women gained weight more consistently throughout the course of pregnancy rather than later in pregnancy. Furthermore, the researchers note that among non-African-American women weight gain during the latter part of pregnancy strongly influenced birth weight, whereas among African-American women variation in maternal weight gain during the first half of pregnancy was more closely associated with a variation in birth weight.

FIRST WEEK OF LIFE MAY DETERMINE ADULT OBESITY. Research demonstrates that LBW and low weight gain during infancy are associated with coronary heart disease. Similarly, research indicates that rapid weight gain in infancy is shown to predict obesity in childhood. In 2004 a landmark study funded by the National Institutes of Health and conducted at the Children's Hospital of Philadelphia, the University of Pennsylvania School of Medicine, and the University of Iowa Fomon Infant Nutrition Unit sought to determine which periods of weight gain in infancy might be associated with adult obesity.

In "Weight Gain in the First Week of Life and Overweight in Adulthood: A Cohort Study of European American Subjects Fed Infant Formula" (*Circulation*, vol. 111, no. 15, April 19, 2005), Nicolas Stettler et al. review the data for 653 subjects who had been weighed on seven occasions during infancy and were contacted when they were young adults, aged 20 to 32 years, when they again reported their height and weight. The researchers pinpointed the period between birth and age eight days as potentially critical because weight gain during the first week of life was associated with adulthood overweight status. The formula-fed babies who gained weight rapidly during their first week of life were significantly more likely to be overweight decades later. Stettler et al. conclude that "in formula-fed infants, weight gain during the first week of life may be a critical determinant for the development of obesity several decades later." The researchers also observe that their findings reinforce the recommendation by the American Academy of Pediatrics that infants should be exclusively breast-fed for the first six months of life. Among the many health benefits associated with breast-feeding is the fact that breast-fed babies are much less likely than formula-fed babies to become obese adults.

Ellen W. Demerath et al. report in "Rapid Postnatal Weight Gain and Visceral Adiposity in Adulthood: The Fels Longitudinal Study" (*Obesity*, vol. 17, no. 11,

November 2009) that rapid infant weight gain is associated not only with an increased risk for obesity but also with excess deposits of fat in the abdomen and in the abdomen surrounding internal organs. Abdominal obesity is associated with an increased risk for heart disease, diabetes, fatty liver, and other health problems.

A high-calorie diet in infancy predicts not only faster early weight gain but also greater fat mass in childhood, which in turn increases the risk of obesity in adulthood. In "Nutrition in Infancy and Long-Term Risk of Obesity: Evidence from 2 Randomized Controlled Trials" (*American Journal of Nutrition*, vol. 92, no. 5, November 2010), Atul Singhal et al. report the results of a rigorous long-term study that followed infants randomly assigned to receive either a control formula or a formula containing more protein and calories than the control formula. When the children were examined at ages five and eight, those who had received the nutrient-rich formula had increased fat mass.

DEFINING AND ASSESSING IDEAL WEIGHT, OVERWEIGHT, AND OBESITY

Historically, the determination of desirable, healthy, or ideal weights have been derived from demographic and actuarial statistics (data compiled to assess insurance risk and formulate insurance premiums). The National Center for Health Statistics (NCHS) compiles and analyzes demographic data (the heights and weights of a representative sample of the U.S. population) to develop standards for desirable weight. In 1943 the Metropolitan Life Insurance Company (MetLife) introduced standard weight-for-height tables for men and women based on an analysis of actuarial data. The MetLife weight-for-height tables assisted adults in determining if their weight was within an appropriate range for height and frame size. Revised in 1959 and 1983, the tables were based on actuarial data, in which desirable or ideal weight was defined as the weight for height that was associated with the lowest mortality rate, or longest life span, among the client population of adults (policyholders) insured by MetLife.

Even though the MetLife and other weight-for-height tables remained in use in 2011, many health professionals and medical researchers believe these tables have limited utility. Nearly every weight-for-height table shows different acceptable weight ranges for men and women, and considerable debate continues among health professionals over which table to use. The tables lack information about body composition, such as the ratio of fat to lean muscle mass; their data are derived primarily from white populations and do not represent the entire U.S. population; they generally do not take age into consideration; and it is often unclear how the frame size is determined. Furthermore, it is now known that ideal, healthy, or low-risk weight varies for different populations and varies for the same population at different times and in relation to different causes of morbidity and mortality.

The limitations of weight-for-height tables have prompted health care practitioners and researchers to adopt other measures that allow comparison of weight independent of height and frame across populations to define desirable or healthy weight as well as overweight and obesity. For example, the *Dietary Guidelines for Americans, 2010* (December 2010, http://health.gov/dietaryguidelines/dga2010/DietaryGuidelines2010.pdf), which is published jointly by the U.S. Department of Health and Human Services and the U.S. Department of Agriculture (USDA), uses the body mass index (BMI), a measure that incorporates height and weight to categorize adult body weight as underweight, healthy weight, overweight, or obese. Because children and adolescents are growing, their BMIs are plotted on a curve that compares them to children of the same age and sex. (See Table 1.4.) A child's relative position on this curve indicates whether he or she is underweight, healthy weight, overweight, or obese.

Overweight is generally defined as excess body weight in relation to height, when compared with a predetermined standard of acceptable, desirable, or ideal weight. One definition characterizes individuals as overweight if they are between 10 and 30 pounds (4.5 and 13.6 kg) heavier than the desirable weight for height. Overweight does not necessarily result from excessive body fat; people may become overweight as the result of an increase in lean muscle. For example, even though muscular bodybuilders with minimal body fat frequently weigh more than nonathletes of the same height, they are overweight because of their increased muscle mass rather than increased fat.

Rather than viewing overweight and obesity as distinct conditions, many researchers prefer to consider weight as a curve or continuum with obesity at the far end of the curve. People who are obese constitute a subset of the overweight population. In this definition, only some overweight people are obese, but all obese people are overweight.

Similarly, there is still no uniform definition of obesity. Some health professionals describe anyone who is more than 30 pounds (13.6 kg) above his or her desirable weight for height as obese. Others assert that body weight 20% or more above desirable or ideal body weight constitutes obesity. Extreme or clinically severe obesity is often defined as weight twice the desirable weight or 100 pounds (45.4 kg) more than the desirable weight. Obesity is also defined as an excessively high amount of adipose tissue (body fat) in relation to lean body mass such as muscle and bone. The amount of body fat (also known as adiposity), the distribution of fat throughout the body, and the size of the adipose tissue deposits are also used

TABLE 1.4

Defining overweight and obesity, 2010

Body weight status can be categorized as underweight, healthy weight, overweight, or obese. Body mass index (BMI) is a useful tool that can be used to estimate an individual's body weight status. BMI is a measure of weight in kilograms (kg) relative to height in meters (m) squared. The terms overweight and obese describe ranges of weight that are greater than what is considered healthy for a given height, while underweight describes a weight that is lower than what is considered healthy for a given height. These categories are a guide, and some people at a healthy weight also may have weight-responsive health conditions. Because children and adolescents are growing, their BMI is plotted on growth charts for sex and age. The percentile indicates the relative position of the child's BMI among children of the same sex and age.

Category	Children and adolescents (BMI for age percentile range)	Adults (BMI)
Underweight	Less than the 5th percentile	Less than 18.5 kg/m^2
Healthy weight	5th percentile to less than the 85th percentile	18.5 to 24.9 kg/m^2
Overweight	85th percentile to less than the 95th percentile	25.0 to 29.9 kg/m^2
Obese	Equal to or greater than the 95th percentile	30.0 kg/m^2 or greater

SOURCE: "Overweight and Obese: What Do They Mean?" in *Dietary Guidelines for Americans, 2010*, 7th ed., U.S. Department of Health and Human Services and U.S. Department of Agriculture, December 2010, http://health.gov/dietaryguidelines/dga2010/DietaryGuidelines2010.pdf (accessed September 26, 2011)

to assess obesity because the location and distribution of body fat are considered to be important predictors of the health risks that are associated with obesity. The location and distribution of body fat may be measured by the ratio of waist-to-hip circumference. High ratios have been associated with higher risks of morbidity and mortality.

Historically, overweight and obese body types have been characterized as apple- or pear-shaped, depending on the anatomical site where fat is more prominent. In the apple or android type of obesity, fat is mainly located in the trunk (upper body, nape of the neck, shoulder, and abdomen). Gynoid obesity, or the pear-shape, features rounded hips and more fat located in the buttocks, thighs, and lower abdomen. Fat cells around the waist, flank, and abdomen are more active metabolically than those in the thighs, hips, and buttocks. This increased metabolic activity is thought to produce the increased health risks that are associated with android obesity. In general, women are more likely to have gynoid obesity.

Research reported in the March 26, 2011, issue of the *Lancet* disputes the relationship between abdominal obesity (android obesity) and the increased risk for cardiovascular disease. In "Separate and Combined Associations of Body-Mass Index and Abdominal Adiposity with Cardiovascular Disease: Collaborative Analysis of 58 Prospective Studies" (vol. 377, no. 9771), investigators in the Emerging Risk Factors Collaboration who tracked 221,934 adults for nearly a decade find that even though obesity (BMI greater than 30) significantly increases the risk for cardiovascular disease, the distribution of the excess fat does not appear to influence this risk. The investigators deemed all distributions of body fat equally harmful in terms of heart health and suggest that in addition to obesity, high blood pressure and cholesterol and a history of diabetes are important predictors of future risk of developing cardiovascular disease.

There are many ways to measure body fat. Weighing an individual underwater in a laboratory with specialized equipment provides a highly accurate assessment of body fat. By performing hydrostatic or underwater weighing, an examiner obtains an estimate of whole-body density and uses this to calculate the percentage of the body that is fat. First, the subject is weighed on a land scale. The subject then puts on a diver's belt with weights to prevent floating during the weighing procedure, sits on a chair that is suspended from a precision scale, and is completely submerged. When maximum expiration of breath is achieved, the subject remains in this submerged position for about 10 seconds while the investigator reads the scale. This procedure is repeated as many as 10 times to obtain reliable, consistent values. The weight of the diver's belt and chair are subtracted from this weight to obtain the true value of the subject's mass in water.

Simpler, but potentially less accurate assessments of body fat include skinfold thickness measurements, which involve measuring subcutaneous (immediately below the skin) fat deposits using an instrument called a caliper in locations such as the upper arm. Skinfold thickness measurements rely on the fact that a certain fraction of total body fat is subcutaneous and by using a representative sample of that fat, the overall body fatness (density) may be predicted. Several skinfold measurements are obtained, and the values are used in equations to calculate body density. Using a caliper, the examiner grasps a fold of skin and subcutaneous fat firmly, pulling it away from the underlying muscle tissue that follows the natural contour of the skin. The caliper jaws exert a relatively constant tension at the point of contact and measure skinfold thickness in millimeters. Most obesity researchers believe there is an acceptable correlation between skinfold thickness and body fat—that it is possible to estimate body fatness from the use of skinfold calipers. Skinfold thickness measurements are considered more subjective than underwater weights because the accuracy of measurements of skinfold thickness depends on the skill and technique of the examiner, and there may be variations in readings from one examiner to another.

Another technique used to evaluate body fat is bioelectric impedance analysis (BIA). BIA offers an indirect estimate of body fat and lean body mass. It entails passing an electrical current through the body and assessing the body's ability to conduct the current. It is based on the principle that resistance is inversely proportional to total body water when an electrical current (with a frequency of 70 megahertz) is applied through several electrodes that are placed on body extremities. Because greater conductivity occurs when there is a higher percentage of body water and because a higher percentage of body water indicates larger amounts of muscle and other lean tissue (fat cells contain less water than muscle cells), people with less fat are better able to conduct electrical current. BIA has been shown to correlate well with total body fat that has been assessed by other methods.

Other means of estimating the location and distribution of body fat include waist-to-hip circumference ratios and imaging techniques such as ultrasound, computed tomography, or magnetic resonance imaging.

Waist Circumference and Waist-to-Hip Ratio

Along with height and weight, waist circumference is a common measure used to assess abdominal fat content. An excess of body fat in the abdomen or upper body is considered to increase the risk of developing heart disease, high blood pressure, diabetes, stroke, and certain cancers. Like body fat, health risks increase as the waist circumference increases. For men, a waist circumference greater than 40 inches (101.6 cm) is considered to confer increased health risks. Women are considered at increased risk when a waist measurement is 35 inches (88.9 cm) or greater. Waist-circumference measures lose their incremental predictive value in people with a BMI greater than or equal to 35 because these individuals generally exceed the cutoff points for increased risk. Table 1.5 shows the relationship between BMI, waist circumference, and dis-

ease risk for people who are underweight, normal weight, overweight, obese, and extremely obese.

In fact, research demonstrates that clothing size, which serves as a surrogate for waist circumference, can help predict disease risk. Laura A. E. Hughes et al. find that skirt and trouser sizes correlate well with waist-circumference measurements and that bigger skirt and trouser sizes are associated with a greater risk of developing selected cancers. In "Self-Reported Clothing Size as a Proxy Measure for Body Size" (*Epidemiology*, vol. 20, no. 5, September 2009), Hughes et al. indicate that the skirt size predicts the risk for endometrial cancer (cancer of the lining of the uterus) and the trouser size predicts the risk for renal cell carcinoma (kidney cancer).

The waist-to-hip ratio is the ratio of waist circumference to hip circumference, which is calculated by dividing waist circumference by hip circumference. For men and women, a waist-to-hip ratio of 1 or more is considered to place them at greater risk. Most people store body fat at the waist and abdomen (android body fat distribution) or at the hips (gynoid body fat distribution).

Body Mass Index

BMI is a single number that evaluates an individual's weight status in relation to height. It does not directly measure the percent of body fat; however, it offers a more accurate assessment of overweight and obesity than weight alone. It is a direct calculation based on height and weight, and it is not gender specific. BMI is the preferred measurement of health care professionals and obesity researchers to assess body fat and is the most common method of tracking overweight and obesity among adults. BMI, which is calculated by dividing weight in kilograms by the square of height in meters, classifies people as underweight, normal weight, overweight, or

TABLE 1.5

Classification of overweight and obesity by body mass index (BMI), waist circumference, and associated disease risk

	BMI (kg/m^2)	Obesity class	Men ≤ 102 cm (≤ 40 in) Women ≤ 88 cm (≤ 35 in)	> 102 cm (> 40 in) > 88 cm (> 35 in)
			Disease risk[a] relative to normal weight and waist circumference	
Underweight	<18.5		—	—
Normal[b]	18.5–24.9		—	—
Overweight	25.0–29.9		Increased	High
Obesity	30.0–34.9	I	High	Very high
	35.0–39.9	II	Very high	Very high
Extreme obesity	≥40	III	Extremely high	Extremely high

[a]Disease risk for type 2 diabetes, hypertension, and cardiovascular disease.
[b]Increased waist circumference can also be a marker for increased risk even in persons of normal weight.

SOURCE: "Table ES-4. Classification of Overweight and Obesity by BMI, Waist Circumference, and Associated Disease Risk," in *Clinical Guidelines on the Identification, Evaluation, and Treatment of Overweight and Obesity in Adults: The Evidence Report*, National Institutes of Health, National Heart, Lung, and Blood Institute in cooperation with The National Institute of Diabetes and Digestive and Kidney Diseases, September 1998, http://www.ncbi.nlm.nih.gov/books/NBK2003/pdf/TOC.pdf (accessed September 28, 2011)

TABLE 1.6

How to calculate body mass index (BMI)

You can calculate BMI as follows

$$BMI = \frac{Weight\ (kg)}{Height\ squared\ (m^2)}$$

If pounds and inches are used

$$BMI = \frac{Weight\ (pounds) \times 703}{Height\ squared\ (inches^2)}$$

Calculation directions and sample

Here is a shortcut method for calculating BMI. (Example: for a person who is 5 feet 5 inches tall weighing 180 lbs.)

1. Multiply weight (in pounds) by 703

$$180 \times 703 = 126,540$$

2. Multiply height (in inches) by height (in inches)

$$65 \times 65 = 4,225$$

3. Divide the answer in step 1 by the answer in step 2 to get the BMI.

$$126,540/4,225 = 29.9$$

$$BMI = 29.9$$

SOURCE: "You Can Calculate BMI As Follows," in *The Practical Guide: Identification, Evaluation, and Treatment of Overweight and Obesity in Adults*, National Institutes of Health, National Heart, Lung, and Blood Institute, North American Association for the Study of Obesity, October 2000, http://www.nhlbi.nih.gov/guidelines/obesity/prctgd_b.pdf (accessed September 28, 2011)

obese. Table 1.6 shows the formula used to calculate BMI when height is measured in either inches or centimeters and weight is measured in either pounds or kilograms.

The World Health Organization and the National Institutes of Health consider individuals overweight when their BMI is between 25 and 29.9, and they are classified as obese when their BMI exceeds 30. Table 1.7 shows the relationship between height, weight, and BMI. Table 1.5 shows the classification of overweight and obesity by BMI and distinguishes between three levels of obesity. Table 1.8 shows weights in pounds and kilograms that represent the three levels of obesity at two different heights: 5 feet, 4 inches and 5 feet, 9 inches.

BMI is a simple, inexpensive tool for assessing weight, but it has several limitations. BMI may deem muscular athletes overweight when they are extremely fit and excess weight is the result of a larger amount of lean muscle. It may similarly misrepresent the health of older adults who as the result of muscle wasting (loss of muscle mass) may be considered to have a normal or healthy weight when they may actually be nutritionally depleted or overweight in terms of body fat composition. Even though it is an imperfect method for assessing individuals, BMI is extremely useful for tracking weight trends in the population.

BMI AND WAIST CIRCUMFERENCE ARE USEFUL MEASURES. In late 2011 the American Heart Association (AHA) issued a statement that was published by Marc-Andre Cornier et al. in "Assessing Adiposity: A Scientific Statement from the American Heart Association" (*Circulation*, vol. 124, no. 18, November 1, 2011). The AHA endorses the use of BMI and waist-circumference measurements as the primary tools for assessing adiposity largely because they are simple, reliable clinical tools. It acknowledges other methods of evaluating overweight and obesity, such as skin-fold thickness, underwater weighing, and imaging methods (e.g., computed tomography, which is used primarily in research settings to produce multiple sliced images of the body and identify deposits of fat in various locations in the body), but states that there is insufficient evidence to advocate these and other methods in daily clinical practice.

Definitions and Estimates of Prevalence Vary

Historically, varying definitions of, and criteria for, overweight and obesity have affected prevalence statistics and made it difficult to compare data. Some overweight- and obesity-related prevalence rates are crude or unadjusted estimates; others are age-adjusted estimates that offer different values. Early efforts to track overweight and obesity in the U.S. population relied on the 1943, 1959, and 1983 MetLife tables of desirable weight-for-height as the reference standard for overweight. During the last three decades, most government agencies and public health organizations have estimated overweight using data from a series of surveys conducted by the NCHS. These surveys include the National Health Examination Surveys, the National Health and Nutrition Examination Surveys (NHANES), and the BRFSS.

Despite changing definitions of overweight and obesity and various methods to track changes in the U.S. population, there is irrefutable evidence that the prevalence of overweight and obesity has steadily increased among people of both genders, all ages, all racial and ethnic groups, all educational levels, and all smoking levels. The prevalence of obesity in the United States was first reported in the 1960 National Health Examination Survey, and subsequent reports were derived from three NHANES: NHANES I, 1971; NHANES II, 1976–80; and NHANES III, 1988–94. Most obesity data referenced in the medical literature in 2011 were drawn from the NHANES study conducted between 2003 and 2008 and the 1997 to 2011 National Health Interview Studies, along with several other national studies. Data from the 1960 National Health Examination Survey, NHANES I, and NHANES II indicated that the prevalence of obesity was relatively constant between 1960 and 1980; however, the results of the NHANES III and the NHANES conducted between 2003 and 2008 indicated a sharp increase

TABLE 1.7

Adult BMI (body mass index) chart

BMI	19	20	21	22	23	24	25	26	27	28	29	30	31	32	33	34	35
Height	Healthy weight						Overweight (Weight in pounds)					Obese					
4'10"	91	96	100	105	110	115	119	124	129	134	138	143	148	153	158	162	167
4'11"	94	99	104	109	114	119	124	128	133	138	143	148	153	158	163	168	173
5'	97	102	107	112	118	123	128	133	138	143	148	153	158	163	168	174	179
5'1"	100	106	111	116	122	127	132	137	143	148	153	158	164	169	174	180	185
5'2"	104	109	115	120	126	131	136	142	147	153	158	164	169	175	180	186	191
5'3"	107	113	118	124	130	135	141	146	152	158	163	169	175	180	186	191	197
5'4"	110	116	122	128	134	140	145	151	157	163	169	174	180	186	192	197	204
5'5"	114	120	126	132	138	144	150	156	162	168	174	180	186	192	198	204	210
5'6"	118	124	130	136	142	148	155	161	167	173	179	186	192	198	204	210	216
5'7"	121	127	134	140	146	153	159	166	172	178	185	191	198	204	211	217	223
5'8"	125	131	138	144	151	158	164	171	177	184	190	197	203	210	216	223	230
5'9"	128	135	142	149	155	162	169	176	182	189	196	203	209	216	223	230	236
5'10"	132	139	146	153	160	167	174	181	188	195	202	209	216	222	229	236	243
5'11"	136	143	150	157	165	172	179	186	193	200	208	215	222	229	236	243	250
6'	140	147	154	162	169	177	184	191	199	206	213	221	228	235	242	250	258
6'1"	144	151	159	166	174	182	189	197	204	212	219	227	235	242	250	257	265
6'2"	148	155	163	171	179	186	194	202	210	218	225	233	241	249	256	264	272
6'3"	152	160	168	176	184	192	200	208	216	224	232	240	248	256	264	272	279

Notes: Locate the height of interest in the left-most column and read across the row for that height to the weight of interest. Follow the column of the weight up to the top row that lists the BMI. BMI of 18.5–24.9 is the healthy range, BMI of 25–29.9 is the overweight range, and BMI of 30 and above is the obese range.

SOURCE: "Figure 2. Adult BMI Chart," in *Dietary Guidelines for Americans, 2005*, 6th ed., U.S. Department of Health and Human Services and U.S. Department of Agriculture, January 2005, http://www.health.gov/dietaryguidelines/dga2005/document/pdf/DGA2005.pdf (accessed September 28, 2011)

TABLE 1.8

Obesity cut points for adults 5'4" and 5'9"

Height	Obesity class I	Obesity class II	Obesity class III
5'4"	174 pounds	204 pounds	232 pounds
5'4"	79 kilograms	93 kilograms	105 kilograms
5'9"	203 pounds	236 pounds	270 pounds
5'9"	92 kilograms	107 kilograms	123 kilograms

SOURCE: Margot Shields, Margaret D. Carroll, and Cynthia L. Ogden, "Table. Obesity Cut Points for Adults 5'4" and 5'9," in "Adult Obesity Prevalence in Canada and the United States," *NCHS Data Brief*, no. 56, National Center for Health Statistics, March 2011, http://www.cdc.gov/nchs/data/databriefs/db56.pdf (accessed September 30, 2011).

FIGURE 1.2

Overweight and obesity in adults age 20 and older by sex, 1988–2008

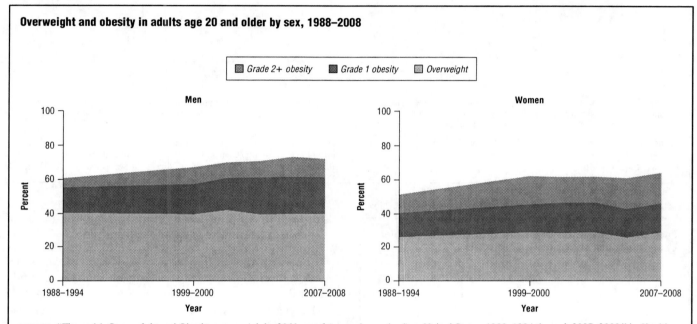

SOURCE: "Figure 14. Overweight and Obesity among Adults 20 Years of Age and over, by Sex: United States, 1988–1994 through 2007–2008," in *Health, United States, 2010: With Special Feature on Death and Dying*, Centers for Disease Control and Prevention, National Center for Health Statistics, 2011, http://www.cdc.gov/nchs/data/hus/hus10.pdf#listtables (accessed September 30, 2011)

in the prevalence of obesity between the late 1980s and 2008.

Overweight and obesity have steadily progressed at an alarming rate over the course of the past three decades. Margot Shields, Margaret D. Carroll, and Cynthia L. Ogden observe in "Adult Obesity Prevalence in Canada and the United States" (*NCHS Data Brief*, no. 56, March 2011) that in the United States the prevalence of obesity in 2007–09 was 34.4%. Between 1988 and 2008 the prevalence of obesity rose among people of all ages.

The NHANES findings reported by the NCHS in *Health, United States, 2010* (2011, http://www.cdc.gov/nchs/data/hus/hus10.pdf) reveal that even though the proportion of American adults who are overweight but not obese held steady at about 40% of men aged 20 years and older from 1988–94 to 2007–08, the prevalence of grade-1 obesity (BMI greater than or equal to 30 but less than

35) rose from 15% to 22% and grade-2 obesity (BMI greater than 35) rose from 5% to 11%. (See Figure 1.2.) Among women aged 20 years and older during this same period, the prevalence of overweight rose from 26% to 29%, grade-1 obesity grew from 15% to 18%, and grade-2 obesity increased from 11% to 18%.

Data from the National Health Interview Study (NHIS) reveal that the prevalence of obesity among adults aged 20 years and older has increased over time, from 19.4% in 1997 to 29.5% in March 2011. (See Figure 1.3.) The prevalence of overweight and obesity generally increases with advancing age, then starts to decline among people over the age of 60 years. In 2011 for men and women combined, the prevalence of obesity was highest among adults aged 40 to 59 years (32.4%) and lowest among adults aged 60 years and older (27.5%). (See Figure 1.4.) There was no significant

FIGURE 1.3

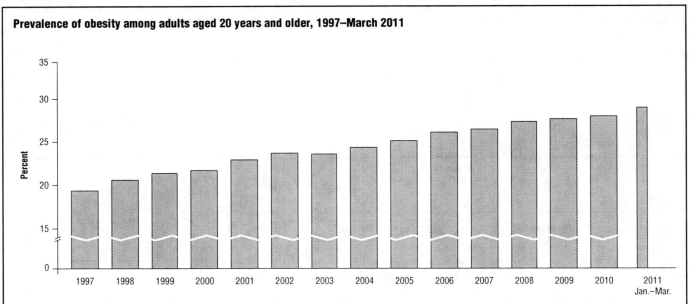

Prevalence of obesity among adults aged 20 years and older, 1997–March 2011

Notes: Data are based on household interviews of a sample of the civilian noninstitutionalized population. Obesity is defined as a body mass index (BMI) of 30 kg/m² or more. The measure is based on self-reported height (m) and weight (kg). Estimates of obesity are restricted to adults aged 20 and over for consistency with the *Healthy People 2010* (3) program. The analyses excluded people with unknown height or weight (about 6% of respondents each year).

SOURCE: P. M. Barnes et al., "Figure 6.1. Prevalence of Obesity among Adults Aged 20 Years and over: United States, 1997–March 2011," in *Early Release of Selected Estimates Based on Data from the January–March 2011 National Health Interview Survey,* Centers for Disease Control and Prevention, National Center for Health Statistics, September 2011, http://www.cdc.gov/nchs/data/nhis/earlyrelease/201109_06.pdf (accessed September 30, 2011)

FIGURE 1.4

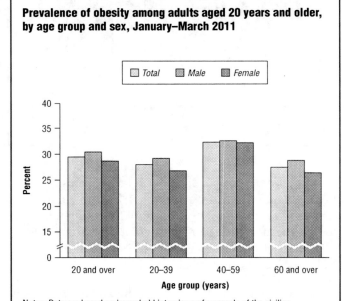

Prevalence of obesity among adults aged 20 years and older, by age group and sex, January–March 2011

Notes: Data are based on household interviews of a sample of the civilian noninstitutionalized population. Obesity is defined as a body mass index (BMI) of 30 kg/m² or more. The measure is based on self-reported height (m) and weight (kg). Estimates of obesity are restricted to adults aged 20 and over for consistency with the *Healthy People 2010* (3) program. The analyses excluded 4.2% of persons with unknown height or weight.

SOURCE: P. M. Barnes et al., "Figure 6.2. Prevalence of Obesity among Adults Aged 20 Years and over, by Age Group and Sex: United States, January–March 2011," in *Early Release of Selected Estimates Based on Data from the January–March 2011 National Health Interview Survey,* Centers for Disease Control and Prevention, National Center for Health Statistics, September 2011, http://www.cdc.gov/nchs/data/nhis/earlyrelease/201109_06.pdf (accessed September 30, 2011)

difference in the prevalence of obesity between men and women in all four age groups.

The age-adjusted prevalence of obesity in racial and ethnic minorities, especially minority women, is generally higher than in whites in the United States. According to P. M. Barnes et al. of the NCHS, in *Early Release of Selected Estimates Based on Data from the January–March 2011 National Health Interview Survey* (September 2011, http://www.cdc.gov/nchs/data/nhis/earlyrelease/201109_06.pdf), in 2011 for both genders, non-Hispanic African-Americans were more likely than Hispanics and non-Hispanic whites to be obese. The age-adjusted prevalence of obesity was highest among non-Hispanic African-American women (45.2%) and lowest among non-Hispanic white women (25.6%). (See Figure 1.5.) Earlier studies, including the NHANES, reported a higher prevalence of overweight and obesity among Hispanics and Native Americans and a lower prevalence of overweight and obesity in Asian-Americans than in the U.S. population as a whole.

WHY ARE SO MANY AMERICANS OVERWEIGHT?

Historically, overweight and obesity were largely attributed to gluttony—solely the result of inappropriate eating. The scientific study of obesity has identified genetic, biochemical, viral, and metabolic alterations in humans and experimental animals, as well as the complex interactions of psychosocial and cultural factors that

FIGURE 1.5

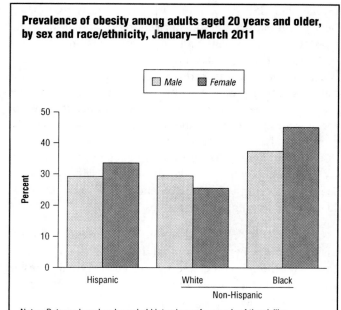

Prevalence of obesity among adults aged 20 years and older, by sex and race/ethnicity, January–March 2011

Notes: Data are based on household interviews of a sample of the civilian noninstitutionalized population. Obesity is defined as a body mass index (BMI) of 30 kg/m² or more. The measure is based on self-reported height (m) and weight (kg). Estimates of obesity are restricted to adults aged 20 and over for consistency with the *Healthy People 2010* (3) program. The analyses excluded 4.2% of persons with unknown height or weight. Estimates are age adjusted using the projected 2000 U.S. population as the standard population and using five age groups: 20–24, 25–34, 35–44, 45–64, and 65 and over.

SOURCE: P. M. Barnes et al., "Figure 6.3. Age-Adjusted Prevalence of Obesity among Adults Aged 20 Years and over, by Sex and Race/ Ethnicity: United States, January–March 2011," in *Early Release of Selected Estimates Based on Data from the January–March 2011 National Health Interview Survey,* Centers for Disease Control and Prevention, National Center for Health Statistics, September 2011, http://www.cdc.gov/nchs/data/nhis/earlyrelease/201109_06.pdf (accessed September 30, 2011)

create susceptibility to overweight and obesity. Even though overweight and obesity are thought to result from multiple causes, for the overwhelming majority of Americans overweight and obesity result from excessive consumption of calories and inadequate physical activity—eating too much and exercising too little.

Some observers maintain that Americans were destined to become overweight when their diets remained unchanged even as the inventions of the industrial revolution such as cars, automation, and a variety of laborsaving devices sharply reduced levels of physical activity. The widespread availability of high-calorie foods and less physically demanding jobs conspired to make Americans fatter. Others contend that the rise in overweight and obesity began during the 1970s, when Americans came to rely on processed, convenient, and calorie-dense, saturated-fat-laden fast foods. In "The Epidemic of Childhood Obesity: A Case for Primary Prevention and Action" (*Bariatric Nursing and Surgical Patient Care,* vol. 4, no. 3, September 2009), Renee Ellen Fox and Deborah E. Trautman cite the interaction of myriad biological and social factors including "dramatic decreases

in the amount of calories expended daily, increases in calorie intake and portion sizes, societal changes such as women entering the workforce in large numbers, more meals eaten in restaurants, and changes in television and video game viewing patterns."

Recent research even implicates a viral cause of obesity. Vincent van Ginnekan, Laura Sitnyakowsky, and Jonathan E. Jeffery note in "Infectobesity: Viral Infections (Especially with Human Adenovirus-36: Ad-36) May Be a Cause of Obesity" (*Medical Hypotheses,* vol. 72, no. 4, April 2009) that the human adenovirus-36 (Ad-36) is capable of inducing adiposity in experimentally infected animals and is known to increase the replication, differentiation, lipid accumulation, and insulin sensitivity in fat cells. (Adenoviruses typically produce respiratory infections.) Recent research finds that in the United States antibodies to Ad-36 are more prevalent in obese subjects (30%) than in nonobese subjects (11%).

Research also confirms genetic origins of obesity. In "Genes and Obesity: A Cause and Effect Relationship" (*Endocrinology Nutrition,* vol. 58, no. 9, November 2011), Emilio González Jiménez asserts that even though obesity usually results from an interaction of specific gene polymorphisms and environmental triggers, about 5% of obesity is attributable to mutations in specific genes. More than 100 genes linked to obesity have been reported. Some of these genes govern hunger and satiety signals, some are involved in the development and growth of fat cells, and others are involved in energy expenditure.

The American Diet Has Changed

The American diet has changed dramatically since the mid-20th century. According to the USDA, in *Agriculture Fact Book, 2001–2002* (March 2003, http:// www.usda.gov/factbook/2002factbook.pdf), during the 1950s food production in the United States provided about 800 fewer calories per person per day than in 2000. Of the 3,800 calories produced per person per day in 2000, the USDA estimates that about 1,100 calories were wasted, either through spoilage, plate waste, or cooking, leaving an average of about 2,700 calories per person per day. The USDA data reveal that between 1970 and 2000 the average number of calories consumed daily rose by 530 calories, an increase of 24.5%. This 24.5% increase consisted of 9.5 percentage points of grains (primarily refined grain products), 9 percentage points of added fats and oils, 4.7 percentage points of added sugars, 1.5 percentage points of fruits and vegetables, and 1 percentage point of meats and nuts. There was a 1.5 percentage point decline in dairy product and egg consumption.

The USDA states that Americans consumed an average of 4 pounds (1.8 kg) more fish and shellfish,

7 pounds (3.2 kg) more red meat, and 46 pounds (20.9 kg) more poultry per person per year in 2000 than they did during the 1950s. Americans consumed more meat—57 pounds (25.9 kg) more per year in 2000 than they did during the 1950s. Despite record-high per capita (per person) consumption of meat in 2000, the proportion of fat in the U.S. food supply from meat, poultry, and fish declined from one-third (33%) during the 1950s to a quarter (24%) in 2000. This decline resulted from the marketing of lower-fat ground and processed meat products, a shift away from red meat to poultry, and closer trimming of outside fat on meat, which commenced in 1986.

According to the USDA, the consumption of milk dropped from an annual average of 36.4 gallons (137.8 L) per person during the 1950s to 22.6 gallons (85.6 L) in 2000, a decrease of 38%. The USDA posits a link between the trend toward dining out and the reduction in beverage milk consumption. According to the USDA, soft drinks, fruit drinks, and flavored teas appear to be displacing milk as the beverages of choice for Americans. By contrast, Americans ate more cheese, from 7.7 pounds (3.5 kg) during the 1950s to 29.8 pounds (13.5 kg) in 2000.

The average use of added fats and oils increased 67%, from 44.6 pounds (20.2 kg) during the 1950s to 74.5 pounds (33.8 kg) in 2000. Added fats include butter, shortenings, and oils used in commercially prepared foods. All fats that naturally occur in foods, such as those in milk and meat, were excluded from the USDA analysis. Americans consumed an average of 23% more salad and cooking oil in 2000 than they did during the 1950s, and more than twice as much shortening. During the same period the consumption of butter and margarine declined by about the same proportion—25%. During the 1950s added fats and oils accounted for the largest proportion of fat in the food supply (41%), followed by animal proteins—meat, poultry, and fish (32%). By 2000 added fats and oils accounted for 53% of total fat consumption, most likely because Americans' appetites for fried foods in fast-food outlets and high-fat snack foods grew, as did the use of salad dressings. USDA food consumption surveys, which assess the prevalence of discretionary fats in the American diet, continue to find that margarine, salad dressing, and mayonnaise, along with cakes and other sweet baked goods, are among the top-10 food sources of fat in the American diet.

The USDA indicates that the consumption of fruit and vegetables increased 20%, from 587.5 pounds (266.5 kg) during the 1970s to 707.7 pounds (321 kg) in 2000. The USDA attributes some of the increase to the introduction of convenient, ready-to-eat, precut, and packaged fruit and vegetables and to increasing consumer health awareness. Despite these gains, the CDC explains in

State Indicator Report on Fruits and Vegetables, 2009 (September 25, 2009, http://www.fruitsandveggiesmatter .gov/downloads/StateIndicatorReport2009.pdf), a state-by-state study of fruit and vegetable consumption, that no state met the national objectives for fruit and vegetable consumption outlined in Healthy People 2010, the nation's framework for health priorities. The CDC finds that just 32.8% of adults met the recommended two or more servings of fruit and only 27.4% consumed the recommended three or more servings of vegetables in 2009. (See Figure 1.6.) Fruit and vegetable consumption by adolescents was even worse—32.2% said they ate at least two servings of fruit daily and 13.2% said they ate at least three servings of vegetables per day.

The BRFSS reveals declining consumption of fruits and vegetables between 2000 and 2009. Table 1.9 shows that even though some states reported marginal gains in fruit and vegetable consumption during this period, most reported declines.

The consumption of fresh produce continued to decline in 2010 and 2011. Dan Witters of the Gallup Organization reports in *Americans' Eating Habits Worse This Year Compared with Last* (June 9, 2011, http:// www.gallup.com/poll/147989/americans-eating-habits-worse-year-compared-last.aspx) on a poll comparing Americans' health behaviors in 2010 and 2011. Witters indicates that fewer Americans reported healthy eating in 2011. Overall fruit and vegetable consumption declined with notable decreases among Hispanics, young adults, older adults, and women. (See Table 1.10.)

FIGURE 1.6

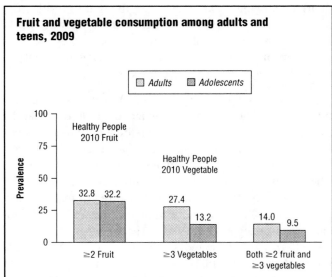

Fruit and vegetable consumption among adults and teens, 2009

SOURCE: "U.S. Fruit and Vegetable Consumption: Daily Frequency among Adults and Adolescents," in *State Indicator Report on Fruits and Vegetables, 2009*, Centers for Disease Control and Prevention, September 29, 2009, http://www.fruitsandveggiesmatter.gov/downloads/StateIndicatorReport2009.pdf (accessed October 1, 2011)

TABLE 1.9

Fruit and vegetable consumption among adults, 2000–09

State	Fruit two or more times per day						Vegetables three or more times per day					
	2000	2002	2003	2005	2007	2009	2000	2002	2003	2005	2007	2009
Overall	34.4	33.5	32.2	32.8	32.9	32.5[a]	26.7	26.3	26.2	27.1	27.4	26.3
Alabama	25.6	24.0	25.7	23.5	23.9	24.6	30.1	27.8	28.5	27.9	28.5	26.9[a]
Alaska	31.0	30.6	31.4	33.5	29.9	30.8	25.4	23.8	26.3	24.6	27.7	27.5
Arizona	43.2	31.0	30.8	33.3	33.5	33.7[a]	38.4	27.1	25.1	26.9	29.9	24.4[a]
Arkansas	23.5	23.1	22.4	23.3	24.3	24.5	29.4	29.4	28.7	29.1	29.2	26.9
California	40.7	40.4	39.3	40.1	40.6	40.1	23.3	23.5	24.6	26.5	25.6	26.8[b]
Colorado	33.3	34.6	34.1	33.7	35.4	35.5	25.6	23.6	25.7	25.3	26.5	25.3
Connecticut	43.5	42.2	41.8	37.6	38.6	37.6[a]	29.2	31.0	30.1	29.9	29.3	28.5
Delaware	34.2	31.9	31.1	28.8	28.9	32.5[a]	29.8	25.5	26.9	26.5	26.1	27.7
District of Columbia	45.7	43.7	38.3	38.8	41.2	40.2[a]	26.1	32.5	29.2	31.3	32.8	32.3[b]
Florida	36.1	36.7	34.5	35.4	36.1	33.3	24.4	27.9	27.4	28.2	29.2	28.3[b]
Georgia	28.2	27.5	26.2	28.0	27.6	29.9	29.2	29.5	29.8	30.9	30.4	29.5
Hawaii	32.6	29.4	33.1	32.6	39.0	32.9[b]	27.0	25.7	36.1	29.5	29.6	26.8
Idaho	27.9	28.4	27.9	30.1	29.3	32.9[b]	24.7	25.1	22.8	27.4	25.2	27.8[b]
Illinois	33.3	33.0	34.7	34.8	36.9	32.4	25.8	22.6	25.4	24.0	23.3	23.3
Indiana	27.7	28.4	29.0	29.2	30.4	28.1	25.5	24.2	25.0	25.2	26.5	23.7
Iowa	28.4	28.5	27.5	28.9	29.9	27.5	21.4	22.6	21.3	23.4	22.4	21.9
Kansas	30.4	24.1	24.9	25.3	23.9	23.8[a]	29.8	25.9	26.8	26.5	27.2	26.0[a]
Kentucky	25.0	23.7	22.5	20.5	24.4	24.4	35.5	32.4	31.4	30.2	28.8	29.4[a]
Louisiana	24.2	23.5	21.5	28.7	28.5	24.6[b]	22.8	25.4	25.3	25.9	26.1	21.3
Maine	37.3	37.5	35.9	35.1	36.6	36.0	29.6	30.7	27.9	32.5	31.6	30.6
Maryland	39.0	39.3	37.8	37.6	35.8	36.9[a]	29.6	31.5	31.4	30.6	28.9	28.7[a]
Massachusetts	42.7	41.8	39.9	38.9	39.0	36.8[a]	29.4	29.1	28.2	29.8	28.9	28.1
Michigan	37.3	33.0	29.5	32.2	31.7	32.1[a]	21.3	21.3	20.5	24.3	23.2	23.9[b]
Minnesota	37.2	35.2	35.1	36.1	27.2	31.2[a]	23.3	21.9	23.9	23.1	25.9	26.4[b]
Mississippi	24.1	22.6	22.1	22.1	24.1	22.9	25.1	25.7	24.0	22.6	22.2	21.6[a]
Missouri	28.4	23.5	25.2	28.8	25.1	27.3	26.1	26.7	25.7	25.7	26.2	23.0[a]
Montana	35.4	32.2	29.6	30.6	29.7	33.5[a]	27.4	26.4	24.1	28.6	28.6	28.0
Nebraska	33.1	31.2	28.5	29.1	33.8	30.2	24.0	22.5	23.0	24.6	26.3	24.3[b]
Nevada	27.8	33.2	31.0	31.4	30.4	30.3	24.7	21.2	20.8	23.5	24.3	25.5
New Hampshire	39.1	37.7	37.6	37.7	36.3	36.2[a]	28.5	29.0	28.5	32.3	30.5	30.4
New Jersey	40.3	37.7	37.1	37.4	36.7	36.6[a]	28.0	27.5	26.3	27.4	29.5	26.2
New Mexico	30.4	30.3	30.1	29.4	27.4	29.8[a]	23.5	24.8	25.1	26.8	26.3	27.3[b]
New York	40.7	41.0	37.4	37.6	39.1	38.9[a]	27.7	24.5	24.2	25.3	27.2	24.7
North Carolina	27.7	28.2	26.9	26.5	25.4	25.0[a]	32.1	31.2	32.6	32.0	29.7	27.5[a]
North Dakota	32.2	30.1	30.6	30.4	29.3	31.1	23.8	22.6	22.3	23.8	24.5	24.6
Ohio	30.9	28.6	29.7	30.0	28.5	29.3	24.6	24.5	25.8	25.1	25.2	24.6
Oklahoma	23.3	19.3	17.4	19.6	20.6	18.1[a]	27.8	25.0	27.4	23.7	24.2	23.5[a]
Oregon	36.2	35.5	32.5	34.1	33.8	33.0[a]	27.4	28.2	25.9	29.0	29.8	30.5[b]
Pennsylvania	33.7	36.9	35.2	33.8	34.9	35.5	25.3	25.0	23.6	26.2	27.1	25.1
Rhode Island	42.8	39.7	37.8	36.3	36.5	36.7[a]	29.3	27.1	27.7	27.3	26.4	25.9[a]
South Carolina	29.4	28.5	27.8	25.6	23.8	23.3[a]	29.9	29.1	26.8	26.2	25.6	22.9[a]
South Dakota	31.3	30.8	29.2	29.2	25.8	25.2[a]	25.7	23.4	23.7	24.5	23.9	19.6[a]
Tennessee	33.8	29.9	25.7	27.2	26.1	26.4[a]	43.5	39.8	35.3	39.0	37.9	33.0[a]
Texas	29.1	30.8	28.9	29.4	29.4	30.4	27.4	26.6	26.2	28.5	29.7	27.2
Utah	30.9	31.2	28.5	30.8	32.2	31.5	21.0	20.8	20.4	22.8	24.9	24.4[a]
Vermont	39.9	39.6	41.6	39.2	38.6	38.9[a]	29.6	29.4	32.3	31.2	31.8	30.3
Virginia	35.5	33.8	32.6	33.4	33.3	33.7	28.1	31.8	30.0	29.7	30.5	30.3
Washington	35.1	32.9	32.7	34.4	33.8	33.9	23.0	24.8	25.4	27.4	29.2	28.3[b]
West Virginia	30.0	25.4	23.4	24.7	24.7	25.3[a]	29.9	29.1	27.7	30.6	25.9	22.1[a]
Wisconsin	34.0	35.7	32.7	33.4	35.2	34.9	20.3	22.7	20.7	21.1	23.6	23.2[b]
Wyoming	27.3	29.2	27.8	29.0	32.1	30.3[b]	25.6	24.7	26.1	25.9	26.8	26.9

[a]Significant decreased linear trend (p<0.05).
[b]Significant increased linear trend (p<0.05).
Notes: Results presented are weighted for age, race/ethnicity, and sex. Linear trend analysis includes age-standardized data in the analytic sample from 2000 (Population = 174,012), 2002 (Population = 232,743), 2003 (Population = 248,255), 2005 (Population = 333,032), 2007 (Population = 401,450), and 2009 (Population = 396,316).

SOURCE: "Table 1. Percentage of U.S. Adults Aged ≥18 Years Who Consumed Fruit Two or More Times per Day and Vegetables Three or More Times per Day, by State—Behavioral Risk Factor Surveillance System, 2000–2009," in "State-Specific Trends in Fruit and Vegetable Consumption among Adults—United States, 2000–2009," *Morbidity and Mortality Weekly Report*, vol. 59, no. 35, September 10, 2010, http://www.cdc.gov/mmwr/pdf/wk/mm5935.pdf (accessed October 9, 2011)

According to the USDA, the per capita use of flour and cereal products reached 199.9 pounds (90.7 kg) in 2000, from an annual average of 155.4 pounds (70.5 kg) during the 1950s and 138.2 pounds (62.7 kg) during 1970s, when grain consumption was at a record low. This increase reflects plentiful grain stocks, robust consumer demand for store-bought bakery items and grain-based snack foods, and increased consumption of fast-food products such as buns, pizza dough, and tortillas. Despite the overall increase in grain consumption, the average

TABLE 1.10

Poll respondents' fruit and vegetable consumption by demographics, 2010 and 2011

FRUITS AND VEGETABLES CONSUMPTION, BY DEMOGRAPHIC GROUP

Percentage who report having had at least five servings of fruits and vegetables at least four days in last week

	2010	2011	Change (in pct. pts.)
Gender			
Women	63.5	61.3	−2.2
Men	51.7	50.1	−1.6
Age			
18–29	49.9	47.3	−2.6
30–44	54.8	54.0	−0.8
45–64	58.4	57.3	−1.1
65+	67.3	64.8	−2.5
Race/ethnicity			
Hispanic	50.8	47.9	−2.9
White	58.4	56.6	−1.8
Asian	58.7	57.2	−1.5
Black	58.7	58.1	−0.6

SOURCE: Dan Witters, "Fruits and Vegetables Consumption, by Demographic Group," in *Americans' Eating Habits Worse This Year Compared with Last*, The Gallup Organization, June 9, 2011, http://www.gallup.com/poll/147989/americans-eating-habits-worse-year-compared-last.aspx (accessed October 1, 2011). Copyright © 2011 by the Gallup Organization. Reproduced by permission of The Gallup Organization.

American's diet contained mostly refined grain products and fell short of the recommended minimum three daily servings of whole-grain products.

The NPD Group notes in *Are We There Yet? Measuring Progress on Making at Least Half Our Grains Whole* (http://www.wholegrainscouncil.org/files/3.AreWeThereYet.pdf) that Americans' consumption of whole grains was unchanged between 1998 and 2005 but increased 20% between 2005 and 2008. During this period whole-grain consumption increased the most (38%) among young adults aged 18 to 34 years. Despite this increase, American adults consumed less than one serving of whole grains per day instead of the recommended three to five servings per day and in 2008 just 11% were adhering to the advice to "make at least half their grains whole."

The USDA cites a variety of factors that have contributed to the changes in the American diet over the past 50 years, including fluctuations in food prices and availability, increases in real (adjusted for inflation) disposable income, and more food assistance for the poor. New products, particularly the expanding array of convenience foods, also alter patterns of consumption, as do more imports, growth in the away-from-home food market, intensified advertising campaigns, and increases in nutrient-enrichment standards and food fortification. The social and demographic trends driving changes in food choices include smaller households, more two-wage earner households, more single-parent households, an aging population, and increased ethnic diversity.

Americans Enjoy Eating Out

A variety of societal trends are thought to contribute to Americans' propensity to overeat, including eating outside the home, as well as ready access to and preference for sugar- and fat-laden foods. Table 1.11 shows how expenditures for eating away from home have steadily increased, and more than doubled from $245.2 billion in 1990 to $594.3 billion in 2010. Purchases of food away from home rose between 2003 and 2008; however, the economic recession that lasted from late 2007 to mid-2009 prompted Americans to limit their eating out. Aylin Kumcu and Phil Kaufman of the Economic Research Service note in "Food Spending Adjustments during Recessionary Times" (*Amber Waves*, September 2011) that there was a 5% decline in food spending during the recession—the largest decrease in 25 years. They indicate that this decline was largely attributable to reductions in food-away-from-home spending, such as at fast-food and sit-down restaurants. (See Figure 1.7.)

Many nutritionists and obesity researchers assert that controlling portion size, which is key to controlling calorie consumption, is more difficult in restaurants, where portions are frequently quite large. Increasingly, restaurants have translated consumer demand for value into more food for less money. Because humans are genetically programmed to eat when food is abundant, larger portions trigger the natural impulse to eat more.

In "External Cues in the Control of Food Intake in Humans: The Sensory-Normative Distinction" (*Physiology & Behavior*, vol. 94, no. 5, August 6, 2008), C. Peter Herman and Janet Polivy confirm that external cues such as portion size exert a strong influence on food intake—when presented with larger portions, people will generally consume more. The problem of portion size is compounded by the observation that Americans are eating larger portions of foods that are high in calories and fat. Furthermore, Herman and Polivy assert that most people are affected by external cues such as portion size, but that sensory cues, such as the extent to which the food is perceived as tasty, have a more powerful effect on people who are obese than they do on people who have a healthy weight.

BIGGER PORTIONS IN RESTAURANTS. Samara Joy Nielsen and Barry M. Popkin of the University of North Carolina, Chapel Hill, looked at portion sizes consumed in the United States to determine whether average portion sizes had increased over time and reported their findings in "Patterns and Trends in Food Portion Sizes, 1977–1998" (*Journal of the American Medical Association*, vol. 289, no. 4, January 22, 2003). In this landmark study, Nielsen and Popkin analyze data collected by national

TABLE 1.11

Food away from home, total expenditures, selected years 1929–2010

Year	Eating and drinking places[a]	Hotels and motels[a]	Retail stores, direct selling[b]	Recreational places[c]	Schools and colleges[d]	All other[e]	Total[f]
			Million dollars				
1929	2,101	362	—	—	175	1,483	4,121
1933	1,235	250	—	—	105	869	2,459
1935	1,257	271	—	—	161	1,145	2,834
1936	1,430	320	—	—	175	1,236	3,161
1937	1,696	351	—	—	194	1,375	3,616
1938	1,626	312	—	—	191	1,260	3,389
1939	1,782	321	—	—	203	1,307	3,613
1940	1,938	353	—	—	219	1,385	3,895
1941	2,369	386	—	—	263	1,781	4,799
1942	2,992	453	—	—	310	2,539	6,294
1943	3,837	604	—	—	332	3,572	8,345
1944	4,471	681	—	—	326	4,415	9,893
1945	5,218	736	—	—	373	4,908	11,235
1946	5,859	846	—	—	525	3,802	11,032
1947	6,243	854	—	—	842	3,864	11,803
1948	6,338	846	—	—	983	4,069	12,236
1949	6,294	786	—	—	979	3,943	12,002
1950	6,472	774	—	—	1,051	4,172	12,469
1951	7,172	783	—	—	1,124	5,167	14,246
1952	7,549	805	—	—	1,138	5,435	14,927
1953	7,834	790	—	—	1,215	5,392	15,231
1954	8,008	752	1,416	274	1,311	3,676	15,437
1955	8,490	809	1,468	313	1,390	3,539	16,009
1956	8,992	875	1,534	354	1,530	3,506	16,791
1957	9,409	932	1,592	342	1,661	3,609	17,545
1958	9,447	922	1,599	356	1,809	3,756	17,889
1959	10,102	982	1,677	385	1,949	3,739	18,834
1960	10,505	1,028	1,716	421	2,082	3,855	19,607
1961	10,907	1,061	1,740	452	2,264	3,961	20,385
1962	11,624	1,134	1,812	472	2,463	4,090	21,595
1963	12,247	1,200	1,854	484	2,624	4,148	22,557
1964	13,156	1,289	1,988	496	2,814	4,279	24,022
1965	14,444	1,409	2,162	522	3,062	4,598	26,197
1966	15,768	1,541	2,346	544	3,329	5,173	28,701
1967	16,595	1,623	2,436	563	3,632	5,570	30,419
1968	18,695	1,703	2,713	616	3,903	5,830	33,460
1969	20,207	1,716	2,984	661	4,256	6,291	36,115
1970	22,617	1,894	3,325	721	4,475	6,551	39,583
1971	24,166	2,086	3,626	762	4,990	6,621	42,251
1972	27,167	2,390	3,811	832	5,370	7,017	46,587
1973	31,265	2,639	4,218	963	5,605	7,960	52,650
1974	34,029	2,864	4,520	1,167	6,287	9,178	58,045
1975	41,384	3,199	4,952	1,369	7,060	10,145	68,109
1976	47,536	3,769	5,341	1,511	7,854	10,822	76,833
1977	52,491	4,115	5,663	2,606	8,413	11,547	84,835
1978	60,042	4,863	6,323	2,810	9,034	13,012	96,084
1979	68,872	5,551	7,157	2,921	9,914	14,756	109,171
1980	75,883	5,906	8,158	3,040	11,115	16,194	120,296
1981	83,358	6,639	8,830	2,979	11,357	17,751	130,914
1982	90,390	6,888	9,256	2,887	11,692	18,663	139,776
1983	98,710	7,660	9,827	3,271	12,338	19,077	150,883
1984	105,836	8,409	10,315	3,489	12,950	20,047	161,046
1985	111,760	9,168	10,499	3,737	13,534	20,133	168,831
1986	121,699	9,665	11,116	4,059	14,401	20,755	181,695
1987	137,190	11,117	9,302	4,396	13,470	21,119	196,594
1988	150,724	11,905	10,359	5,082	13,889	22,474	214,434
1989	160,226	12,179	11,369	6,089	14,609	24,016	228,488
1990	171,616	12,508	12,786	7,206	15,299	25,756	245,172
1991	180,062	12,460	13,515	7,936	16,186	26,369	256,527
1992	184,855	13,204	9,988	8,511	17,666	27,736	261,960
1993	197,987	13,362	10,485	9,364	18,330	28,003	277,531
1994	207,545	13,880	10,633	10,106	19,271	28,597	290,032
1995	216,091	14,211	10,370	11,080	20,064	29,290	301,105
1996	223,546	14,553	10,373	11,515	20,867	29,825	310,679
1997	237,475	15,381	10,695	12,129	21,901	32,136	329,717
1998	250,467	16,069	11,353	12,795	23,053	32,606	346,342

nutrition surveys (the Nationwide Food Consumption Survey and the Continuing Survey of Food Intakes by Individuals) that were conducted in the United States in 1977, 1989, 1994, and 1996, detailing the consumption habits of more than 63,000 people. For each survey year, the researchers analyze the average portion sizes that

TABLE 1.11

Food away from home, total expenditures, selected years 1929–2010 [CONTINUED]

Year	Eating and drinking places[a]	Hotels and motels[a]	Retail stores, direct selling[b]	Recreational places[c]	Schools and colleges[d]	All other[e]	Total[f]
				Million dollars			
1999	261,473	16,710	12,469	13,500	23,920	34,269	362,342
2000	282,153	18,003	13,699	14,232	24,468	36,098	388,652
2001	289,223	20,813	14,618	14,964	25,394	36,747	401,760
2002	300,706	21,513	17,364	16,095	26,735	37,512	419,924
2003	319,097	21,914	18,366	17,325	28,077	39,009	443,787
2004	341,624	23,462	19,655	18,229	30,185	40,417	473,572
2005	363,917	24,570	20,958	19,958	31,521	42,305	503,228
2006	388,671	25,328	21,998	22,253	31,478	43,486	533,214
2007	410,521	26,048	22,784	23,804	32,437	45,634	561,229
2008	422,159	25,961	23,466	24,179	33,647	47,530	576,941
2009	419,639	25,872	22,539	23,979	34,965	47,650	574,645
2010	433,497	25,784	24,147	25,417	36,543	48,881	594,269

— = Not available.
[a]Includes tips.
[b]Includes vending machine operators but not vending machines operated by organizations.
[c]Motion picture theaters, bowling alleys, pool parlors, sports arenas, camps, amusement parks, golf and country clubs (includes concessions beginning in 1977).
[d]Includes school food subsidies.
[e]Military exchanges and clubs; railroad dining cars; airlines; food service in manufacturing plants, institutions, hospitals, boarding houses, fraternities and sororities, and civic and social organizations; and food supplied to military forces, civilian employees and child day care centers.
[f]Computed from unrounded data.

SOURCE: "Table 3. Food away from Home: Total Expenditures," in *Food CPI and Expenditures: Food Expenditure Tables*, U.S. Department of Agriculture, Economic Research Service, July 13, 2011, http://www.ers.usda.gov/briefing/cpifoodandexpenditures/Data/Expenditures_tables/table3.htm (accessed October 1, 2011)

FIGURE 1.7

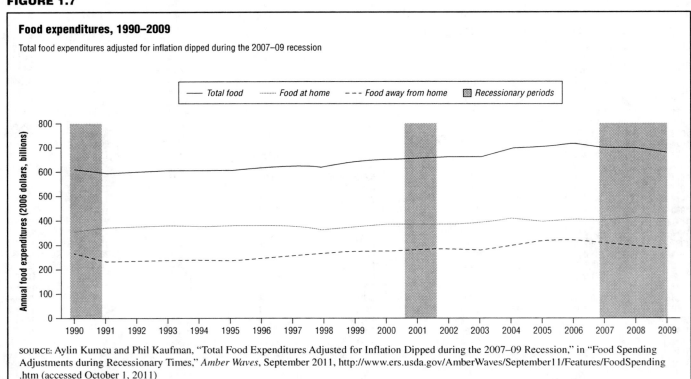

Food expenditures, 1990–2009

Total food expenditures adjusted for inflation dipped during the 2007–09 recession

SOURCE: Aylin Kumcu and Phil Kaufman, "Total Food Expenditures Adjusted for Inflation Dipped during the 2007–09 Recession," in "Food Spending Adjustments during Recessionary Times," *Amber Waves*, September 2011, http://www.ers.usda.gov/AmberWaves/September11/Features/FoodSpending .htm (accessed October 1, 2011)

were consumed of specific food items (salty snacks, desserts, soft drinks, fruit drinks, french fries, hamburgers, cheeseburgers, pizza, and Mexican food) by eating location (home, restaurant, and fast-food outlet). Nielsen and Popkin report that between 1977 and 1996 the aver-

age portions of salty snacks such as chips increased by 60% and soft drinks grew by 50%. The average bag of chips grew from 1 ounce (28.4 g) in 1977 to 1.6 ounces (45.4 g) in 1996. During this same period an average dispensed soft drink increased from 13.1 ounces

(387.4 mL) to 19.9 ounces (588.4 mL). As a result, the average chips-and-soda snack in 1996 contained 150 more calories than it did in 1977.

The portion-size changes were observed with many fast-food offerings. During the 20 years studied the size of the average hamburger grew by 23%, to 7 ounces (198.4 g), and the servings of fries grew by 16%, to 3.5 ounces (99.2 g). In 1996 a regular-sized burger-and-fries meal contained 155 more calories than it did in 1977. Worse still, Nielsen and Popkin find that portion size had also expanded in Americans' homes, indicating widespread ignorance about appropriate portion size. Interestingly, portion sizes were smallest in restaurants, although they, too, had increased during the study period. For example, the average restaurant portion of spaghetti with tomato sauce and meatballs doubled in size from 500 to 1,025 calories.

BIGGER PORTIONS AT HOME. Increased portion sizes at home are reflected in recipes and cookbooks. Lisa R. Young notes in *The Portion Teller: Smartsize Your Way to Permanent Weight Loss* (2005) that recipes call for bigger portions using the same ingredients than they did in past decades. For example, a brownie recipe from Irma S. Rombauer and Marion Rombauer Becker's *Joy of Cooking* (1964) recommended dividing it into 30 servings, whereas the same recipe in the 1997 edition of the book was divided into only 16 servings. Similarly, a 1987 recipe for Toll House cookies yielded 60 servings, whereas in earlier decades the same recipe yielded 100 servings. Other popular food items have increased in size and caloric content. In "Portion Distortion" (2010, http://hp2010.nhlbihin.net/portion/), the National Heart, Lung, and Blood Institute compares portion sizes and the corresponding calories of several popular foods between 1983 and 2003. Researchers find that two decades earlier a bagel measured 3 inches (7.6 cm) in diameter and contained 140 calories. In 2003 a 6-inch (15.2 cm) bagel contained 350 calories.

Nielsen and Popkin also note other changes in eating behavior. For example, they find that in 1996 Americans obtained 19% of their total calories from snacks—double the amount of 1977—and 81% from meals. They conclude that "control of portion size must be systematically addressed both in general and as it relates to fast-food pricing and marketing. The best way to encourage people to eat smaller portions is if food portions served inside and outside the home are smaller."

Even though the Nationwide Food Consumption Survey and the Continuing Survey of Food Intakes by Individuals have not been repeated since 1996, there is no evidence that portion sizes have returned to their previous sizes or have even decreased in size. In a review of research about portion size, Ingrid H. M. Steenhuis and

Willemijn M. Vermeer of Vrije Universiteit Amsterdam observe in "Portion Size: Review and Framework for Interventions" (*International Journal of Behavioral Nutrition and Physical Activity*, vol. 6, no. 58, August 21, 2009) that since the 1970s portion sizes, especially of high energy-dense (high-calorie) foods eaten at home and in restaurants, have increased. The researchers confirm that "portion distortion," a term that is used to describe the phenomenon of people becoming acclimated to larger portions so that they not only do not view them as excessive but also have more difficulty selecting appropriate amounts of food, definitely increases consumption by at least 30%.

The contribution of increased portion size to increased daily intake of energy from food and drink was confirmed by research conducted by Kiyah J. Duffey and Barry M. Popkin and reported in "Energy Density, Portion Size, and Eating Occasions: Contributions to Increased Energy Intake in the United States, 1977–2006" (*PLoS Medicine*, vol. 8, no. 6, June 2011). The researchers analyze data from the Nationwide Food Consumption Survey (1977–78), the Continuing Survey of Food Intakes by Individuals (1989–91), and the NHANES (1994–98 and 2003–06) to determine the contribution of changes in the energy density of foods consumed, the portion size, and the number of meals and snacks per day. They find that the daily total energy intake increased by 570 calories between 1977 and 2006. Duffey and Popkin indicate that even though all three factors contributed to changes in the average daily total energy intake over the past 30 years, increases in the number of eating occasions and portion size accounted for most of the change. In fact, the consumption of food and beverage portions increased across all eating and drinking occasions (meals and snacks).

Is the Food Industry the Culprit?

In "The Perils of Ignoring History: Big Tobacco Played Dirty and Millions Died. How Similar Is Big Food?" (March 2009, http://vancouver.ca/parks/active community/pdf/FoodTobacco_YaleUni.pdf), Kelly D. Brownell and Kenneth E. Warner implicate marketing strategies employed by the food industry as a significant factor in the rise of obesity. Furthermore, they liken food industry practices to those of the tobacco industry, concluding that:

> The tobacco industry had a playbook, a script, that emphasized personal responsibility, paying scientists who delivered research that instilled doubt, criticizing the "junk" science that found harms associated with smoking, making self-regulatory pledges, lobbying with massive resources to stifle government action, introducing "safer" products, and simultaneously manipulating and denying both the addictive nature of their products and their marketing to children. The

script of the food industry is both similar to and different from the tobacco industry script.... Because obesity is now a major global problem, the world cannot afford a repeat of the tobacco history, in which industry talks about the moral high ground but does not occupy it.

In "Personal Responsibility and Obesity: A Constructive Approach to a Controversial Issue" (*Health Affairs*, vol. 29, no. 3, March–April 2010), Kelly D. Brownell et al. explain that people gain weight when their environment promotes highly palatable food and cite research suggesting that some foods can trigger symptoms of addiction. The researchers aver that the traditional approach to diet and obesity has been one of rugged individualism—educating individuals and exhorting them to alter their behavior, often without regard to environmental influences. Instead of focusing solely on personal responsibility, Brownell et al. propose efforts on the part of government and the food industry to create conditions that encourage responsible choices. Furthermore, they call on the food industry to limit its "relentless" and often "stealth" marketing techniques such as food marketing that is incorporated into video games.

David A. Kessler also implicates the food industry in *The End of Overeating: Taking Control of the Insatiable American Appetite* (2009). He asserts that conditioned overeating is not a personal character flaw; rather, it is a biological response to the widespread availability of foods that are high in salt, fat, and sugar. Kessler blames the food industry for engineering highly processed industrial foods that use salt, fat, and added sugar to trigger cravings in some people and addiction in other people who are susceptible.

Some industry observers believe that one ingredient in particular triggers cravings: high-fructose corn syrup. In "Brain Functional Magnetic Resonance Imaging Response to Glucose and Fructose Infusions in Humans" (*Diabetes, Obesity, and Metabolism*, vol. 13, no. 3, March 2011), Jonathan Q. Purnell et al. explain that the brain responds differently to glucose (sugar) than it does to fructose. Consuming glucose increases responses in the reward- and executive-function parts of the brain, whereas fructose inhibits these responses. This action may explain why fructose consumption appears to promote obesity—it actually stimulates hunger, which in turn increases consumption and weight gain.

Fructose also appears to trigger fat storage more efficiently than other sugars do. New studies show that the body does not metabolize high-fructose corn syrup well. Even though all sugars are stored in the body as fat, some researchers think that fructose is more readily converted into fat than other sugars. The fructose encourages the liver to promote fat by activating enzymes that create higher levels of cholesterol and triglycerides (fatty substances that are normally present in the bloodstream and all the cells of the body) and make muscles more insulin resistant. Elevated levels of cholesterol and triglycerides increase the risk of coronary heart disease, and insulin resistance can lead to diabetes.

High-fructose corn syrup does more than sweeten; it also acts as a preservative, giving sweet foods a longer shelf life. Since the 1970s high-fructose corn syrup has been used to sweeten nearly every product on supermarket shelves, from cereal to soda. Some researchers feel that because it is so ubiquitous, many Americans are unknowingly consuming excessive amounts of fructose. Table 1.12 shows the per capita consumption of high-fructose corn syrup, which peaked in 1999 and has since slowly declined.

During the first decade of the 21st century high-fructose corn syrup received negative publicity, and as a result consumption continued to decline. In response, the Corn Refiners Association launched a controversial advertising campaign in 2009 that was intended to rebrand high-fructose corn syrup as "corn sugar." In April 2011 the noncorn sugar companies Western Sugar Cooperative, the Michigan Sugar Company, and the C&H Sugar Company Inc. filed suit against the Corn Refiners Association, asserting that renaming high-fructose corn syrup as "corn sugar" is misleading advertising that is intended to induce consumers to equate the two products. In September a federal judge in Los Angeles, California, heard arguments from both sides before ruling on a motion made by the Corn Refiners Association to dismiss the lawsuit. The following month the judge ruled that the case would go forward.

In *The Fattening of America: How the Economy Makes Us Fat, if It Matters, and What to Do about It* (2008), Eric A. Finkelstein and Laurie Zuckerman observe that Americans consumed 1,000 calories more per week in 2008 than they did in 1985. Finkelstein and Zuckerman describe how declining food costs, especially for high-calorie, low-nutrient foods, and modern technology combined to reduce the cost of producing higher-calorie processed food products. They note that when the staples used to produce fast foods became cheaper, the food industry intensified marketing efforts to induce consumers to buy and eat more. Table 1.13 shows that food expenditures have consistently decreased as a percentage of disposable personal income, declining from 23.4% of personal disposable income in 1929 to just 9.4% in 2010.

TABLE 1.12

Estimated number of per capita calories of high fructose corn syrup consumed daily, 1970–2010[a]

Year	Primary weight (market level)[b] lb/yr	Loss from primary to retail weight percent	Weight at retail level lb/yr	Loss from retail/institutional to consumer level percent	Weight at consumer level lb/yr	Loss at consumer level Nonedible share percent	Other (uneaten food, spoilage, etc.) percent	Per capita consumption (adjusted for loss) lbs/yr	oz/daily	g/daily	Calories per serving number	Serving weight grams	Calories consumed daily[c] number	Servings (teaspoons) consumed daily[d] teaspoons
1970	0.5	0.0	0.5	11.0	0.5	0.0	20.0	0.4	0.0	0.5	16.0	4.2	2	0.1
1971	0.8	0.0	0.8	11.0	0.7	0.0	20.0	0.6	0.0	0.7	16.0	4.2	3	0.2
1972	1.2	0.0	1.2	11.0	1.0	0.0	20.0	0.8	0.0	1.0	16.0	4.2	4	0.2
1973	2.1	0.0	2.1	11.0	1.8	0.0	20.0	1.5	0.1	1.8	16.0	4.2	7	0.4
1974	2.8	0.0	2.8	11.0	2.5	0.0	20.0	2.0	0.1	2.4	16.0	4.2	9	0.6
1975	4.9	0.0	4.9	11.0	4.3	0.0	20.0	3.5	0.2	4.3	16.0	4.2	16	1.0
1976	7.2	0.0	7.2	11.0	6.4	0.0	20.0	5.1	0.2	6.4	16.0	4.2	24	1.5
1977	9.6	0.0	9.6	11.0	8.5	0.0	20.0	6.8	0.3	8.5	16.0	4.2	32	2.0
1978	10.8	0.0	10.8	11.0	9.6	0.0	20.0	7.7	0.3	9.5	16.0	4.2	36	2.3
1979	14.8	0.0	14.8	11.0	13.1	0.0	20.0	10.5	0.5	13.1	16.0	4.2	50	3.1
1980	19.0	0.0	19.0	11.0	16.9	0.0	20.0	13.5	0.6	16.8	16.0	4.2	64	4.0
1981	22.8	0.0	22.8	11.0	20.3	0.0	20.0	16.3	0.7	20.2	16.0	4.2	77	4.8
1982	26.6	0.0	26.6	11.0	23.7	0.0	20.0	19.0	0.8	23.6	16.0	4.2	90	5.6
1983	31.2	0.0	31.2	11.0	27.8	0.0	20.0	22.2	1.0	27.6	16.0	4.2	105	6.6
1984	37.2	0.0	37.2	11.0	33.1	0.0	20.0	26.5	1.2	32.9	16.0	4.2	125	7.8
1985	45.2	0.0	45.2	11.0	40.2	0.0	20.0	32.2	1.4	40.0	16.0	4.2	152	9.5
1986	45.7	0.0	45.7	11.0	40.7	0.0	20.0	32.5	1.4	40.4	16.0	4.2	154	9.6
1987	47.7	0.0	47.7	11.0	42.5	0.0	20.0	34.0	1.5	42.2	16.0	4.2	161	10.1
1988	49.0	0.0	49.0	11.0	43.6	0.0	20.0	34.9	1.5	43.3	16.0	4.2	165	10.3
1989	48.2	0.0	48.2	11.0	42.9	0.0	20.0	34.3	1.5	42.6	16.0	4.2	162	10.2
1990	49.6	0.0	49.6	11.0	44.1	0.0	20.0	35.3	1.5	43.9	16.0	4.2	167	10.4
1991	50.3	0.0	50.3	11.0	44.8	0.0	20.0	35.8	1.6	44.5	16.0	4.2	170	10.6
1992	51.8	0.0	51.8	11.0	46.1	0.0	20.0	36.9	1.6	45.8	16.0	4.2	175	10.9
1993	54.5	0.0	54.5	11.0	48.5	0.0	20.0	38.8	1.7	48.2	16.0	4.2	184	11.5
1994	56.2	0.0	56.2	11.0	50.0	0.0	20.0	40.0	1.8	49.7	16.0	4.2	189	11.8
1995	57.6	0.0	57.6	11.0	51.3	0.0	20.0	41.0	1.8	51.0	16.0	4.2	194	12.1
1996	57.8	0.0	57.8	11.0	51.4	0.0	20.0	41.1	1.8	51.1	16.0	4.2	195	12.2
1997	60.4	0.0	60.4	11.0	53.7	0.0	20.0	43.0	1.9	53.4	16.0	4.2	204	12.7
1998	61.9	0.0	61.9	11.0	55.1	0.0	20.0	44.1	1.9	54.8	16.0	4.2	209	13.0
1999	63.7	0.0	63.7	11.0	56.7	0.0	20.0	45.4	2.0	56.4	16.0	4.2	215	13.4
2000	62.7	0.0	62.7	11.0	55.8	0.0	20.0	44.6	2.0	55.5	16.0	4.2	211	13.2
2001	62.6	0.0	62.6	11.0	55.7	0.0	20.0	44.6	2.0	55.4	16.0	4.2	211	13.2
2002	62.9	0.0	62.9	11.0	56.0	0.0	20.0	44.8	2.0	55.6	16.0	4.2	212	13.2
2003	61.0	0.0	61.0	11.0	54.3	0.0	20.0	43.4	1.9	54.0	16.0	4.2	206	12.8
2004	59.9	0.0	59.9	11.0	53.3	0.0	20.0	42.7	1.9	53.0	16.0	4.2	202	12.6
2005	59.2	0.0	59.2	11.0	52.7	0.0	20.0	42.2	1.8	52.4	16.0	4.2	200	12.5
2006	58.3	0.0	58.3	11.0	51.9	0.0	20.0	41.5	1.8	51.6	16.0	4.2	197	12.3
2007	56.3	0.0	56.3	11.0	50.1	0.0	20.0	40.1	1.8	49.8	16.0	4.2	190	11.9
2008	53.1	0.0	53.1	11.0	47.3	0.0	20.0	37.8	1.7	47.0	16.0	4.2	179	11.2

TABLE 1.12

Estimated number of per capita calories of high fructose corn syrup consumed daily, 1970–2010[a] [CONTINUED]

Year	Primary weight (market level)[b]	Loss from primary to retail weight	Weight at retail level	Loss from retail/institutional to consumer level	Weight at consumer level	Loss at consumer level — Nonedible share	Loss at consumer level — Other (uneaten food, spoilage, etc.)		Per capita consumption (adjusted for loss)		Calories per serving	Serving weight	Calories consumed daily[c]	Servings (teaspoons) consumed daily[d]
	lb/yr	percent	lb/yr	percent	lb/yr	percent	percent	lbs/yr	oz/daily	g/daily	number	grams	number	teaspoons
2009	50.2	0.0	50.2	11.0	44.7	0.0	20.0	35.7	1.6	44.4	16.0	4.2	169	10.6
2010	48.9	0.0	48.9	11.0	43.5	0.0	20.0	34.8	1.5	43.3	16.0	4.2	165	10.3

[a]Estimated number of daily per capita calories calculated by adjusting HFCS deliveries for domestic food and beverage use for food losses.
[b]U.S. per capita high fructose corn syrup (HFCS) estimated deliveries for domestic food and beverage use, calendar year.
[c]Number of daily teaspoons multiplied by calories per serving.
[d]Grams per day divided by serving weight.
Note: Some data are preliminary.

SOURCE: "Table 52. High Fructose Corn Syrup: Estimated Number of per Capita Calories Consumed Daily, by Calendar Year," in *Sugar and Sweeteners: Recommended Data*, U.S. Department of Agriculture, Economic Research Service, July 25, 2011, http://www.ers.usda.gov/Briefing/Sugar/Data.htm (accessed October 1, 2011)

TABLE 1.13

Food expenditures by families and individuals as a share of disposable personal income, 1929–2010

Year	Disposable personal income	Expenditures for food					
		At home[a]		Away from home[b]		Total[c]	
	Billion dollars	Billion dollars	Percent	Billion dollars	Percent	Billion dollars	Percent
1929	83.4	16.9	20.3	2.6	3.1	19.5	23.4
1930	74.7	15.8	21.2	2.3	3.1	18.1	24.2
1931	64.3	12.7	19.8	2.1	3.3	14.8	23.0
1932	49.2	9.6	19.5	1.7	3.5	11.3	23.0
1933	46.1	10.1	21.9	1.5	3.3	11.6	25.2
1934	52.8	11.1	21.0	1.7	3.2	12.8	24.2
1935	59.3	12.1	20.4	1.8	3.0	13.9	23.4
1936	67.4	12.7	18.8	2.0	3.0	14.7	21.8
1937	72.2	13.3	18.4	2.2	3.0	15.5	21.5
1938	66.6	12.6	18.9	2.1	3.2	14.7	22.1
1939	71.4	13.0	18.1	2.3	3.2	15.2	21.3
1940	76.8	13.5	17.6	2.4	3.1	15.9	20.7
1941	93.8	15.3	16.3	2.9	3.1	18.2	19.4
1942	118.6	18.5	15.6	3.6	3.0	22.1	18.6
1943	135.4	20.7	15.3	4.5	3.3	25.2	18.6
1944	148.3	22.1	14.9	5.1	3.4	27.2	18.4
1945	152.2	23.6	15.5	5.7	3.7	29.3	19.2
1946	161.4	28.4	17.6	6.5	4.0	34.9	21.6
1947	171.2	32.8	19.2	7.4	4.3	40.2	23.5
1948	190.6	34.9	18.3	7.5	3.9	42.4	22.3
1949	190.4	34.3	18.0	7.8	4.1	42.0	22.1
1950	210.1	35.7	17.0	7.6	3.6	43.3	20.6
1951	231.0	40.0	17.3	8.4	3.6	48.4	20.9
1952	243.4	41.8	17.2	8.8	3.6	50.6	20.8
1953	258.6	42.3	16.4	9.0	3.5	51.3	19.9
1954	264.3	42.4	16.0	9.3	3.5	51.7	19.6
1955	283.3	42.9	15.1	9.8	3.5	52.7	18.6
1956	303.0	44.4	14.7	10.4	3.4	54.8	18.1
1957	319.8	48.1	15.0	10.9	3.4	59.0	18.4
1958	330.5	49.8	15.1	11.1	3.4	60.9	18.4
1959	350.5	50.1	14.3	12.1	3.5	62.3	17.8
1960	365.4	51.5	14.1	12.6	3.4	64.0	17.5
1961	381.8	52.0	13.6	13.1	3.4	65.1	17.1
1962	405.1	52.9	13.1	13.9	3.4	66.8	16.5
1963	425.1	53.3	12.5	14.5	3.4	67.9	16.0
1964	462.5	55.5	12.0	15.7	3.4	71.2	15.4
1965	498.1	58.4	11.7	16.9	3.4	75.4	15.1
1966	537.5	61.0	11.3	18.6	3.5	79.6	14.8
1967	575.3	61.4	10.7	19.8	3.4	81.1	14.1
1968	625.0	64.5	10.3	21.7	3.5	86.2	13.8
1969	674.0	69.0	10.2	23.4	3.5	92.3	13.7
1970	735.7	75.5	10.3	26.4	3.6	102.0	13.9
1971	801.8	79.5	9.9	28.1	3.5	107.6	13.4
1972	869.1	86.0	9.9	31.3	3.6	117.3	13.5
1973	978.3	94.9	9.7	34.9	3.6	129.8	13.3
1974	1,071.6	107.3	10.0	38.5	3.6	145.8	13.6
1975	1,187.4	117.4	9.9	45.9	3.9	163.3	13.8
1976	1,302.5	125.1	9.6	52.6	4.0	177.7	13.6
1977	1,435.7	133.8	9.3	58.5	4.1	192.3	13.4
1978	1,608.3	147.3	9.2	67.5	4.2	214.8	13.4
1979	1,793.5	164.0	9.1	76.9	4.3	240.9	13.4
1980	2,009.0	180.8	9.0	85.2	4.2	266.0	13.2
1981	2,246.1	195.5	8.7	95.8	4.3	291.3	13.0
1982	2,421.2	201.0	8.3	104.5	4.3	305.5	12.6
1983	2,608.4	211.4	8.1	113.7	4.4	325.1	12.5
1984	2,912.0	224.0	7.7	121.9	4.2	345.8	11.9
1985	3,109.3	234.0	7.5	128.6	4.1	362.6	11.7
1986	3,285.1	242.7	7.4	137.9	4.2	380.6	11.6
1987	3,458.1	252.7	7.3	144.4	4.2	397.1	11.5
1988	3,726.3	271.7	7.2	155.5	4.1	427.2	11.4
1989	4,021.7	290.1	7.2	163.3	4.1	453.4	11.3
1990	4,285.8	314.5	7.3	175.2	4.1	489.6	11.4
1991	4,464.3	328.6	7.4	184.0	4.1	512.6	11.5
1992	4,751.4	324.4	6.8	189.5	4.0	513.9	10.8
1993	4,911.9	333.1	6.8	203.8	4.1	537.0	10.9
1994	5,151.8	345.5	6.7	214.4	4.2	559.9	10.9

TABLE 1.13

Food expenditures by families and individuals as a share of disposable personal income, 1929–2010 [CONTINUED]

Year	Disposable personal income	Expenditures for food					
		At home[a]		Away from home[b]		Total[c]	
	Billion dollars	Billion dollars	Percent	Billion dollars	Percent	Billion dollars	Percent
1995	5,408.2	351.7	6.5	223.9	4.1	575.6	10.6
1996	5,688.5	365.8	6.4	231.0	4.1	596.7	10.5
1997	5,988.8	388.1	6.5	244.4	4.1	632.5	10.6
1998	6,395.9	396.8	6.2	257.0	4.0	653.8	10.2
1999	6,695.0	414.5	6.2	268.9	4.0	683.5	10.2
2000	7,327.2	433.0	5.9	288.8	3.9	721.9	9.9
2001	7,648.5	454.4	5.9	298.5	3.9	752.8	9.8
2002	8,009.7	475.3	5.9	312.2	3.9	787.5	9.8
2003	8,377.8	491.0	5.9	330.7	3.9	821.8	9.8
2004	8,889.4	510.9	5.7	353.5	4.0	864.4	9.7
2005	9,277.3	535.9	5.8	376.6	4.1	912.5	9.8
2006	9,915.7	555.2	5.6	399.9	4.0	955.0	9.6
2007	10,423.6	583.1	5.6	420.8	4.0	1,003.9	9.6
2008	10,952.9	611.7	5.6	431.9	3.9	1,043.6	9.5
2009	11,034.9	609.2	5.5	429.6	3.9	1,038.8	9.4
2010	11,379.9	630.1	5.5	443.9	3.9	1,074.0	9.4

[a]Food-at-home includes cash purchases from grocery stores and other retail outlets, including purchases with food stamps and Women, Infants, and Children (WIC) vouchers and food produced and consumed on farms (valued at farm prices), but excludes government-donated foods.
[b]Food-away-from-home includes meals and snacks purchased by families and individuals and food furnished to employees, but excludes food paid for by government and business, such as donated foods to schools, meals in prisons and other institutions, and expense-account meals.
[c]Total may not add due to rounding.

SOURCE: "Table 7. Food Expenditures by Families and Individuals As a Share of Disposable Personal Income," in *Food CPI and Expenditures: Food Expenditure Tables*, U.S. Department of Agriculture, Economic Research Service, July 13, 2011, http://www.ers.usda.gov/briefing/cpifoodandexpenditures/data/Expenditures_tables/table7.htm (accessed October 1, 2011)

CHAPTER 2
WEIGHT AND PHYSICAL HEALTH

If we could give every individual the right amount of nourishment and exercise, not too little and not too much, we would have found the safest way to health.

—Hippocrates

During the 20th century and the first decade of the 21st century, advances in public health and medical care helped Americans lead longer, healthier lives. Two important measures of the health of the population are infant mortality (death) rates and life expectancy at birth rates. By the end of the 20th century, infant mortality rates had significantly decreased and life expectancy had increased by 29.4 years. Table 2.1 shows the long-term upward trend in life expectancy as well as recent gains. In 2007 life expectancy at birth for the total population reached a record high of 77.9 years, up from 75.4 years in 1990. The Central Intelligence Agency estimates in *World Factbook: United States* (November 17, 2011, https://www.cia.gov/library/publications/the-world-factbook/geos/us.html) that in 2011 life expectancy at birth increased to 78.4 years (80.9 years for females and 75.9 years for males).

As deaths from infectious diseases declined during the second half of the 20th century, mortality from chronic diseases, such as heart disease and cancer, increased. Table 2.2 displays the 10 leading causes of death in the United States in 1980 and 2007. Overweight and obesity are considered contributing factors to at least four of the 10 leading causes of death in 2007: diseases of the heart, malignant neoplasms (tumors), cerebrovascular diseases (diseases affecting the supply of blood to the brain), and diabetes mellitus. Obesity may also be implicated in some deaths attributable to another leading cause of death: nephritis, nephrotic syndrome, and nephrosis (kidney disease or chronic renal failure). Table 2.2 also reveals the rise of diabetes as a cause of death. In 1980 it was the seventh-leading cause of death, claiming 34,851 lives. By 2007 it was the underlying cause of 71,382

deaths. Epidemiologists (scientists who study the occurrence and distribution of diseases and the factors that govern their spread) and medical researchers believe the increasing prevalence of diabetes in the U.S. population and the resultant rise in deaths attributable to diabetes are direct consequences of the obesity epidemic in the United States.

Overweight and obesity increase not only the risk of morbidity (illness or disease) and mortality but also the severity of diseases such as hypertension (high blood pressure), arthritis, and other musculoskeletal problems. Table 2.3 lists the health consequences that may result from overweight and obesity among adults and children. It also estimates the likelihood of these health consequences. For example, adults who are obese are twice as likely to suffer from high blood pressure than adults who have a healthy weight.

In "Contribution of Obesity to International Differences in Life Expectancy" (*American Journal of Public Health*, vol. 101, no. 11, November 2011), Samuel H. Preston and Andrew Stokes examine the relationship between obesity and life expectancy in the United States. The researchers observe that "the United States has the highest prevalence of obesity and one of the lowest life expectancies among high-income countries." By estimating the fraction of deaths attributable to obesity by country, Preston and Stokes find that the high prevalence of obesity in the United States not only reduces life expectancy but also strongly contributes to its low rank in international comparisons of life expectancy.

IS OBESITY A DISEASE?

Researchers now recognize that obesity does not simply result from willful overeating and laziness, but from a complex combination of genetic, metabolic, behavioral, and environmental factors. Rather than viewing it as a lifestyle choice or personal failing, several

TABLE 2.1

Life expectancy at birth, at 65 years of age, and at 75 years of age, according to race and sex, selected years 1900–2007

[Data are based on death certificates]

Specified age and year	All races Both sexes	All races Male	All races Female	White Both sexes	White Male	White Female	Black or African American[a] Both sexes	Black or African American[a] Male	Black or African American[a] Female
				Remaining life expectancy in years					
At birth									
1900[b, c]	47.3	46.3	48.3	47.6	46.6	48.7	33.0	32.5	33.5
1950[c]	68.2	65.6	71.1	69.1	66.5	72.2	60.8	59.1	62.9
1960[c]	69.7	66.6	73.1	70.6	67.4	74.1	63.6	61.1	66.3
1970	70.8	67.1	74.7	71.7	68.0	75.6	64.1	60.0	68.3
1980	73.7	70.0	77.4	74.4	70.7	78.1	68.1	63.8	72.5
1990	75.4	71.8	78.8	76.1	72.7	79.4	69.1	64.5	73.6
1995	75.8	72.5	78.9	76.5	73.4	79.6	69.6	65.2	73.9
1999	76.7	73.9	79.4	77.3	74.6	79.9	71.4	67.8	74.7
2000	76.8	74.1	79.3	77.3	74.7	79.9	71.8	68.2	75.1
2001	76.9	74.2	79.4	77.4	74.8	79.9	72.0	68.4	75.2
2002	76.9	74.3	79.5	77.4	74.9	79.9	72.1	68.6	75.4
2003	77.1	74.5	79.6	77.6	75.0	80.0	72.3	68.8	75.6
2004	77.5	74.9	79.9	77.9	75.4	80.4	72.8	69.3	76.0
2005	77.4	74.9	79.9	77.9	75.4	80.4	72.8	69.3	76.1
2006	77.7	75.1	80.2	78.2	75.7	80.6	73.2	69.7	76.5
2007	77.9	75.4	80.4	78.4	75.9	80.8	73.6	70.0	76.8
At 65 years									
1950[c]	13.9	12.8	15.0	—	12.8	15.1	13.9	12.9	14.9
1960[c]	14.3	12.8	15.8	14.4	12.9	15.9	13.9	12.7	15.1
1970	15.2	13.1	17.0	15.2	13.1	17.1	14.2	12.5	15.7
1980	16.4	14.1	18.3	16.5	14.2	18.4	15.1	13.0	16.8
1990	17.2	15.1	18.9	17.3	15.2	19.1	15.4	13.2	17.2
1995	17.4	15.6	18.9	17.6	15.7	19.1	15.6	13.6	17.1
1999	17.7	16.1	19.1	17.8	16.1	19.2	16.0	14.3	17.3
2000	17.6	16.0	19.0	17.7	16.1	19.1	16.1	14.1	17.5
2001	17.7	16.2	19.0	17.8	16.3	19.1	16.2	14.2	17.6
2002	17.8	16.2	19.1	17.9	16.3	19.2	16.3	14.4	17.7
2003	17.9	16.4	19.2	18.0	16.5	19.3	16.4	14.5	17.9
2004	18.2	16.7	19.5	18.3	16.8	19.5	16.7	14.8	18.2
2005	18.2	16.8	19.5	18.3	16.9	19.5	16.8	14.9	18.2
2006	18.5	17.0	19.7	18.6	17.1	19.8	17.1	15.1	18.6
2007	18.6	17.2	19.9	18.7	17.3	19.9	17.2	15.2	18.7
At 75 years									
1980	10.4	8.8	11.5	10.4	8.8	11.5	9.7	8.3	10.7
1990	10.9	9.4	12.0	11.0	9.4	12.0	10.2	8.6	11.2
1995	11.0	9.7	11.9	11.1	9.7	12.0	10.2	8.8	11.1
1999	11.2	10.0	12.1	11.2	10.0	12.1	10.4	9.2	11.1
2000	11.0	9.8	11.8	11.0	9.8	11.9	10.4	9.0	11.3
2001	11.1	9.9	11.9	11.1	9.9	11.9	10.5	9.1	11.4
2002	11.0	9.9	11.9	11.1	9.9	11.9	10.5	9.2	11.4
2003	11.1	10.0	11.9	11.1	10.0	11.9	10.6	9.3	11.5
2004	11.4	10.3	12.2	11.4	10.3	12.2	10.8	9.5	11.7
2005	11.3	10.2	12.1	11.4	10.3	12.1	10.8	9.5	11.7
2006	11.6	10.5	12.3	11.5	10.5	12.3	11.1	9.8	12.0
2007	11.7	10.6	12.5	11.7	10.6	12.4	11.2	9.9	12.1

—Data not available.
[a]Data shown for 1900–1960 are for the nonwhite population.
[b]Death registration area only. The death registration area increased from 10 states and the District of Columbia (D.C.) in 1900 to the coterminous United States in 1933.
[c]Includes deaths of persons who were not residents of the 50 states and D.C.
Notes: Populations for computing life expectancy for 1991–1999 are 1990-based postcensal estimates of U.S. resident population. In 1997, life table methodology was revised to construct complete life tables by single years of age that extend to age 100. Previously, abridged life tables were constructed for 5-year age groups ending with 85 years and over. Life table values for 2000 and later years were computed using a slight modification of the new life table method due to a change in the age detail of populations received from the U.S. Census Bureau. Values for data years 2000–2007 are based on a newly revised methodology that uses vital statistics death rates for ages under 66 and modeled probabilities of death for ages 66 to 100 based on blended vital statistics and Medicare probabilities of dying and may differ from figures previously published. The revised methodology is similar to that developed for the 1999–2001 decennial life tables. Starting with 2003 data, some states allowed the reporting of more than one race on the death certificate. The multiple-race data for these states were bridged to the single-race categories of the 1977 Office of Management and Budget Standards for comparability with other states.

SOURCE: "Table 22. Life Expectancy at Birth, at 65 Years of Age, and at 75 Years of Age, by Race and Sex: United States, Selected Years 1900–2007," in *Health, United States, 2010: With Special Feature on Death and Dying*, Centers for Disease Control and Prevention, National Center for Health Statistics, 2011, http://www.cdc.gov/nchs/data/hus/hus10.pdf#listtables (accessed September 30, 2011)

groups favor declaring obesity a disease. Proponents assert that many public health benefits would result from designating obesity as a disease, including:

• Reducing the social stigma and prejudice that are associated with obesity, and promoting attitudinal changes to reduce weight-based discrimination

TABLE 2.2

Leading causes of death and numbers of deaths, according to sex and race, 1980 and 2007

[Data are based on death certificates]

Sex, race, Hispanic origin, and rank order	1980 Cause of death	Deaths	2007 Cause of death	Deaths
All persons				
Rank	All causes	1,989,841	All causes	2,423,712
1	Diseases of heart	761,085	Diseases of heart	616,067
2	Malignant neoplasms	416,509	Malignant neoplasms	562,875
3	Cerebrovascular diseases	170,225	Cerebrovascular diseases	135,952
4	Unintentional injuries	105,718	Chronic lower respiratory diseases	127,924
5	Chronic obstructive pulmonary diseases	56,050	Unintentional injuries	123,706
6	Pneumonia and influenza	54,619	Alzheimer's disease	74,632
7	Diabetes mellitus	34,851	Diabetes mellitus	71,382
8	Chronic liver disease and cirrhosis	30,583	Influenza and pneumonia	52,717
9	Atherosclerosis	29,449	Nephritis, nephrotic syndrome and nephrosis .	46,448
10	Suicide	26,869	Septicemia	34,828
Male				
Rank	All causes	1,075,078	All causes	1,203,968
1	Diseases of heart	405,661	Diseases of heart	309,821
2	Malignant neoplasms	225,948	Malignant neoplasms	292,857
3	Unintentional injuries	74,180	Unintentional injuries	79,827
4	Cerebrovascular diseases	69,973	Chronic lower respiratory diseases	61,235
5	Chronic obstructive pulmonary diseases	38,625	Cerebrovascular diseases	54,111
6	Pneumonia and influenza	27,574	Diabetes mellitus	35,478
7	Suicide	20,505	Suicide	27,269
8	Chronic liver disease and cirrhosis	19,768	Inluenza and pneumonia	24,071
9	Homicide	18,779	Nephritis, nephrotic syndrome and nephrosis	22,616
10	Diabetes mellitus	14,325	Alzheimer's disease	21,800
Female				
Rank	All causes	914,763	All causes	1,219,744
1	Diseases of heart	355,424	Diseases of heart	306,246
2	Malignant neoplasms	190,561	Malignant neoplasms	270,018
3	Cerebrovascular diseases	100,252	Cerebrovascular diseases	81,841
4	Unintentional injuries	31,538	Chronic lower respiratory diseases	66,689
5	Pneumonia and influenza	27,045	Alzheimer's disease	52,832
6	Diabetes mellitus	20,526	Unintentional injuries	43,879
7	Atherosclerosis	17,848	Diabetes mellitus	35,904
8	Chronic obstructive pulmonary diseases	17,425	Influenza and pneumonia	28,646
9	Chronic liver disease and cirrhosis	10,815	Nephritis, nephrotic syndrome and nephrosis	23,832
10	Certain conditions originating in the perinatal period	9,815	Septicemia	18,989
White				
Rank	All causes	1,738,607	All causes	2,074,151
1	Diseases of heart	683,347	Diseases of heart	531,636
2	Malignant neoplasms	368,162	Malignant neoplasms	483,939
3	Cerebrovascular diseases	148,734	Chronic lower respiratory diseases	118,081
4	Unintentional injuries	90,122	Cerebrovascular diseases	114,695
5	Chronic obstructive pulmonary diseases	52,375	Unintentional injuries	106,252
6	Pneumonia and influenza	48,369	Alzheimer's disease	68,933
7	Diabetes mellitus	28,868	Diabetes mellitus	56,390
8	Atherosclerosis	27,069	Influenza and pneumonia	45,947
9	Chronic liver disease and cirrhosis	25,240	Nephritis, nephrotic syndrome and nephrosis	36,871
10	Suicide	24,829	Suicide	31,348

- Enabling more people to seek treatment for obesity by providing health insurance coverage for treatment

- Increasing public awareness of the severity of obesity as a threat to health and longevity

- Stimulating scientific and medical research on the prevention and treatment of the condition and speeding approval of new antiobesity drugs

Advocates of classifying obesity as a disease, including the World Health Organization (WHO), the National Institutes of Health, the National Academy of Sciences, the Federal Trade Commission, the Maternal and Child Health Bureau, the American Heart Association, the American Academy of Family Physicians, the American Society for Bariatric Surgery, the American Society of Bariatric Physicians, and the American Obesity Association (AOA), observe that in the past, alcoholism was viewed as a personal choice or moral weakness, whereas in the 21st century it is considered a disease. They also note that eating disorders such as anorexia nervosa (intense fear of becoming fat even when dangerously underweight) and bulimia nervosa (recurrent episodes of binge eating followed by purging to prevent weight gain) are classified as diseases. In view of the size and scope of the obesity epidemic, proponents argue that the social and financial costs of allowing the problem of obesity to go unchecked

TABLE 2.2

Leading causes of death and numbers of deaths, according to sex and race, 1980 and 2007 [CONTINUED]

[Data are based on death certificates]

Sex, race, Hispanic origin, and rank order	1980		2007	
	Cause of death	Deaths	Cause of death	Deaths
Black or African American				
Rank	All causes	233,135	All causes	289,585
1	Diseases of heart	72,956	Diseases of heart	71,209
2	Malignant neoplasms	45,037	Malignant neoplasms	64,049
3	Cerebrovascular diseases	20,135	Cerebrovascular diseases	17,085
4	Unintentional injuries	13,480	Unintentional injuries	13,559
5	Homicide	10,172	Diabetes mellitus	12,459
6	Certain conditions originating in the perinatal period	6,961	Homicide	8,870
7	Pneumonia and influenza	5,648	Nephritis, nephrotic syndrome and nephrosis	8,392
8	Diabetes mellitus	5,544	Chronic lower respiratory diseases	7,901
9	Chronic liver disease and cirrhosis	4,790	Human immunodeficiency virus (HIV) disease	6,470
10	Nephritis, nephrotic syndrome, and nephrosis	3,416	Septicemia	6,297

Notes: Starting with 2003 data, some states allowed the reporting of more than one race on the death certificate. The multiple-race data for these states were bridged to the single-race categories of the 1977 Office of Management and Budget standards for comparability with other states. The race groups, white, black, Asian or Pacific Islander, and American Indian or Alaska Native, include persons of Hispanic and non-Hispanic origin. Persons of Hispanic origin may be of any race.

SOURCE: Adapted from "Table 26. Leading Causes of Death and Numbers of Deaths, by Sex, Race, and Hispanic Origin: United States, 1980 and 2007," in *Health, United States, 2010: With Special Feature on Death and Dying,* Centers for Disease Control and Prevention, National Center for Health Statistics, 2011, http://www.cdc.gov/nchs/data/hus/hus10.pdf#listtables (accessed September 30, 2011)

will far exceed the costs associated with extending health care coverage for weight-reduction programs.

The AOA contends that obesity meets the criteria for disease because according to *Stedman's Medical Dictionary* (2005) a disease should have at least two of the following three features:

- Recognized etiologic (causative) agents
- Identifiable signs and symptoms
- Consistent anatomical alterations

The AOA describes etiologic agents for obesity as social, behavioral, cultural, physiological, metabolic, and genetic factors. The identifiable signs and symptoms of obesity include an excess accumulation of adipose tissue (fat); an increase in the size or number of fat cells; insulin resistance; decreased levels of high-density lipoprotein and norepinephrine; alterations in the activity of the sympathetic and parasympathetic nervous system; and elevated blood pressure, blood glucose, cholesterol, and triglyceride levels. The consistent anatomical alteration of obesity is the increase in body mass.

Opponents contend that even though obesity increases the risk of developing many diseases, it is not an ailment in itself but an unhealthy consequence of poor lifestyle choices. They liken it to cigarette smoking, a risk factor that predisposes people to disease, and they dispute the notion that labeling obesity as a disease will have a beneficial effect on the ability of public health organizations to alter the course of the obesity epidemic. They maintain the public tends to view diseases as con-

ditions that are contracted or contagious; and with disease comes a victim mentality, rather than an assumption of personal responsibility. Because many health professionals consider the assumption of personal responsibility as being crucial for the long-term success of obesity treatment, any action that releases people from assuming personal responsibility is counterproductive.

Furthermore, because people who are obese often function normally and can perform all the activities of daily living, opponents assert that their lives are not impaired or compromised as they might be by other chronic diseases. Some researchers, such as Silvia Migliaccio et al. of the Università Sapienza di Roma in "Is Obesity in Women Protective against Osteoporosis?" (*Diabetes, Metabolic Syndrome, and Obesity,* vol. 4, July 2011), also point to the fact that in a few instances obesity may even be protective by reducing the risk of osteoporosis.

Opponents to granting disease status to obesity predict that the financial ramifications would be devastating for taxpayers and the health insurance industry. Health care costs, which increase every year, would skyrocket. Antiobesity programs would drive insurance premiums even higher and place unreasonable burdens on the already overburdened Medicare (a medical insurance program for older adults and people with disabilities) and Medicaid (a federal and state health care program for people below the poverty level) programs. Employers, especially small businesses, might be forced by high health care costs to drop employee coverage altogether.

A related concern is the lack of universally accepted, effective treatment for obesity. If obesity is

TABLE 2.3

Health consequences of overweight and obesity

Premature death

- An estimated 300,000 deaths per year may be attributable to obesity.
- The risk of death rises with increasing weight.
- Even moderate weight excess (10 to 20 pounds for a person of average height) increases the risk of death, particularly among adults aged 30 to 64 years.
- Individuals who are obese (body mass index (BMI) > 30) have a 50 to 100% increased risk of premature death from all causes, compared to individuals with a healthy weight.

Heart disease

- The incidence of heart disease (heart attack, congestive heart failure, sudden cardiac death, angina or chest pain, and abnormal heart rhythm) is increased in persons who are overweight or obese (BMI > 25).
- High blood pressure is twice as common in adults who are obese than in those who are at a healthy weight.
- Obesity is associated with elevated triglycerides (blood fat) and decreased high density lipoprotein (HDL) cholesterol ("good cholesterol").

Diabetes

- A weight gain of 11 to 18 pounds increases a person's risk of developing type 2 diabetes to twice that of individuals who have not gained weight.
- Over 80% of people with diabetes are overweight or obese.

Cancer

- Overweight and obesity are associated with an increased risk for some types of cancer including endometrial (cancer of the lining of the uterus), colon, gall bladder, prostate, kidney, and postmenopausal breast cancer.
- Women gaining more than 20 pounds from age 18 to midlife double their risk of postmenopausal breast cancer, compared to women whose weight remains stable.

Breathing problems

- Sleep apnea (interrupted breathing while sleeping) is more common in obese persons.
- Obesity is associated with a higher prevalence of asthma.

Arthritis

- For every 2-pound increase in weight, the risk of developing arthritis is increased by 9 to 13%.
- Symptoms of arthritis can improve with weight loss.

Reproductive complications

Complications of pregnancy
- Obesity during pregnancy is associated with increased risk of death in both the baby and the mother and increases the risk of maternal high blood pressure by 10 times.
- In addition to many other complications, women who are obese during pregnancy are more likely to have gestational diabetes and problems with labor and delivery.
- Infants born to women who are obese during pregnancy are more likely to be high birthweight and, therefore, may face a higher rate of Cesarean section delivery and low blood sugar (which can be associated with brain damage and seizures).
- Obesity during pregnancy is associated with an increased risk of birth defects, particularly neural tube defects, such as spina bifida.
- Obesity in premenopausal women is associated with irregular menstrual cycles and infertility.

Additional health consequences

- Overweight and obesity are associated with increased risks of gall bladder disease, incontinence, increased surgical risk, and depression.
- Obesity can affect the quality of life through limited mobility and decreased physical endurance as well as through social, academic, and job discrimination.

Children and adolescents

- Risk factors for heart disease, such as high cholesterol and high blood pressure, occur with increased frequency in overweight children and adolescents compared to those with a healthy weight.
- Type 2 diabetes, previously considered an adult disease, has increased dramatically in children and adolescents. Overweight and obesity are closely linked to type 2 diabetes.
- Overweight adolescents have a 70% chance of becoming overweight or obese adults. This increases to 80% if one or more parent is overweight or obese.
- The most immediate consequence of overweight, as perceived by children themselves, is social discrimination.

SOURCE: "Overweight and Obesity: Health Consequences," in *The Surgeon General's Call to Action to Prevent and Decrease Overweight and Obesity*, U.S. Department of Health and Human Services, Office of the Surgeon General, 2001, http://www.surgeongeneral.gov/topics/obesity/calltoaction/fact_consequences .htm (accessed October 29, 2011)

---

classified as a disease, which treatment or therapies should be covered? For example, if exercise is deemed beneficial, then health insurers might be required to pay for gym memberships. Furthermore, some opponents believe it is not necessary to designate obesity as a disease to encourage Americans to seek treatment. They cite the more than $50 billion that is spent annually on weight-loss programs and services as evidence that Americans are not reluctant to seek treatment for obesity.

Even though the debate has not been fully resolved, obesity is rapidly acquiring recognition as a disease. In 2002 the Internal Revenue Service ruled that for tax purposes obesity is a disease, allowing Americans for the first time to claim a deduction for some health care expenses that are related to obesity, just as they can for expenditures that are related to cancer, diabetes, heart disease, and other illnesses.

In 2004 the federal Medicare program discarded its long-standing position that obesity is not a disease, which effectively removed a major roadblock for people seeking coverage for treatment of obesity. After years of review, the Centers for Medicare and Medicaid Services, which administers the health program for older adults and people who are disabled, announced in *CMS Manual System: Pub. 100-03 Medicare National Coverage Determinations* (October 1, 2004, http://www.cms.hhs.gov/ transmittals/downloads/R23NCD.pdf) that it eliminated the phrase "obesity itself cannot be considered an illness" from its policy that had been used to deny coverage for weight-loss treatment. Even though the decision stopped short of declaring obesity a disease and did not automatically imply coverage for any specific treatment, it enabled individuals, physicians, and companies to apply to Medicare for reimbursement for a variety of weight-loss therapies. Medicare coverage for selected weight-loss procedures took effect in February 2006.

Because private insurance companies often use Medicare as a model for their coverage and benefits, the Medicare decision prompted them to expand coverage for weight-loss procedures. As of January 2012, private health insurance coverage for weight-loss therapies and surgical procedures varied widely. In "Health Insurance FAQ Regarding Weight Loss" (September 13, 2011, http://www.ksdk.com/news/health/cuttingedge/article/276519/219/Health-insurance-FAQ-regarding-weight-loss), Patricia T. Horvath, the executive director of United-Healthcare Employer and Individual in Northern Ohio, explained to Kevin Held that "insurance coverage for weight loss surgery varies by state and insurance provider. Many insurance companies—both public and private—now offer coverage, including gastric bypass insurance. While some insurers may foot the entire bill, many public or private insurance companies that cover weight loss surgery will pay 80 percent of what is considered 'customary and usual' for the surgery."

THE GENETICS OF BODY WEIGHT AND OBESITY

Genetics, the study of single genes and their effects, explains how and why traits such as hair color and blood types run in families. In the early 21st century the scientific community agreed that body shape and body weight are also regulated traits, that genes govern much of this regulation, and that altering genetically predetermined set points for body weight is often difficult. Genomics, a discipline that emerged during the 1980s, is the study of more than single genes; it considers the functions and interactions of all the genes in the genome. In terms of understanding genetics as a risk factor for obesity, genomics has broader applicability than does genetics because it is likely that humans carry dozens of genes that are directly related to body size and that most obesity is multifactorial—resulting from the complex interactions of multiple genes and environmental factors.

Because genomics is a relatively new discipline, many questions are still unanswered about how genes influence the ability to balance energy input and energy expenditure, and why individuals vary in their abilities to perform this critical body function. Table 2.4 summarizes what is known and what remains to be learned about variations in body weight, energy metabolism, and inherited obesity syndromes.

TABLE 2.4

Obesity and genetics

What we know:	What we don't know:
Biological relatives tend to resemble each other in many ways, including body weight. Individuals with a family history of obesity may be predisposed to gain weight and interventions that prevent obesity are especially important.	Why are biological relatives more similar in body weight? What genes are associated with this observation? Are the same genetic associations seen in every family? How do these genes affect energy metabolism and regulation?
In an environment made constant for food intake and physical activity, individuals respond differently. Some people store more energy as fat in an environment of excess; others lose less fat in an environment of scarcity. The different responses are largely due to genetic variation between individuals.	Why are interventions based on diet and exercise more effective for some people than others? What are the biological differences between these high and low responders? How do we use these insights to tailor interventions to specific needs?
Fat stores are regulated over long periods of time by complex systems that involve input and feedback from fatty tissues, the brain, and endocrine glands like the pancreas and the thyroid. Overweight and obesity can result from only a very small positive energy input imbalance over a long period of time.	What elements of energy regulation feedback systems are different in individuals? How do these differences affect energy metabolism and regulation?
Rarely, people have mutations in single genes that result in severe obesity that starts in infancy. Studying these individuals is providing insight into the complex biological pathways that regulate the balance between energy input and energy expenditure.	Do additional obesity syndromes exist that are caused by mutations in single genes? If so, what are they? What are the natural history, management strategy, and outcome for affected individuals?
Obese individuals have genetic similarities that may shed light on the biological differences that predispose to gain weight. This knowledge may be useful in preventing or treating obesity in predisposed people.	How do genetic variations that are shared by obese people affect gene expression and function? How do genetic variation and environmental factors interact to produce obesity? What are the biological features associated with the tendency to gain weight? What environmental factors are helpful in countering these tendencies?
Pharmaceutical companies are using genetic approaches (pharmacogenomics) to develop new drug strategies to treat obesity.	Will pharmacologic approaches benefit most people affected with obesity? Will these drugs be accessible to most people?
The tendency to store energy in the form of fat is believed to result from thousands of years of evolution in an environment characterized by tenuous food supplies. In other words, those who could store energy in times of plenty were more likely to survive periods of famine and to pass this tendency to their offspring.	How can thousands of years of evolutionary pressure be countered? Can specific factors in the modern environment (other than the obvious) be identified and controlled to more effectively counter these tendencies?

SOURCE: "Obesity and Genetics: What We Know, What We Don't Know and What It Means," in *Public Health Genomics*, Centers for Disease Control and Prevention, National Office of Public Health Genomics, July 21, 2009, http://www.cdc.gov/genomics/resources/diseases/obesity/obesknow.htm (accessed October 2, 2011)

Single Mutant Genes Cause Obesity

Even though most obesity in humans is not due to mutations (alterations or changes) in single genes, there are obesity syndromes caused by variations in single genes. According to Alexandra I. F. Blakemore and Philippe Froguel of the Imperial College of London, in "Investigation of Mendelian Forms of Obesity Holds out the Prospect of Personalized Medicine" (*Annals of the New York Academy of Sciences*, vol. 1214, no. 1, December 2010), these mutations occur in genes that encode proteins that are related to the regulation of food intake and account for approximately 5% of all obesity.

The Centers for Disease Control and Prevention (CDC) reports in "Genomics and Health: Obesity and Genomics" (January 20, 2011, http://www.cdc.gov/genomics/resources/diseases/obesity/obesedit.htm) that as of October 2005, when the obesity gene map was completed, single gene mutations in 11 genes were believed to be responsible for 176 cases of obesity worldwide. One example is a mutation of the leptin gene (on chromosome 7) and its receptor. The circulating hormone leptin (leptos means thin) sends the brain a satiety signal to decrease appetite. Obese mice of the ob/ob strain produce no leptin and tend to overeat; when given leptin, the mice stop eating and lose weight. However, experiments have failed to replicate these findings in humans. Blood concentrations of leptin are usually elevated in obese people, suggesting that they may be insensitive or resistant to leptin, rather than leptin deficient. Most obese individuals appear to have normal genetic sequences for leptin and its receptor, although people with a demonstrable genetic leptin deficiency suffer from extreme obesity.

Melanocortin 4 receptor (MC4R) deficiency is the most commonly occurring monogenic (single gene) form of obesity. Inheriting one copy of certain variants of the gene causes obesity in some families. In "Melanocortin-4 Receptor Mutations in Obesity" (*Advances in Clinical Chemistry*, vol. 48, 2009), Ferruccio Santini et al. report that mutations in MC4R produce a distinct obesity syndrome that is inherited. The researchers observe that these mutant receptors play a pivotal role in the control of eating behavior—that the regulation of body weight in humans is sensitive to variations in the amount of functional MC4R and are present in about 6% of people who are obese.

Blakemore and Froguel observe that recent research on genome-wide single nucleotide polymorphisms (SNPs) associated with obesity, particularly the role of the FTO (fat mass and obesity-associated) gene, has outpaced research concentrating on a single gene that determines the occurrence of obesity. The focus on the FTO gene may be warranted because common variants of the FTO gene, which are located on chromosome 16, may be implicated in as much as 22% of obesity, according to the CDC. The FTO gene is also associated with an increased risk for diabetes.

In "Pediatric Obesity: Etiology and Treatment" (*Endocrinology and Metabolism Clinics*, vol. 58, no. 5, October 2011), Melissa K. Crocker and Jack A. Yanovski of the U.S. Public Health Service summarize what is known about the genetic underpinnings of obesity. The researchers observe that "most of the known genetic causes of obesity primarily increase energy intake. Genes regulating the leptin signaling pathway are particularly important for human energy homeostasis." Crocker and Yanovski report that SNPs of many genes and chromosomal regions have been found to be associated with body weight or body composition; however, mechanisms explaining how such SNPs exert an influence on energy balance are often not fully understood. The researchers reiterate one of the challenges of clinical genetic research: "Even in studies including thousands of genotyped people, such SNPs can be linked to body weight only when they are relatively common in the population."

Multiple Gene Variants Involved in Body Weight and Obesity

Heritability studies seek to determine the proportion of variance of a particular trait that is attributable to genetic factors and the proportion that is attributable to environmental factors. Such studies indicate that genetic factors may account for as much as 75% of the variability in human body weight and approximately 33% of the variation in the overall body mass index (BMI; body weight in kilograms divided by height in meters squared). Genetic factors affect variations in the resting metabolic rate, body fat distribution, and weight gain related to overfeeding, which explains in part why some individuals are more susceptible than others to weight gain or weight loss. To ensure survival in times of scarce food supplies, the human body has evolved to resist any loss of body fat. This biological drive to maintain weight is coordinated through central nervous system pathways, with the involvement of many neuropeptides. (Neuropeptides are released by neurons as intercellular messengers. Many neuropeptides are also hormones outside of the nervous system.) Evidence from twin, adoption, and family studies reveals that biological relatives exhibit similarities in the maintenance of body weight. First-degree relatives of moderately obese people are at three to four times the risk of obesity relative to the general population. First-degree relatives of severely obese people are at five times greater risk. Genetic predisposition to obesity does not mean that developing the condition is inevitable; however, research indicates that inherited genetic variation is an important risk factor for obesity.

Genetic factors have been implicated in the development of eating disorders such as anorexia and bulimia and appear to be involved in the extent to which diet and exercise are effective strategies for weight reduction. Furthermore, genetic variations among individuals may promote different food preferences and eating patterns that interact with environmental conditions to maintain healthy body weight or promote obesity.

These genetic risk factors tend to be familial but are not inherited in a simple manner; they may reflect many genetic variations, and each variation may contribute a small amount of risk and may interact with environmental elements to produce obesity. Tuomo Rankinen et al. present in "The Human Obesity Gene Map: The 2005 Update" (*Obesity*, vol. 14, no. 4, April 2006) the 12th update of the human obesity gene map by the Pennington Biomedical Research Center, which was completed in October 2005. This map contains over 600 genes, markers, and chromosomal regions that are associated with or linked to human obesity. Besides offering direction for future efforts to prevent and treat obesity, mounting genetic evidence offers a compelling argument that obesity is not a personal failing and that in most cases obesity involves multiple genetic and environmental components that affect endocrine, metabolic, and regulatory mechanisms.

Extra Genes Point to a Genetic Cause of Thinness

Unlike obesity, few genetic variants associated with underweight have been identified. Sébastien Jacquemont et al. report in "Mirror Extreme BMI Phenotypes Associated with Gene Dosage at the Chromosome 16p11.2 Locus" (*Nature*, vol. 478, no. 7367, August 31, 2011) that duplication of a portion of chromosome 16 is associated with being very thin (BMI less than 18.5). The researchers analyzed the deoxyribonucleic acid of more than 95,000 people and find that more than half of children with this duplication had significantly lower than normal weight gain. Jacquemont et al. also note that people missing this gene have an increased risk for obesity.

Genetic Susceptibility and Environmental Influences

Even though genetics may largely predetermine adult body weight absent specific environmental triggers or influences, genetic destiny in terms of body weight may not necessarily be realized. For example, an individual with a strong genetic predisposition for obesity will not become obese in the absence of sufficient food (caloric) intake. Similarly, when people who are genetically predisposed to normal body weight consume a largely high-fat diet, they may become overweight or obese because they may be more inclined to overeat. This is in part because the brain has difficulty conveying the satiety signal (the message to stop eating) when fatty foods are being consumed.

Besides caloric intake and physical activity, both of which are able to modify body weight, environmental influences before birth also significantly influence adult health and body weight. Research demonstrates that the pregnant mother's nutritional status affects the metabolism of her unborn child. Women who are severely malnourished during pregnancy stimulate the fetus to modify its metabolism to conserve and store energy, a survival practice that can promote overweight when the food supply is ample.

Societal and cultural norms can also cause environmental influences such as lifestyle and behavior to override genetic programming. For example, in the United States many young women with genetic predisposition to normal body weight or even overweight sharply limit their caloric intake and exercise vigorously to achieve "model thin" bodies. Similarly, in cultures where overweight is perceived as an indication of prosperity and is admired and coveted, people may override genetic tendencies to be normal weight by increasing caloric intake in an effort to achieve the culturally established ideal.

HEALTH RISKS AND CONSEQUENCES OF OVERWEIGHT AND OBESITY

People who are overweight or obese are at higher risk of developing one or more serious medical conditions, and obesity is associated with increases in deaths from all causes. Overweight and obesity significantly increase the risk for hypercholesterolemia (high cholesterol), hypertension, heart disease, and stroke; type 2 diabetes; osteoarthritis and chronic joint pain; gallbladder disease; fatty liver disease; several types of cancers; and sleep apnea (interrupted breathing while sleeping) and sleep disorders.

According to Neil K. Mehta and Virginia W. Chang, in "Mortality Attributable to Obesity among Middle-Aged Adults in the United States" (*Demography*, vol. 46, no. 4, November 2009), there are divergent estimates of deaths attributable to obesity and the differences are largely explained by the studies' varying methodological approaches. For example, in 2004 one study analyzing data from 2000 reported that obesity was second only to smoking as a cause of preventable deaths and deemed obesity a contributing cause in 435,000 deaths per year. The following year other researchers estimated that fewer than 30,000 deaths in 2000 were attributable to overweight or obesity because they attributed 86,000 fewer deaths to overweight, which they considered to be protective against mortality. Mehta and Chang analyzed mortality data of middle-aged adults, a group that is experiencing improving mortality and increasing obesity. They find that being overweight or having class I obesity (BMI 30 to 35) is not associated with increased mortality risk compared with normal BMI but that class

II/III (BMI 35 to 40 for class II and BMI greater than 40 for class III) obesity does confer significantly higher mortality—about 40% for females and 62% for males, compared with people with normal BMI.

The CDC observes in "Frequently Asked Questions about Calculating Obesity-Related Risk" (May 25, 2005, http://www.cdc.gov/PDF/Frequently_Asked_Questions _About_Calculating_Obesity-Related_Risk.pdf) that "because obesity has so many different effects on so many diseases, it is extremely difficult for doctors to identify obesity-related deaths reliably on death certificates. So, instead, scientists use complex modeling techniques to estimate deaths related to obesity," which in turn produce varying estimates of the annual number of obesity-related deaths. The CDC states that in the United States, an estimated 112,000 deaths per year are associated with obesity.

Hypercholesterolemia, Hypertension, Heart Disease, and Stroke

Overweight, obesity, and excess abdominal fat are directly related to cardiovascular risk factors, including high levels of total serum cholesterol, LDL cholesterol (low-density lipoprotein; a fatlike substance often called bad cholesterol because high levels increase the risk for heart disease), triglycerides, blood pressure, fibrinogen, and insulin, and low levels of HDL cholesterol (high-density lipoprotein; often called good cholesterol because high levels appear to protect against heart disease). The association between total serum cholesterol and coronary heart disease is largely due to LDL. A high-risk LDL cholesterol is greater than or equal to 160 milligrams per deciliter (mg/dL) with a 10 mg/dL rise in LDL cholesterol corresponding to approximately a 10% increase in risk. High-risk total serum cholesterol is greater than or equal to 240 mg/dL. The age-adjusted percentage of the population aged 20 years and older suffering from high serum cholesterol levels fell from 20.8% in 1988–94 to 14.9% in 2005–08. (See Table 2.5.) The overall decline in high total serum cholesterol occurred in response to the increasing use of effective cholesterol-lowering statin drugs.

The percentage of the population suffering from hypertension (people with elevated blood pressure and those taking antihypertensive medication) increased between 1988–94 and 2005–08, from 25.5% to 30.9% of the population. (See Table 2.6.) The highest rates for those aged 20 years and older during the 2005–08 period were reported among African-American females (44%). Both men and women were increasingly likely to have hypertension as they aged. Hypertension is approximately three times more common in obese than in normal-weight people, and the relationship between weight and blood pressure is clearly one of cause and effect, because when weight increases, so does blood pressure, and when weight decreases, blood pressure falls.

The physiological processes that produce the hypertension associated with obesity include sodium retention and increases in vascular resistance, blood volume, and cardiac output (the volume of blood pumped, measured in liters per minute). Even though it is not known precisely how weight loss results in a decrease in blood pressure, it is known that weight loss is associated with a reduction in vascular resistance and total blood volume and cardiac output. Weight loss also results in an improvement in insulin resistance, a reduction in sympathetic nervous system activity, and the suppression of the renin-angiotensin-aldosterone system, a group of hormones that are responsible for the opening and narrowing of blood vessels and the retention of fluids.

Obesity increases the risk for coronary artery disease, which in turn increases the risk for future heart failure. Congestive heart failure is not a disease but a condition that occurs when the heart is unable to pump enough blood to meet the needs of the body's tissues. When the heart fails, it is unable to pump out all the blood that enters its chambers. Congestive heart failure is a frequent complication of severe obesity and a major cause of death. The duration of obesity is a strong predictor of congestive heart failure because over time elevated total blood volume and high cardiac output cause the left ventricle of the heart to increase in size (known as left ventricular hypertrophy) beyond that expected from normal growth. Left ventricular hypertrophy is frequently identified in cardiac patients with obesity and in part results from hypertension, but abnormalities in left ventricular mass and function also occur in the absence of hypertension and may be related to the severity of obesity.

Inflammation in blood vessels and throughout the body is thought to increase the risk for heart disease and stroke (sudden injury to the brain due to a compromised blood and oxygen supply). People with more body fat have higher blood levels of substances such as plasminogen activator inhibitor-1, an enzyme produced in the kidneys that inhibits the conversion of plasminogen to plasmin and initiates fibrinolysis. Fibrinolysis leads to the breakdown of fibrin, which is responsible for the semi-solid character of a blood clot that can occlude (block) blood vessels. This is the mechanism believed to account for the finding that obesity is associated with an increased risk of blood clot formation. Occluded arteries may produce myocardial infarction (heart attack) or stroke. Overweight increases the risk for ischemic stroke—resulting from a clot or blockage—but does not appear to increase the risk for hemorrhagic stroke (bleeding inside the brain), which, in general, is associated with more fatality. According to the National Heart, Lung, and Blood Institute (NHLBI), in *The Clinical Guidelines on the Identification,*

TABLE 2.5

Cholesterol levels among persons 20 years of age and older, by selected characteristics, selected years 1988–2008

[Data are based on interviews and laboratory data of a sample of the civilian noninstitutionalized population]

Sex, age, race and Hispanic origin[a], and percent of poverty level	1988–1994	1999–2002	2005–2008
	Percent of population with high serum total cholesterol (greater than or equal to 240 mg/dL)[e]		
20 years and over, age-adjusted[b]			
Both sexes[c]	20.8	17.3	14.9
Male	19.0	16.4	13.4
Female	22.0	17.8	16.0
Not Hispanic or Latino:			
White only, male	18.8	16.5	13.5
White only, female	22.2	18.1	16.8
Black or African American only, male	16.9	12.4	9.5
Black or African American only, female	21.4	17.7	13.2
Mexican male	18.5	17.4	16.8
Mexican female	18.7	13.8	13.9
Percent of poverty level:[d]			
Below 100%	20.6	18.3	15.6
100%–199%	20.6	19.1	15.0
200%–399%	20.8	18.9	16.1
400% or more	19.5	14.4	14.0
20 years and over, crude			
Both sexes[c]	19.6	17.3	15.2
Male	17.7	16.5	13.8
Female	21.3	18.0	16.6
Not Hispanic or Latino:			
White only, male	18.0	16.9	14.0
White only, female	22.5	19.1	17.8
Black or African American only, male	14.7	12.2	9.6
Black or African American only, female	18.2	16.1	12.8
Mexican male	15.4	15.0	15.5
Mexican female	14.3	10.7	13.0
Percent of poverty level:[d]			
Below 100%	17.6	16.4	14.0
100%–199%	19.8	18.2	14.8
200%–399%	19.3	18.7	16.0
400% or more	19.9	15.5	15.3
Male			
20–34 years	8.2	9.8	9.1
35–44 years	19.4	19.7	16.0
45–54 years	26.6	23.6	19.8
55–64 years	28.0	19.9	16.2
65–74 years	21.9	13.7	7.9
75 years and over	20.4	10.2	8.6
Female			
20–34 years	7.3	8.9	8.4
35–44 years	12.3	12.4	13.7
45–54 years	26.7	21.4	18.6
55–64 years	40.9	25.6	27.1
65–74 years	41.3	32.3	21.8
75 years and over	38.2	26.5	19.4

[a]Persons of Mexican origin may be of any race. Starting with 1999 data, race-specific estimates are tabulated according to the 1997 Revisions to the Standards for the Classification of Federal Data on Race and Ethnicity and are not strictly comparable with estimates for earlier years. The two non-Hispanic race categories shown in the table conform to the 1997 Standards. Starting with 1999 data, race-specific estimates are for persons who reported only one racial group. Prior to data year 1999, estimates were tabulated according to the 1977 Standards. Estimates for single-race categories prior to 1999 included persons who reported one race or, if they reported more than one race, identified one race as best representing their race.
[b]Age-adjusted to the 2000 standard population using five age groups: 20–34 years, 35–44 years, 45–54 years, 55–64 years, and 65 years and over. Age-adjusted estimates may differ from other age-adjusted estimates based on the same data and presented elsewhere if different age groups are used in the adjustment procedure.
[c]Includes persons of all races and Hispanic origins, not just those shown separately.
[d]Percent of poverty level is based on family income and family size. Persons with unknown percent of poverty level are excluded (4% in 2005–2008).
[e]High serum total cholesterol is defined as greater than or equal to 240 mg/dL (6.20 mmol/L), regardless of whether the respondent reported taking cholesterol-lowering medications.

SOURCE: Adapted from "Table 68. Cholesterol among Persons 20 Years of Age and over, by Selected Characteristics: United States, 1988–1994 through 2005–2008," in *Health, United States, 2010: With Special Feature on Death and Dying*, Centers for Disease Control and Prevention, National Center for Health Statistics, 2011, http://www.cdc.gov/nchs/data/hus/hus10.pdf#listtables (accessed September 30, 2011)

Evaluation, and Treatment of Overweight and Obesity in Adults: The Evidence Report (June 1998, http://www.nhlbi.nih.gov/guidelines/obesity/e_txtbk/index.htm),

the risk of stroke increases as BMI rises. For example, the risk of ischemic stroke is 75% higher in women with a BMI greater than 27 and 137% higher in women with a

TABLE 2.6

Hypertension and elevated blood pressure among persons 20 years of age and older, by selected characteristics, selected years 1988–2008

[Data are based on interviews and physical examinations of a sample of the civilian noninstitutionalized population]

Sex, age, race and Hispanic origin[a], and percent of poverty level	Hypertension[b, c] (high blood pressure and/or taking antihypertensive medication)			Uncontrolled high blood pressure among persons with hypertension[d]		
	1988–1994	1999–2002	2005–2008	1988–1994	1999–2002	2005–2008
	Percent of population					
20 years and over, age-adjusted[e]						
Both sexes[f]	25.5	30.0	30.9	77.2	70.6	59.4
Male	26.4	28.8	31.6	83.2	73.3	63.8
Female	24.4	30.6	29.8	68.5	61.8	48.5
Not Hispanic or Latino:						
White only, male	25.6	27.6	31.5	82.6	70.3	60.8
White only, female	23.0	28.5	28.1	67.0	63.6	47.4
Black or African American only, male	37.5	40.6	41.4	84.0	74.3	70.6
Black or African American only, female	38.3	43.5	44.4	71.1	67.2	51.5
Mexican male	26.9	26.8	26.3	87.9	89.5	68.8
Mexican female	25.0	27.9	26.2	77.6	71.5	65.3
Percent of poverty level:[g]						
Below 100%	31.7	33.9	33.8	75.0	71.2	57.7
100%–199%	26.6	33.5	33.7	76.0	73.4	65.7
200%–399%	24.7	30.1	31.8	76.2	67.8	58.8
400% or more	22.6	26.4	28.7	81.5	70.3	56.7
20 years and over, crude						
Both sexes[f]	24.1	30.2	32.1	73.9	67.3	54.1
Male	23.8	27.6	31.4	79.3	67.1	56.3
Female	24.4	32.7	32.8	68.8	67.4	52.1
Not Hispanic or Latino:						
White only, male	24.3	28.3	33.2	78.0	64.0	53.6
White only, female	24.6	32.8	33.4	67.8	66.9	51.1
Black or African American only, male	31.1	35.9	38.9	83.3	71.3	64.2
Black or African American only, female	32.5	41.9	44.0	70.0	67.5	51.8
Mexican male	16.4	16.5	17.7	86.5	86.9	64.0
Mexican female	15.9	18.8	19.2	80.6	74.5	62.8
Percent of poverty level:[g]						
Below 100%	25.7	30.3	28.5	74.0	71.3	58.8
100%–199%	26.7	34.8	37.0	75.1	70.7	61.9
200%–399%	22.4	29.9	33.7	73.4	64.4	52.0
400% or more	22.0	26.8	29.0	74.3	63.8	49.5
Male						
20–34 years	7.1	*8.1	9.1	92.6	89.9	81.4
35–44 years	17.1	17.1	21.1	89.0	73.3	66.9
45–54 years	29.2	31.0	33.6	76.2	66.4	55.4
55–64 years	40.6	45.0	51.3	70.3	55.9	50.0
65–74 years	54.4	59.6	64.0	74.3	59.1	47.7
75 years and over	60.4	69.0	67.2	82.5	74.3	53.5

BMI greater than 32, compared with women having a BMI less than 21.

In "Inflammation, a Link between Obesity and Cardiovascular Disease" (*Mediators of Inflammation*, August 2010), Zhaoxia Wang and Tomohiro Nakayama confirm that obesity is associated with increased morbidity and mortality from cardiovascular disease—heart disease, stroke and other vascular disease, and atherosclerosis (the deposit of fatty plaque in the walls of arteries that impede blood flow). The researchers posit that obesity induces inflammation, which accelerates atherosclerosis. Wang and Nakayama believe that advancing the understanding of inflammation and the relationship between obesity and cardiovascular disease will help enhance the biological, physical, and functional changes that are associated with obesity.

Figure 2.1 shows the process, known as a treatment algorithm, that is used to assess and treat overweight individuals, based on their body weight, abdominal fat, and the risk factors for cardiovascular morbidity and mortality.

Type 2 Diabetes

Diabetes is a disease that affects the body's use of food, causing blood glucose (sugar levels in the blood) to become too high. Normally, the body converts sugars, starches, and proteins into a form of sugar called glucose. The blood then carries glucose to all the cells throughout the body. In the cells, with the help of the hormone insulin, the glucose is either converted into energy for use immediately or stored for the future. Beta cells of the pancreas, a small organ located behind the stomach,

TABLE 2.6

[Data are based on interviews and physical examinations of a sample of the civilian noninstitutionalized population]

Sex, age, race and Hispanic origin[a], and percent of poverty level	Hypertension[b, c] (high blood pressure and/or taking antihypertensive medication)			Uncontrolled high blood pressure among persons with hypertension[d]		
	1988–1994	1999–2002	2005–2008	1988–1994	1999–2002	2005–2008
	Percent of population					
Female						
20–34 years	2.9	*2.7	3.2	82.2	56.9	49.1
35–44 years	11.2	15.1	13.8	56.8	58.6	40.9
45–54 years	23.9	31.8	33.0	58.5	61.1	46.3
55–64 years	42.6	53.9	52.7	64.3	60.0	52.4
65–74 years	56.2	72.7	68.4	68.7	73.5	51.2
75 years and over	73.6	83.1	80.4	81.9	78.1	62.9

*Estimates are considered unreliable. Data preceded by an asterisk have a relative standard error (RSE) of 20%–30%.
[a]Persons of Mexican origin may be of any race. Starting with 1999 data, race-specific estimates are tabulated according to the 1997 Revisions to the Standards for the Classification of Federal Data on Race and Ethnicity and are not strictly comparable with estimates for earlier years. The two non-Hispanic race categories shown in the table conform to the 1997 Standards. Starting with 1999 data, race-specific estimates are for persons who reported only one racial group. Prior to data year 1999, estimates were tabulated according to the 1977 Standards. Estimates for single-race categories prior to 1999 included persons who reported one race or, if they reported more than one race, identified one race as best representing their race.
[b]Hypertension is defined as having measured high blood pressure and/or taking antihypertensive medication. High blood pressure is defined as having a measured systolic pressure of at least 140 mmHg or diastolic pressure of at least 90 mmHg. Those with high blood pressure also may be taking prescribed medicine for high blood pressure. Those taking antihypertensive medication may not have measured high blood pressure but are still classified as having hypertension.
[c]Respondents were asked, "Are you now taking prescribed medicine for your high blood pressure?"
[d]Uncontrolled high blood pressure among hypertensives is defined as measured systolic pressure of at least 140 mmHg or diastolic pressure of at least 90 mmHg, among those with measured high blood pressure or reporting taking antihypertensive medication.
[e]Age-adjusted to the 2000 standard population using five age groups: 20–34 years, 35–44 years, 45–54 years, 55–64 years, and 65 years and over. Age-adjusted estimates may differ from other age-adjusted estimates based on the same data and presented elsewhere if different age groups are used in the adjustment procedure.
[f]Includes persons of all races and Hispanic origins, not just those shown separately.
[g]Percent of poverty level is based on family income and family size. Persons with unknown percent of poverty level are excluded (5% in 2005–2008).
Notes: Percentages are based on the average of blood pressure measurements taken. In 2005–2008, 81% of participants had three blood pressure readings. Excludes pregnant women.

SOURCE: "Table 67. Hypertension and High Blood Pressure among Persons 20 Years of Age and over, by Selected Characteristics: United States, 1988–1994 through 2005–2008," in *Health, United States, 2010: With Special Feature on Death and Dying*, Centers for Disease Control and Prevention, National Center for Health Statistics, 2011, http://www.cdc.gov/nchs/data/hus/hus10.pdf#listtables (accessed September 30, 2011)

---

manufacture the insulin. The process of turning food into energy via glucose (blood sugar) is important because the body depends on glucose for every function.

With diabetes, the body can convert food to glucose, but there is a problem with insulin. In one type of diabetes (insulin-dependent diabetes or type 1), the pancreas does not manufacture enough insulin, and in another type (noninsulin dependent or type 2), the body has insulin but cannot use the insulin effectively (this latter condition is called insulin resistance). When insulin is either absent or ineffective, glucose cannot get into the cells to be used for energy. Instead, the unused glucose builds up in the bloodstream and circulates through the kidneys. If a person's blood-glucose level rises high enough, the excess glucose "spills" over into the urine, causing frequent urination. This, in turn, leads to an increased feeling of thirst as the body tries to compensate for the fluid that is lost through urination.

Type 2 diabetes is most often seen in adults and is the most common type of diabetes in the United States. In this type, the pancreas produces insulin, but it is not used effectively because the body resists responding to it. Heredity may be a predisposing factor in the genesis of type 2 diabetes, but because the pancreas continues to produce insulin, the disease is considered more of a problem of insulin resistance, in which the body is not using the hormone efficiently.

Because diabetes deprives body cells of the glucose needed to function properly, several complications can develop to threaten the lives of diabetics. The healing process of the body is slowed or impaired and the risk of infection increases. Complications of diabetes include higher risk and rates of heart disease; circulatory problems, especially in the legs, are often severe enough to require surgery or even amputation; diabetic retinopathy, a condition that can cause blindness; kidney disease that may require dialysis; dental problems; and problems with pregnancy.

The National Institutes of Health's Weight-Control Information Network (WIN) observes in *Do You Know the Health Risks of Being Overweight?* (December 2007, http://win.niddk.nih.gov/Publications/health_risks.htm) that over 85% of people with type 2 diabetes are overweight, and in people who are prone to type 2 diabetes, becoming overweight can trigger the onset of the disease. It is not known precisely how overweight contributes to

FIGURE 2.1

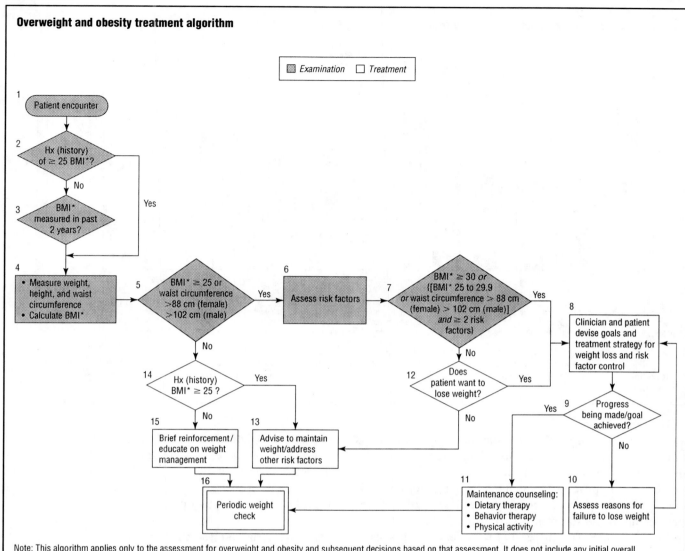

Overweight and obesity treatment algorithm

Note: This algorithm applies only to the assessment for overweight and obesity and subsequent decisions based on that assessment. It does not include any initial overall assessment for cardiovascular risk factors or diseases that are indicated.
*BMI = body mass index.

SOURCE: "Treatment Algorithm," in *Clinical Guidelines on the Identification, Evaluation, and Treatment of Overweight and Obesity in Adults: The Evidence Report*, National Institutes of Health, National Heart, Lung, and Blood Institute in cooperation with The National Institute of Diabetes and Digestive and Kidney Diseases, 2005, http://hp2010.nhlbihin.net/oei_ss/download/pdf/CORESET2.pdf (accessed October 6, 2011)

the causation of this disease. One hypothesis is that being overweight causes cells to change, making them less effective at using glucose. This then stresses the cells that produce insulin, causing them to fail gradually. Maintaining a healthy weight and keeping physically fit can usually prevent or delay the onset of type 2 diabetes.

From 1997 to March 2011 the percentage of Americans diagnosed with diabetes rose from 5.1% to 8.8%. (See Figure 2.2.) These numbers may significantly underestimate the true prevalence of diabetes in the United States in view of National Health and Nutrition Examination Survey findings that show sizable numbers of adults have undiagnosed diabetes.

"DIABESITY" AND "DOUBLE DIABETES." The recognition of obesity-dependent diabetes prompted scientists and physicians to coin a new term to describe this condition: diabesity. The term was first used during the 1990s and has gained widespread acceptance. Even though diabesity is attributed to the same causes as type 2 diabetes (insulin resistance and pancreatic cell dysfunction), researchers are beginning to link the inflammation that is associated with obesity to the development of diabetes and cardiovascular disease.

Qudsia Anjum of the International Medical Center in Rabigh, Saudi Arabia, contends in "Diabesity—A Future Pandemic" (*Journal of Pakistan Medical Association*,

FIGURE 2.2

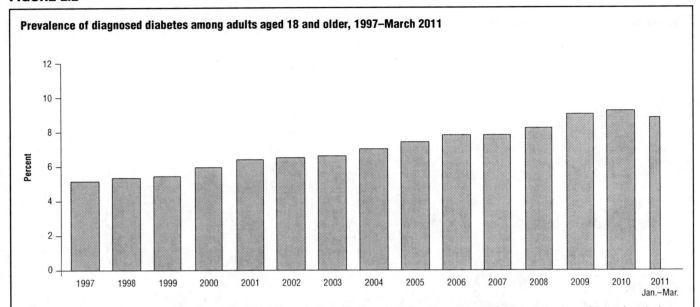

Prevalence of diagnosed diabetes among adults aged 18 and older, 1997–March 2011

Notes: Data are based on household interviews of a sample of the civilian noninstitutionalized population. Prevalence of diagnosed diabetes is based on self-report of ever having been diagnosed with diabetes by a doctor or other health professional. Persons reporting "borderline" diabetes status and women reporting diabetes only during pregnancy were not coded as having diabetes in the analyses. The analyses excluded persons with unknown diabetes status (about 0.1% of respondents each year).

SOURCE: P. M. Barnes et al., "Figure 14.1. Prevalence of Diagnosed Diabetes among Adults Aged 18 Years and over: United States, 1997–March 2011," in *Early Release of Selected Estimates Based on Data from the January–March 2011 National Health Interview Survey*, Centers for Disease Control and Prevention, National Center for Health Statistics, September 2011, http://www.cdc.gov/nchs/data/nhis/earlyrelease/201109_14.pdf (accessed September 30, 2011)

vol. 61, no. 4, April 2011) that the diabesity epidemic is the "tip of the iceberg; the impending threat is yet to be dealt. The combination and interdependence of diabetes and obesity imposes a therapeutic challenge to the clinicians." Anjum observes that global estimates of diabetes project an increase from 171 million in 2000 to 366 million in 2030. The increasing prevalence of diabesity has prompted the development of new treatment strategies to address both problems. In "Emerging Therapies in the Treatment of 'Diabesity': Beyond GLP-1" (*Trends in Pharmacological Sciences*, vol. 32, no. 1, January 2011), George Tharakan, Tricia Tan, and Stephen Bloom of the Imperial College of London explain that even though weight-loss surgery has proven to be an effective treatment for diabesity, "finding a pharmaceutical alternative that mimics the benefits of surgery without surgical complications has become the 'holy grail' of the twenty-first century."

Another recent phenomenon is the growing number of patients who are diagnosed with both type 1 and type 2 diabetes simultaneously. Dubbed "double diabetes," it has been reported in both children and adults. Paolo Pozzilli et al. explain in "Obesity, Autoimmunity, and Double Diabetes in Youth" (*Diabetes Care*, vol. 34, suppl. 2, May 2011) that the increase in double diabetes, also known as type 1.5, has gained the attention of the medical community. People with double diabetes have characteristics of both type 1 and type 2 diabetes. When

children and adolescents with type 1 diabetes become overweight or obese, they are at increased risk for double diabetes. Pozzilli et al. do not believe that double diabetes is a new or emerging form of diabetes; they opine that it reflects the increasing prevalence of obesity.

Osteoarthritis and Joint Injury

Being only 10 pounds overweight increases the force on the knee by 30–60 pounds with each step.... Even small amounts of weight loss reduce the risk of developing knee OA [osteoarthritis]. Preliminary studies suggest weight loss decreases pain substantially in those with knee OA.

—Susan Bartlett, "Osteoarthritis Weight Management" (2010)

The word *arthritis* literally means joint inflammation. The name applies to more than 100 related diseases that are known as rheumatic diseases. A joint is any point where two bones meet. When a joint becomes inflamed, swelling, redness, pain, and loss of motion occur. In the most serious forms of the disease, the loss of motion can be physically disabling. Arthritis is the leading cause of disability and the leading cause of limitation of activity among working-age adults (aged 18 to 64 years) in the United States. In 2009 approximately 21% of adults aged 18 to 44 years, 42% of those aged 45 to 64 years, and about half of people aged 65 years and older said they suffered from joint pain in the 30 days preceding the survey. (See Figure 2.3.)

FIGURE 2.3

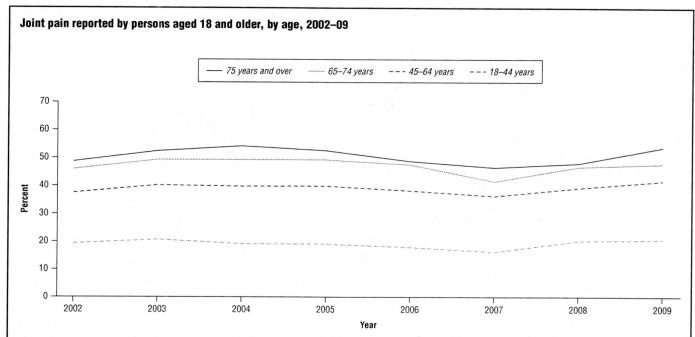

Joint pain reported by persons aged 18 and older, by age, 2002–09

——— 75 years and over   ·········· 65–74 years   - - - 45–64 years   – – – 18–44 years

SOURCE: "Figure 7. Joint Pain in the Past 30 Days among Adults 18 Years of Age and over, by Age: United States, 2002–2009," in *Health, United States, 2010: With Special Feature on Death and Dying*, Centers for Disease Control and Prevention, National Center for Health Statistics, 2011, http://www.cdc.gov/nchs/data/hus/hus10.pdf#listtables (accessed September 30, 2011)

People who are overweight or obese are at increased risk for osteoarthritis, which is not an inflammatory arthritis. Osteoarthritis, sometimes called degenerative arthritis, causes the breakdown of bones and cartilage (connective tissue attached to bones) and usually causes pain and stiffness in the fingers, knees, feet, hips, and back. Extra weight places extra pressure on joints and cartilage, causing them to erode. Furthermore, people with more body fat may have higher blood levels of substances that cause inflammation. Inflammation at the joints may increase the risk for osteoarthritis.

According to the CDC, in "Prevalence of Doctor-Diagnosed Arthritis and Arthritis-Attributable Activity Limitation—United States, 2007–2009" (*Morbidity and Mortality Weekly Report*, vol. 59, no. 39, October 8, 2010), during the 2007–09 period physician-diagnosed arthritis increased significantly with increasing BMI. The age-adjusted prevalence among people who were obese (25.2% for men, 33.8% for women) was nearly twice that for people who were normal or underweight (13.8% for men, 18.9% for women). (See Figure 2.4.)

In "Osteoarthritis Weight Management" (2010, http://www.hopkins-arthritis.org/patient-corner/disease-management/osteoandweight.html), Susan Bartlett of Johns Hopkins University indicates that obese women have about four times the risk of knee osteoarthritis, compared with women of healthy weight, and for obese

FIGURE 2.4

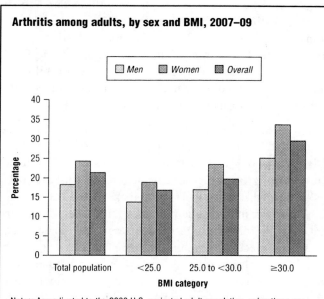

Arthritis among adults, by sex and BMI, 2007–09

☐ Men   ▨ Women   ▨ Overall

Notes: Age adjusted to the 2000 U.S. projected adult population, using three age groups: 18–44 years, 45–64 years, and ≥65 years.
BMI = weight (kg)/height (m²). Categorized as follows: underweight/normal weight (<25.0), overweight (25.0 to <30.0), and obese (≥30.0).

SOURCE: "FIGURE. Age-Adjusted Prevalence of Doctor-Diagnosed Arthritis among Adults, by Sex and Body Mass Index (BMI) Category—National Health Interview Survey, United States, 2007–2009," in "Prevalence of Doctor-Diagnosed Arthritis and Arthritis-Attributable Activity Limitation—United States, 2007–2009," *MMWR*, vol. 59, no. 39, October 8, 2010, http://www.cdc.gov/mmwr/pdf/wk/mm5939.pdf (accessed October 7, 2011) men the risk is five times greater. The CDC observes that even modest weight loss of just 10 pounds (4.5 kg) can reduce the risk for knee osteoarthritis among women by 50% and may also reduce the mortality risk in people with osteoarthritis by half.

By 2011 the relationship between weight loss and improvements in the symptoms of knee pain due to arthritis was clear and definitive enough to warrant classifying it as an effective treatment for this condition. According to Erika Ringdahl and Sandesh Pandit of the University of Missouri School of Medicine, in "Treatment of Knee Osteoarthritis" (*American Family Physician*, vol. 83, no. 11, June 1, 2011), obesity is the strongest modifiable risk factor for knee osteoarthritis. Weight loss is one of the standard nonsurgical treatments for overweight and obese patients suffering from osteoarthritis of the knee because it acts to reduce pain and improve physical function.

Gallbladder Disease

Gallstones are small, hard pellets that can form when bile in the gallbladder (a muscular saclike organ that lies under the liver in the right side of the abdomen) precipitates (becomes solid out of the bile solution). Bile contains water, cholesterol, fats, bile salts, proteins, and bilirubin. The gallbladder stores and concentrates the bile produced in the liver that is not needed immediately for digestion. Bile is released from the gallbladder into the small intestine in response to food. The pancreatic duct joins the common bile duct at the small intestine, adding enzymes to aid in digestion. (See Figure 2.5.) If bile contains too much cholesterol, bile salts, or bilirubin, under certain conditions it can harden into stones. Most gallstones are formed primarily from cholesterol.

The National Digestive Diseases Information Clearinghouse (NDDIC) of the National Institute of Diabetes and Digestive and Kidney Diseases explains in "Gallstones" (July 2007, http://digestive.niddk.nih.gov/ddiseases/pubs/gallstones/) that when gallstones block the flow of bile they can produce inflammation in the gallbladder, liver, and pancreas. When blockage persists, the consequences may be severe infection, which if left untreated may not only be painful but also deadly. When gallstones produce such symptoms, the treatment is generally a surgical procedure, called cholecystectomy, in which the gallbladder is removed. People who are not candidates for surgery may be given prescription drugs to dissolve gallstones; however, it is likely that gallstones will recur in people treated with drugs.

People who are overweight have an increased risk for developing gallstones because the liver overproduces cholesterol and deposits it in the bile, which then becomes supersaturated. The NDDIC indicates that the risk of

FIGURE 2.5

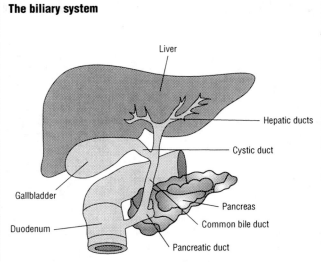

The biliary system

The gallbladder and the ducts that carry bile and other digestive enzymes from the liver, gallbladder, and pancreas to the small intestine are called the biliary system.

SOURCE: "The Gallbladder and the Ducts That Carry Bile and Other Digestive Enzymes from the Liver, Gallbladder, and Pancreas to the Small Intestine Are Called the Biliary System," in *Gallstones*, National Institutes of Health, National Institute of Diabetes and Digestive and Kidney Diseases, National Digestive Diseases Information Clearinghouse, July 2007, http://digestive.niddk.nih.gov/ddiseases/pubs/gallstones/index.htm (accessed October 7, 2011)

gallstones is higher among people who are overweight or obese and among people who fast or lose a large amount of weight very quickly.

Rapid weight loss or weight cycling (the repeated loss and regain of body weight) further increases cholesterol production in the liver, with resulting supersaturation and risk for gallstone formation. Olga N. Tucker et al. of the Bariatric and Metabolic Institute in Weston, Florida, indicate in "Is Concomitant Cholecystectomy Necessary in Obese Patients Undergoing Laparoscopic Gastric Bypass Surgery?" (*Surgical Endoscopy*, vol. 22, no. 11, November 2008) that gallstones develop in approximately 25% of obese patients who undergo strict dietary restriction and in as many as 50% of patients who undergo gastric bypass surgery (one of several surgical weight-loss treatments that may be prescribed for people with clinically severe obesity).

In "Gastrointestinal System and Obesity" (*Critical Care Clinics*, vol. 26, no. 4, October 2010), Doyle D. Ashburn and Mary Jane Reed confirm that obesity increases the risk for development of cholesterol gallstones. The researchers theorize that this occurs in response to the activity of adipose tissue in and around the internal organs. Insulin resistance leads to an excess of insulin called hyperinsulinemia that in turn increases cholesterol excretion from the liver and results in the abnormal function of the gallbladder. These conditions create an environment that is conducive to stone formation. Even though some gallstones produce no symptoms, others cause serious and even life-threatening medical conditions.

Fatty Liver Disease

Fatty liver is defined as an excess accumulation of fat in the liver, usually exceeding 5% of the total liver weight. More than 50% of the excess fat deposit in the liver is triglyceride. The enlargement of the liver is caused by the reduction of fatty acid oxidation (fat metabolism) in the liver, resulting in an excess accumulation of fat. It causes injury and inflammation in the liver and may lead to severe liver damage, cirrhosis (buildup of scar tissue that blocks proper blood flow in the liver), or liver failure. Arthur J. McCullough of the Cleveland Clinic in Cleveland, Ohio, observes in "Epidemiology of the Metabolic Syndrome in the USA" (*Journal of Digestive Diseases*, vol. 12, no. 5, October 2011) that nonalcoholic fatty liver disease (NAFLD) is now recognized as a component of metabolic syndrome, which includes hypertension, diabetes, and elevated triglycerides. Metabolic syndrome is a major risk factor for the development of nonalcoholic steatohepatitis, the most severe form of NAFLD. McCullough estimates that 25% of people in the United States have metabolic syndrome and as such also suffer from NAFLD.

People with diabetes or with higher than normal blood sugar levels (but not yet in the diabetic range) are more likely to have fatty liver disease than those with normal blood sugar levels. It is not known why some people who are overweight or diabetic get fatty liver and others do not. Losing weight reduces the buildup of fat in the liver and prevents further injury; however, weight loss should not exceed 2.2 pounds (1 kg) per week because more rapid weight loss may exacerbate the disease.

Zobair M. Younossi et al. analyzed prevalence data for chronic liver disease over the course of two decades and reported their findings in "Changes in the Prevalence of the Most Common Causes of Chronic Liver Diseases in the United States from 1988 to 2008" (*Clinical Gastroenterology and Hepatology*, vol. 9, no. 6, June 2011). The researchers find that the prevalence of NAFLD rose from 5.5% in 1988 to 11% in 2008. Between 1988 and 1994 NAFLD accounted for 46.8% of chronic liver disease cases; it rose to 62.8% between 1994 and 2004 and then to 75.1% between 2005 and 2008. During these same years there were steady increases in obesity (21.7%, 30%, and 33.2%, respectively). Younossi et al. conclude that "given the increasing rates of obesity, NAFLD prevalence is expected to contribute substantially to the burden of [chronic liver diseases] in the United States."

Cancer

Cancer encompasses a large group of diseases that are characterized by the uncontrolled growth and spread of abnormal cells. These cells may grow into masses of tissue called malignant tumors. The dangerous aspect of cancer is that cancer cells invade and destroy normal tissue.

The spread of cancer cells occurs either by local growth of the tumor or by some of the cells becoming detached and traveling through the blood and lymph systems to start additional tumors in other parts of the body. Metastasis (the spread of cancer cells) may be confined to a region of the body, but if left untreated (and often despite treatment), the cancer cells can spread throughout the entire body, eventually causing death. It is perhaps the rapid, invasive, and destructive nature of cancer that makes it, arguably, the most feared of all diseases, even though it is second to heart disease as the leading cause of death in the United States. (See Table 2.2.)

Kyla King reports in "Obesity: A Preventable Cancer Risk? Promoting Change with Sensitivity" (*Grand Rapids [MI] Press*, March 28, 2011) that in the United States overweight and obesity are responsible for as many as 14% of cancer deaths in men and 20% of cancer deaths in women. King also observes that people with cancer who are overweight or obese face additional challenges, in that surgery may be more complicated and doses of anticancer drugs must be adjusted.

Overweight increases the risk of developing several types of cancer, including cancers of the colon, esophagus, gallbladder, kidney, pancreas, liver, and prostate, as well as uterine (specifically cancer of the lining of the uterus) and postmenopausal breast cancer. Excessive weight gain during adult life increases the risk for several of these cancers. For example, according to the American Cancer Society, in *Cancer Prevention and Early Detection: Facts and Figures, 2011* (2011, http://www.cancer.org/acs/groups/content/@epidemiologysurveilance/documents/document/acspc-029459.pdf), overweight and obesity contribute to between 14% and 20% of all cancer-related deaths, and a full third of the more than 500,000 cancer-related deaths "can be attributed to poor diet and physical inactivity." The American Cancer Society states that losing weight may reduce the risk of developing some cancers such as breast cancer and that diets high in processed and red meat and low in fruits, vegetables, and whole grains are associated with increased cancer risk.

In "Obesity and Cancer Risk: Recent Review and Evidence" (*Current Oncology Reports*, vol. 13, no 1, February 2011), Karen Basen-Engquist and Maria Chang report that 9% of postmenopausal breast cancer, 11% of colon cancer, 25% of kidney cancer, 37% of esophageal cancer, and 39% of cancer of the lining of the uterus are attributable to obesity. The researchers explain that as BMI increases by 1 pound per square foot (5 kg per sq. m), cancer mortality increases by 10%.

Overweight may also increase the risk of dying from some cancers. David P. Rose and Linda Vona-Davis conclude in "Influence of Obesity on Breast Cancer Receptor Status and Prognosis" (*Expert Review of Anticancer Therapy*, vol. 9, no. 8, August 2009) that "pre-existing obesity and postoperative weight gain are related to a poor prognosis in breast cancer.... Weight control is important, not only to target breast cancer progression, but also to reduce the risk of nonbreast cancer mortality risk associated with excess adiposity."

It is not yet known exactly how being overweight increases cancer risk, recurrence, or mortality. It may be that fat cells make or influence hormones such as estrogen, progesterone, and androgens and insulin that affect cell growth and lead to cancer. It is also possible that eating habits—such as a high-fat, high-calorie diet—or physical inactivity that promote overweight contribute to cancer risk.

Sleep Apnea and Sleep Disorders

Sleep apnea is a condition in which breathing becomes shallow or stops completely for short periods during sleep. A pause in breathing can last about 10 to 20 seconds or longer, and pauses can occur 20 times or more an hour. Sleep apnea can increase the risk of developing high blood pressure, heart attack, or stroke. Untreated sleep apnea can increase the risk of diabetes and daytime sleepiness, which can increase the risk for work-related accidents and automobile accidents.

The most common type of sleep apnea, and the type that is linked to overweight and obesity, is obstructive sleep apnea (OSA). During sleep there is insufficient airflow into the lungs through the mouth and nose, and the amount of oxygen in the blood may drop because the airway is transiently occluded. The NHLBI notes in "Who Is at Risk for Sleep Apnea?" (August 1, 2010, http://www.nhlbi.nih.gov/health/health-topics/topics/sleepapnea/atrisk.html) that millions of Americans have OSA and that "more than half of the people who have this condition are overweight."

Obesity, particularly upper-body obesity, is a risk factor for sleep apnea and is related to its severity. Most people with sleep apnea have a BMI greater than 30. In general, men whose neck circumference is 17 inches (43 cm) or greater and women with a neck circumference of 16 inches (41 cm) or greater are at higher risk for sleep apnea. Large neck girth in both men and women who snore is highly predictive of sleep apnea because people with large neck girth store more fat around their neck, which may compromise their airway. A smaller airway can make breathing difficult or stop it altogether. In addition, fat stored in the neck and throughout the body can produce substances that cause inflammation, and inflammation in the neck may be a risk factor for sleep apnea. Weight loss usually resolves or significantly improves sleep apnea by decreasing neck size and reducing inflammation.

Too little sleep is also linked to obesity. Anne G. Wheaton et al. of the CDC note in "Relationship between Body Mass Index and Perceived Insufficient Sleep among U.S. Adults: An Analysis of 2008 BRFSS Data" (*BMC Public Health*, vol. 10, no. 11, May 2011) that people who are overweight or obese report that they sleep less per week than their normal-weight counterparts. The researchers analyzed data from 384,541 participants in the 2008 Behavioral Risk Factor Surveillance System, which asked survey respondents, "During the past 30 days, for about how many days have you felt you did not get enough rest or sleep?" The researchers find a strong association between reported insufficient sleep and BMI-based weight categories from normal-weight through obese class III among both men and women. For example, 35% of people with class III obesity said they had 14 or more days of insufficient sleep, compared with 25% of normal-weight people. Wheaton et al. suggest that "the possible effect of excess weight on sleep should be considered by developers of programs to address sleep disorders and that the possible effect of insufficient sleep on weight should be considered by developers of weight-reduction programs."

Other research confirms the relationship between disordered sleep and BMI and reveals that besides too little sleep, interrupted or discontinuous sleep is also associated with obesity. In "Sleep Discontinuity and Impaired Sleep Continuity Affect Transition to and from Obesity over Time: Results from the Alameda County Study" (*Scandinavian Journal of Public Health*, January 11, 2010), Maria E. Nordin and Robert M. Kaplan examine self-reported changes in sleep and BMI over time, from 1965 to 1994. The researchers find that discontinuous sleep is not only associated with an increased risk for obesity but also lowers the chance for weight loss among people who are obese.

Women's Reproductive Health

Besides increased risk of breast cancer and cancer of the lining of the uterus, women who are overweight or obese may suffer from infertility (difficulty or inability to conceive a child) and other gynecological or pregnancy-related medical problems. Obesity is associated with menstrual irregularities such as abnormally heavy menstrual periods and amenorrhea (cessation of menstruation), and has been found to affect ovulation, response to fertility treatment, pregnancy rates, and pregnancy outcomes.

In "Polycystic Ovary Syndrome and Metabolic Comorbidities: Therapeutic Options" (*Drugs Today*, vol. 45, no. 10, October 2009), Vincenzo De Leo et al. note that abdominal obesity in women is linked to polycystic ovarian syndrome (PCOS), an endocrine condition that afflicts approximately 5% to 10% of premenopausal women. About 60% of women with PCOS are obese. PCOS is characterized by the accumulation of cysts (fluid-filled sacs) on the ovaries, chronic anovulation (absent ovulation), and other metabolic disturbances. Symptoms include excess facial and body hair, acne, obesity, irregular menstrual cycles, insulin resistance, and infertility. A key characteristic of PCOS is hyper-androgenism—excessive production of male hormones (androgens), particularly testosterone, by the ovaries—which is responsible for the acne, male-pattern hair growth, and baldness seen in women with PCOS. Hyper-androgenism has been linked to insulin resistance and hyperinsulinemia, both of which are common in PCOS. Women with PCOS have an increased risk of early-onset heart disease, hypertension, diabetes, and reproductive cancers and a higher incidence of miscarriage and infer-tility. In overweight women, modest weight loss (as little as 5%) through diet and exercise may correct hyperan-drogenism and restore ovulation and fertility.

According to Gabriella G. Gosman et al., in "Repro-ductive Health of Women Electing Bariatric Surgery" (*Fertility and Sterility*, vol. 94, no. 4, September 2010), a study of 1,538 women undergoing weight-loss surgery, women who become obese by age 18 are at greater risk of developing PCOS and infertility than their healthy-weight peers. This finding is of increased significance in view of the growing number of overweight young adults.

Obesity during pregnancy is associated with increased morbidity for both the expectant mother and the unborn child. Obese pregnant women are signifi-cantly more likely to suffer from hypertension and gesta-tional diabetes (glucose intolerance of variable severity that begins during pregnancy and generally resolves after birth) than normal-weight expectant mothers. Obesity is also associated with difficulties in managing labor and delivery, leading to premature births and higher rates of cesarean section (delivery of a fetus by surgical incision through the abdominal wall and uterus). Risks associated with anesthesia are higher in obese women, as there is a greater tendency toward hypoxemia (abnormal lack of oxygen in the blood) and greater difficulty administering local or general anesthesia.

The children of women who are obese during preg-nancy are at increased risk of birth defects—congenital malformations, particularly of neural tube defects. Neural tube defects are abnormalities of the brain and spinal cord that result from the failure of the neural tube to develop properly during early pregnancy. The neural tube is the embryonic nerve tissue that eventually develops into the brain and the spinal cord.

Some research suggests that boys born to higher-weight mothers may be more likely to develop testicular

cancer. Investigators who find a relationship between mothers' weight and risk of testicular cancer, such as Cecilia Høst Ramlau-Hansen et al. in "Perinatal Markers of Estrogen Exposure and Risk of Testicular Cancer: Follow-up of 1,333,873 Danish Males Born between 1950 and 2002" (*Cancer Causes and Control*, vol. 20, no. 9, November 2009), posit that exposure of unborn males to high levels of estrogen is involved in the subse-quent development of testicular cancer. Boys born to higher-weight mothers are more likely to have been exposed to high estrogen levels than boys born to lower-weight mothers because higher weight results in higher insulin levels and lower levels of the protein that normally binds estrogen. As a result, higher levels of estrogen are able to cross the placenta and affect the male fetus.

Other research does not link higher maternal BMI to increased risk for testicular cancer. For example, in "Maternal Body Mass Index (BMI) and Risk of Testicu-lar Cancer in Male Offspring: A Systematic Review and Meta-Analysis" (*Cancer Epidemiology*, vol. 34, no. 5, October 2010), Shama Alam et al. analyze data from seven studies that considered the mother's' BMI and testicular cancer risk in their male offspring. The researchers find that higher maternal weight does not increase the risk of testicular cancer in male offspring. However, Alam et al. caution that their finding may simply reflect the fact that women who have had more than one child tend to weigh more than those who have had just one child, and having multiple children is itself associated with a decreased risk of testicular cancer, compared with women having a first or only child.

Furthermore, women who are obese before preg-nancy appear to have a higher risk of stillbirth and of having an infant die soon after birth. Peter W. Tennant, Judith Rankin, and Ruth Bell of Newcastle University note in "Maternal Body Mass Index and the Risk of Fetal and Infant Death: A Cohort Study from the North of England" (*Human Reproduction*, vol. 26, no. 6, April 2011) that early pregnancy obesity (BMI greater than or equal to 30) carries significant health implications. Ten-nant, Rankin, and Bell find that obese mothers were at increased risk for gestational diabetes and that their infants were at increased risk for stillbirth, early infant death, and birth defects. It is not yet known how obesity increases the risk of stillbirth and early infant death, but one possible explanation may be that obesity influences the hormonal system and the metabolism of blood fats that in turn may compromise blood flow to the placenta (an organ that forms during pregnancy and functions as a filter between the mother and fetus).

Babies born to overweight and obese women are at greater risk of having heart defects. Suzanne M. Gilboa et al. report in "Association between Prepregnancy Body Mass Index and Congenital Heart Defects" (*American*

Journal of Obstetrics and Gynecology, vol. 202, no. 1, January 2010) the results of a study of 6,440 infants born with congenital heart defects and 5,673 infants without birth defects. The researchers find that when compared with babies born to normal-weight women, there was a significant increase in many types of heart defects in babies born to overweight and obese women. Gilboa et al. looked at 25 types of heart defects and found associations with obesity for 10 of them. Five of these 10 types were also associated with overweight prior to pregnancy. Women who were overweight but not obese prior to and during pregnancy had approximately a 15% increased risk of delivering a baby with certain heart defects.

WEIGHT GAIN DURING PREGNANCY. Weight gain during pregnancy is expected and beneficial. The fetus, expanded blood volume, the enlarged uterus, breast tissue growth, and other products of conception generate approximately 13 to 17 pounds (5.9 to 7.7 kg) of extra weight. Weight gain beyond this anticipated amount is largely maternal adipose tissue that is often retained after pregnancy. The challenge health professionals face when developing recommendations about weight gain during pregnancy is achieving a balance between gains intended to produce high-birth-weight infants, who may then require delivery by cesarean section, and low-birth-weight infants with a higher infant mortality rate. Analysis of data from the CDC's Pregnancy Nutrition Surveillance System shows that extremely overweight women benefit from reduced weight gain during pregnancy to help decrease the risk for high-birth-weight infants. Table 2.7 shows the recommended amount of weight gain during pregnancy based on prepregnancy BMI.

In "Risks and Management of Obesity in Pregnancy: Current Controversies" (*Current Opinions in Obstetrics and Gynecology*, vol. 21, no. 2, April 2009), Joseph R. Wax of the Maine Medical Center in Portland, Maine, finds that limiting pregnancy weight gain in obese women to less than 15 pounds (6.8 kg) may reduce some risks such as infants who are large for their gestational age, cesarean delivery, and preeclampsia (high blood pressure and excess protein in the urine), but it also increases the risk for small-for-gestational-age newborns. Infants of obese women are at significantly increased risk for being born with neural tube defects, congenital heart disease, and other anomalies.

Metabolic Syndrome

McCullough estimates in "Epidemiology of the Metabolic Syndrome in the USA" that approximately 25% of Americans exhibit a cluster of medical conditions that are characterized by insulin resistance and the presence of obesity, abdominal fat, high blood sugar and triglycerides, high blood cholesterol, and high blood pressure. This constellation of symptoms, called metabolic syndrome, was first defined in *Third Report of the National Cholesterol Education Program (NCEP) Expert Panel on Detection, Evaluation, and Treatment of High Blood Cholesterol in Adults (Adult Treatment Panel III)* (September 2002, http://www.nhlbi.nih.gov/guidelines/cholesterol/atp3full.pdf). The report concludes that for most affected people, metabolic syndrome results from poor diet and insufficient physical activity.

The diagnosis of metabolic syndrome, which is also known as syndrome X, requires that people meet at least three of the following criteria:

- Waistline measurement (waist circumference) of 40 inches (102 cm) or more for men and 35 inches (89 cm) or more for women
- Blood pressure of 130/85 millimeters of mercury (mmHg) or higher
- Fasting blood glucose level greater than 100 mg/dL
- Serum triglyceride level above 150 mg/dL
- HDL level less than 40 mg/dL for men or under 50 mg/dL for women

According to the American Heart Association, three groups of people are the most likely to be diagnosed with metabolic syndrome: diabetics, people with hypertension and hyperinsulinemia, and people who have suffered heart attacks and have hyperinsulinemia without glucose intolerance.

Even though research shows that the signs of metabolic syndrome are common among family members, until 2003 a definitive genetic link had not been identified. Ruth J. F. Loos et al. demonstrate in "Genome-Wide Linkage Scan for the Metabolic Syndrome in the HERITAGE Family Study" (*Journal of Clinical Endocrinology and Metabolism*, vol. 88, no. 12, December 2003) the existence of genetic regions that may signal a predisposition to metabolic syndrome. The researchers find evidence of genetic linkages to metabolic syndrome in both African-American and white patients.

TABLE 2.7

Recommended weight gain during pregnancy

BMI	Kilograms	Pounds
<19.8	12.5 to 18	28 to 40
>19.8 to 26	11.5 to 16	25 to 35
>26 to 29	7 to 11.5	15 to 25
>29	≤6	≤13

SOURCE: "Weight Gain during Pregnancy," in *Guidelines on Overweight and Obesity: Electronic Textbook*, National Institutes of Health, National Heart, Lung, and Blood Institute in cooperation with The National Institute of Diabetes and Digestive and Kidney Diseases, 1998, http://www.nhlbi.nih.gov/guidelines/obesity/e_txtbk/ratnl/22111.htm (accessed October 7, 2011)

By 2011 additional genetic links had been identified. For example, in "Multivariate Linkage Scan for Metabolic Syndrome Traits in Families with Type 2 Diabetes" (*Obesity*, vol. 19, no. 6, June 2011), Karen L. Edwards et al. report that an evaluation of linkages for traits that are associated with metabolic syndrome finds multiple regions on chromosome 1 that correlate with these traits.

The exact origins of metabolic syndrome are not fully known; regardless, affected individuals experience a series of biochemical changes that, in time, lead to the development of potentially harmful medical conditions. The biochemical changes begin when insulin loses its ability to cause cells to absorb glucose from the blood (insulin resistance). As a result, glucose levels remain high after food is consumed and the pancreas, sensing a high glucose level in the blood, continues to secrete insulin. The loss of insulin sensitivity may be genetic or may be in response to high fat levels with fatty deposits in the pancreas.

Moderate weight loss, in the range of 5% to 10% of body weight, can help restore the body's sensitivity to insulin and greatly reduce the chance that the syndrome will progress into a more serious illness. Increased physical activity alone has also been shown to improve insulin sensitivity.

Giovanni de Simone et al. investigated the relationship between increased prevalence of left ventricular hypertrophy and metabolic syndrome–associated cardiovascular risk and reported their findings in "Metabolic Syndrome and Left Ventricular Hypertrophy in the Prediction of Cardiovascular Events: The Strong Heart Study" (*Nutrition, Metabolism, and Cardiovascular Diseases*, vol. 19, no. 2, February 2009). Using data from the Strong Heart Study, a population-based longitudinal cohort study of cardiovascular risk factors and disease in Native Americans living in communities in Arizona, in southwestern Oklahoma, and in South and North Dakota, the researchers find that 60% of the subjects had metabolic syndrome. Of this group, 25% had left ventricular hypertrophy, compared with 13% of subjects in a control group. About half of the subjects were obese and had diabetes, high blood pressure, and low HDL cholesterol.

After adjusting for age, sex, LDL cholesterol, smoking, and diabetes, the researchers determine that subjects with metabolic syndrome were twice as likely to have left ventricular hypertrophy as those without metabolic syndrome. De Simone et al. conclude, "In this study we demonstrate that a substantial part of the metabolic syndrome–related [cardiovascular] risk is mediated by the metabolic syndrome–associated [left ventricular] hypertrophy."

By 2011 it was widely accepted that metabolic syndrome included vascular risk factors that were associated with cognitive decline and even the development of dementia. In "Metabolic Syndrome and Cognitive Impairment: Current Epidemiology and Possible Underlying Mechanisms" (*Journal of Alzheimer's Disease*, vol. 21, no. 3, September 2010), Francesco Panza et al. assert that even though it not understood how or why metabolic syndrome causes cognitive impairment, early identification and treatment of people who are at risk may offer new ways to delay the onset of cognitive decline and dementia syndromes or to prevent the progression of these syndromes. Panza et al. believe that future clinical research should focus on determining whether modifications of these risk factors, which include inflammation, can reduce the risk of cognitive decline and the development of dementia.

REDEFINING METABOLIC SYNDROME. In an effort to standardize diagnosis, prevention, screening, and treatment, the International Diabetes Federation presents in *The IDF Consensus Worldwide Definition of the Metabolic Syndrome* (2006, http://www.idf.org/webdata/docs/IDF_Meta_def_final.pdf) a new worldwide definition of metabolic syndrome. The diagnostic criteria are central obesity, which is defined as a waist circumference that is equal to or more than 37 inches (94 cm) for males and 31.5 inches (80 cm) for females of European descent, and ethnic-specific measurements for Chinese, Japanese, and South Asians, along with two of the following: triglycerides of at least 150 mg/dL; low HDL cholesterol, which is defined as less than 40 mg/dL in males and less than 50 mg/dL in females; blood pressure of at least 130/85 mmHg; fasting hyperglycemia, which is defined as glucose that is equal to or greater than 100 mg/dL; previous diagnosis of diabetes; or impaired glucose tolerance. This definition of metabolic syndrome, which includes diabetes or prediabetes, abdominal obesity, unfavorable lipid profile, and hypertension, triples the risk of myocardial infarction and stroke and doubles mortality from these conditions. It also increases the risk of developing type 2 diabetes, if not already present, fivefold.

SOME QUESTION THE DIAGNOSIS OF METABOLIC SYNDROME. In 2010 the WHO joined the American Diabetes Association and the European Association for the Study of Diabetes in questioning the utility of the diagnosis of metabolic syndrome. Representatives of these organizations say they feel the syndrome is neither a distinct disease nor well established by scientific research. Rebecca K. Simmons et al. state in "The Metabolic Syndrome: Useful Concept or Clinical Tool? Report of a WHO Expert Consultation" (*Diabetologia*, vol. 53, no. 4, April 2010) that metabolic syndrome has only limited value as a diagnostic or patient management tool. The WHO report questions the existence as well as the utility of the syndrome and observes that different definitions of it create confusion when comparing prevalence rates. Simmons et al. assert that "although the metabolic syndrome can predict diabetes and cardiovascular disease, the construct was never intended for use as a detailed risk predictor, and there are other tools available which provide a measure of absolute risk within defined populations."

Simmons et al. conclude that "in the absence of a clear mechanism, interim definitions of the metabolic syndrome can only be considered provisional rather than definitive," and note that the WHO report calls for:

- Clarifying the metabolic pathways that underlie the development of diabetes and cardiovascular disease
- Understanding early-life determinants of metabolic risk
- Developing strategies for reducing heart disease and diabetes risk
- Developing population-based prevention strategies

CHAPTER 3

THE INFLUENCES OF MENTAL HEALTH AND CULTURE ON WEIGHT AND EATING DISORDERS

That diet and appetite are closely linked to psychological health and emotional well-being is widely recognized. Psychological factors often influence eating habits. Many people overeat when they are bored, stressed, angry, depressed, or anxious. Psychological distress can aggravate weight problems by triggering impulses to overeat. Emotional discomfort drives many people to overeat as a way to relieve anxiety and improve mood. Some people revert to the so-called comfort foods of their youth—the meals or treats that were offered to them when they were sick or the foods that evoke memories of the carefree days of childhood. Others rely on chocolate and other sweets, which actually contain chemicals that are known to have a soothing effect on mood. Over time, the associations between emotions, food, and eating can become firmly fixed.

Emotional arousal may also sabotage healthy self-care efforts such as resolutions to diet and exercise. Anxiety and depression can produce feelings of helplessness and hopelessness about efforts to lose weight that undermine the best intentions, prompt detrimental food choices and inactivity, and over time cause many people to give up trying entirely. Because overweight and obesity often contribute to emotional stress and psychological disorders, a cycle develops that couples increasing weight gain with progressively more severe emotional difficulties.

Emotional disturbance alone is rarely the causative factor of overweight or obesity. However, for people with a genetic susceptibility or predisposition to obesity and exposure to environmental factors that promote obesity, emotional and psychological stress can trigger or exacerbate the problem. Even efforts to lose weight can backfire—serving to increase rather than to alleviate emotional stress. For example, people who fail to lose weight or those who succeed in losing weight only to regain it may suffer from frustration and diminished feelings of competence and self-worth. Similarly, being overweight or obese and feeling self-conscious about it or suffering from weight-based discrimination or prejudice can be ongoing sources of stress and frustration. Feelings of helplessness, frustration, and continuous emotional stress can cause or worsen mental health problems such as anxiety and depression.

Many mental health and medical professionals view overweight as both a cause and a consequence of disturbances in physical and mental health. Even though it may be important to determine whether a metabolic disturbance caused an individual to become overweight or resulted from excessive weight gain, or whether depression triggered behaviors leading to obesity or resulted from problems associated with obesity, it is often impossible to distinguish whether overweight is a symptom of another disorder or the causative factor.

THE ORIGINS OF EATING DISORDERS

Despite the challenges of compromised self-esteem and societal prejudice, the National Institute of Diabetes and Digestive and Kidney Diseases indicates that most overweight people have about the same number of psychological problems as people of average weight. However, the Weight-Control Information Network explains in *Binge Eating Disorder* (April 7, 2010, http://win.niddk.nih.gov/publications/binge.htm) that even though eating disorders affect normal-weight individuals, people who are mildly obese and try to lose weight repetitively may suffer from eating disorders such as binge eating, and most people with binge-eating disorders are overweight or obese. People with the most severe eating disorders are more likely to have symptoms of depression and low self-esteem. Binge eaters have lost control of their eating behaviors and consume abnormal quantities of food in short periods. Binge-eating disorders are thought to be even more common in people who are severely obese.

Even though depression and stress may contribute to a substantial percentage of cases of obesity, they are considered the leading causes of eating disorders. Most mental health professionals concur that the origins of eating disorders can be traced to behavioral or psychological difficulties. Anger and impulsive behavior have been associated with binge-eating disorders, but even mild mental health or social problems such as shyness or lack of self-confidence can lead to social withdrawal, isolation, and a sedentary lifestyle that promotes weight gain and ultimately obesity. Jerica M. Berge et al. report in "Family Life Cycle Transitions and the Onset of Eating Disorders: A Retrospective Grounded Theory Approach" (*Journal of Clinical Nursing*, July 12, 2011) that eating disorders may be precipitated by transitional events in family life, such as school transitions, the death of a family member, relationship changes, illness or hospitalization, home or job changes, and abuse or sexual assault. The risk for eating disorders is greatest when there is a lack of needed support during these stressful life transitions.

At first glance, eating disorders appear to center on preoccupations with food and weight; however, mental health professionals believe these disorders are often about more than simply food. Besides psychological factors that may predispose people to eating disorders, including diminished self-esteem, depression, anxiety, loneliness, or feelings of lack of control, a variety of interpersonal and social factors have been implicated as causal factors for these disorders. Interpersonal issues that may increase the risk for developing eating disorders include troubled family and personal relationships; difficulty expressing emotions; a history of physical or sexual abuse; or the experience of being teased, taunted, or ridiculed about body size, shape, or weight.

In "A 30-Year Follow-up of the Effects of Child Abuse and Neglect on Obesity in Adulthood" (*Obesity*, vol. 17, no. 10, October 2009), Tyrone Bentley and Cathy S. Widom report the results of research considering the relationship between mistreatment of children (physical and sexual abuse and neglect) and the risk for obesity in adulthood. The researchers matched 410 children with court-substantiated cases of physical and sexual abuse and neglect with 303 children of similar ages, sex, race, ethnicity, and social class who had not suffered abuse or neglect. Thirty years later the body mass index (BMI; body weight in kilograms divided by height in meters squared) of each subject was compared with the other subjects. Bentley and Widom find that a history of physical abuse predicted higher adult BMI scores but that histories of sexual abuse or neglect were not predictive of having a higher BMI as an adult. The researchers posit that physical abuse may have activated a hormonal response that resulted in increasing peripheral cortisol, a hormone that is pivotal in mediating responses to stress and metabolism. Alternatively, or in addition to the hormonal imbalance, the subjects may have developed disordered eating as a way to cope with the trauma of physical abuse.

Twin and family studies suggest that the predisposition to develop an eating disorder also has a genetic origin. For example, in "Shared and Unique Genetic and Environmental Influences on Binge Eating and Night Eating: A Swedish Twin Study" (*Eating Behaviors*, vol. 11, no. 2, April 2010), Tammy L. Root et al. analyzed a sample of Swedish twins that were born between 1959 and 1985 and asked questions including, "Have you ever had binges when you ate what most people would regard as an unusually large amount of food in a short period of time?" and "When you were having eating binges, did you feel that your eating was out of control?" Subjects who responded "yes" to the first question and "slightly," "very much," or "extremely" to the second question were considered to have engaged in binge eating. Root et al. find the prevalence of binge eating in their sample (5.8%) to be slightly higher than the U.S. national average (4.9%). They conclude that their findings are consistent with previous studies suggesting that genetic factors make a substantial contribution to risk for binge eating.

Social factors that may contribute to eating disorders include sharply restricted, rigid definitions of beauty that exclude people who do not conform to a particular body weight and shape; cultures that glorify thinness and overemphasize the importance of obtaining a "perfect body"; and cultures that judge and value people based on external physical appearance rather than on internal qualities such as character, intellect, generosity, and kindness. Appearance-driven concerns, rather than health needs, continue to motivate many obese individuals to lose weight. Societal pressures reinforce these appearance-driven concerns by portraying obese individuals in a negative manner.

A related consideration that further complicates pinpointing the origins of eating disorders is the extent to which temperament interacts with genetic predisposition and interpersonal and social factors to promote eating disorders. Researchers and mental health professionals observe that temperamental tendencies such as perfectionism, compulsivity, impulsivity, and other behavioral, cognitive, and emotional leanings seem to predispose to eating disorders.

Binge-Eating Disorders

Binge eating is a common problem among people who are overweight and obese. Besides consuming unusually large amounts of food in a single sitting, binge eaters generally suffer from low mood and low alertness, and experience uncontrollable compulsions to eat. They

FIGURE 3.1

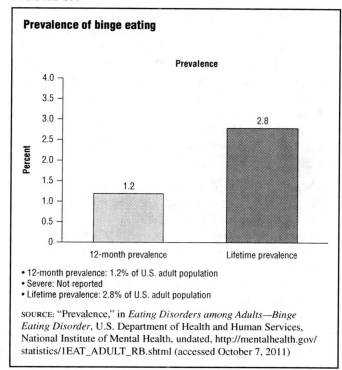

Prevalence of binge eating

Prevalence

- 12-month prevalence: 1.2% of U.S. adult population
- Severe: Not reported
- Lifetime prevalence: 2.8% of U.S. adult population

SOURCE: "Prevalence," in *Eating Disorders among Adults—Binge Eating Disorder*, U.S. Department of Health and Human Services, National Institute of Mental Health, undated, http://mentalhealth.gov/statistics/1EAT_ADULT_RB.shtml (accessed October 7, 2011)

experience food cravings before binge episodes and feelings of discontent, dissatisfaction, and restlessness following binges.

An estimated 2.8% of adults will have a binge-eating disorder at some point during their lifetime. (See Figure 3.1.) In "Eating Disorders among Adults—Binge Eating Disorder" (undated, http://mentalhealth.gov/statistics/1EAT_ADULT_RB.shtml), the National Institute of Mental Health (NIMH) indicates that binge-eating disorder is the most common eating disorder. The average age of onset is 25 and the prevalence of binge eating declines with advancing age—people aged 18 to 59 years are more likely to suffer from it than people aged 60 years and older.

Even though the disorder is more common in people who are overweight or obese, normal-weight people also develop the disorder. People who suffer from binge eating often:

- Feel that eating is out of their ability to control

- Eat amounts of food most people would think are unusually large

- Eat much more quickly than usual during binge episodes

- Eat until the point of physical discomfort

- Consume large amounts of food, even when they are not hungry

- Eat alone because they feel embarrassed about the amount of food they eat

- Feel disgusted, depressed, or guilty after overeating

In an effort to determine whether dietary restraint is a behavioral factor that activates genetic predisposition for binge eating, Sarah E. Racine et al. looked at 1,678 young adolescent and adult same-sex female twins from the Minnesota Twin Family Study and the Michigan State University Twin Registry and published their findings in "Dietary Restraint Moderates Genetic Risk for Binge Eating" (*Journal of Abnormal Psychology*, vol. 120, no. 1, February 2011). The researchers indicate that dietary restraint is an important trigger for people who have a genetic risk for binge eating.

Some Dieters Are Consumed by Eating Disorders

In the 21st century Americans are preoccupied with body image. They are constantly bombarded with images of thin, beautiful young women and lean, muscular men in magazines, on billboards, on the Internet, on television, and in movies. Advertising implies that to be thin and beautiful is to be happy. Many prominent weight-loss programs reinforce this suggestion. Well-balanced, low-fat food plans or other diets that restrict carbohydrates or calories combined with exercise can help many overweight people achieve a healthier weight and lifestyle. Dieting to achieve a healthy weight is quite different from dieting obsessively to become "model thin," which can have consequences that range from mildly harmful to life-threatening. Table 3.1 enumerates the health consequences of eating disorders.

According to the NIMH, dieting plays a role in the onset of two serious eating disorders: anorexia nervosa and bulimia. Preteens, teens, and college-age women are at special risk. In fact, the National Women's Health Resource Center states in "Eating Disorders" (2011, http://www.healthywomen.org/condition/eating-disorders) that between 85% and 95% of people who develop anorexia or bulimia are women. However, researchers are beginning to report rising rates of anorexia and bulimia among men. Studies suggest that for every 10 women with an eating disorder, one male is afflicted.

A 2009 survey of high school students found that 14.5% of teenaged girls and 6.9% of teenaged boys said they had not eaten for 24 or more hours and 6.3% of teenaged girls and 3.8% of teenaged boys reported other behaviors that may be symptoms of eating disorders, such as taking laxatives to lose weight or keep from gaining weight. (See Table 3.2.) In 2009, 5.4% of teenaged girls and 2.6% of teenaged boys admitted that they vomited or took laxatives to lose or maintain their weight. (See Table 3.3.)

Anorexia Nervosa

Anorexia nervosa involves severe weight loss—a minimum of 15% below normal body weight. Anorexic people literally starve themselves, even though they may be very hungry. For reasons that researchers do not yet

TABLE 3.1

Health consequences of eating disorders

- Eating disorders are serious, potentially life-threatening conditions that affect a person's emotional and physical health.
- Eating disorders are not just a "fad" or a "phase." People do not just "catch" an eating disorder for a period of time. They are real, complex, and devastating conditions that can have serious consequences for health, productivity, and relationships.
- People struggling with an eating disorder need to seek professional help. The earlier a person with an eating disorder seeks treatment, the greater the likelihood of physical and emotional recovery.

Health consequences of anorexia nervosa: In anorexia nervosa's cycle of self-starvation, the body is denied the essential nutrients it needs to function normally. Thus, the body is forced to slow down all of its processes to conserve energy, resulting in serious medical consequences:

- Abnormally slow heart rate and low blood pressure, which mean that the heart muscle is changing. The risk for heart failure rises as the heart rate and blood pressure level sink lower and lower.
- Reduction of bone density (osteoporosis), which results in dry, brittle bones.
- Muscle loss and weakness.
- Severe dehydration, which can result in kidney failure.
- Fainting, fatigue, and overall weakness.
- Dry hair and skin; hair loss is common.
- Growth of a downy layer of hair called lanugo all over the body, including the face, in an effort to keep the body warm.

Health consequences of bulimia nervosa: The recurrent binge-and-purge cycles of bulimia can affect the entire digestive system and can lead to electrolyte and chemical imbalances in the body that affect the heart and other major organ functions. Some of the health consequences of bulimia nervosa include:

- Electrolyte imbalances that can lead to irregular heartbeats and possibly heart failure and death. Electrolyte imbalance is caused by dehydration and loss of potassium and sodium from the body as a result of purging behaviors.
- Potential for gastric rupture during periods of bingeing.
- Inflammation and possible rupture of the esophagus from frequent vomiting.
- Tooth decay and staining from stomach acids released during frequent vomiting.
- Chronic irregular bowel movements and constipation as a result of laxative abuse.
- Peptic ulcers and pancreatitis.

Health consequences of binge eating disorder: Binge eating disorder often results in many of the same health risks associated with clinical obesity. Some of the potential health consequences of binge eating disorder include:

- High blood pressure.
- High cholesterol levels.
- Heart disease as a result of elevated triglyceride levels.
- Secondary diabetes.
- Gallbladder disease.

SOURCE: "Health Consequences of Eating Disorders," National Eating Disorders Association, 2002, http://www.nationaleatingdisorders.org/nedaDir/files/documents/handouts/HlthCnsq.pdf (accessed October 7, 2011)

fully understand, anorexics become terrified of gaining weight. Both food and weight become obsessions. They often develop strange eating habits, refuse to eat with other people, and exercise strenuously to burn calories and prevent weight gain. Anorexic individuals continue to believe they are overweight even when they are dangerously thin.

This condition often begins when a young woman who is slightly overweight or normal weight starts to diet to lose weight. After achieving the desired weight loss, she redoubles her efforts to lose more weight, and dieting becomes an obsession that may eclipse other interests. Affected individuals take pleasure in how well they can avoid food consumption and measure their self-worth by their ability to lose weight. Eating and weight gain are perceived as weaknesses and personal failures.

The medical complications of anorexia are similar to starvation. When the body attempts to protect its most vital organs, the heart and the brain, it goes into "slow gear." Menstrual periods stop, and breathing, pulse, blood pressure, and thyroid function slow down. The nails and hair become brittle, the skin dries, and the lack of body fat produces an inability to withstand cold temperatures. Depression, weakness, and a constant obsession with food are also symptoms of the disease. In addition, personality changes may occur. The person suffering from anorexia may have outbursts of anger and hostility or may withdraw socially. In the most serious cases, death can result.

Scientists often describe eating disorders as addictions, and Mario Speranza et al. support this notion in "An Investigation of Goodman's Addictive Disorder Criteria in Eating Disorders" (*European Eating Disorders Review*, August 10, 2011). The researchers find that common addictive personality traits are present in many people suffering from eating disorders and substance use–related disorders. Speranza et al. conclude that "a subgroup of individuals with an eating disorder experiences their disorder as an addiction and may deserve specific therapeutic attention."

Bulimia

People who suffer from bulimia eat compulsively and then purge (get rid of the food) through self-induced vomiting, use of laxatives, diuretics, strict diets, fasts, exercise, or a combination of several of these compensatory behaviors. Bulimia often begins when a person is disgusted with the excessive amount of "bad" food consumed and vomits to rid the body of the calories.

Many bulimics are at a normal body weight or above because of their frequent binge-purge behavior, which can occur from once or twice per week to several times per day. Those bulimics who maintain normal weight may manage to keep their eating disorder a secret for years. As with anorexia, bulimia usually begins during adolescence or early adulthood. According to the NIMH, the average age of onset is 20, but many bulimics do not seek help until they are in their 30s or 40s. Figure 3.2 shows the prevalence and demographics of bulimia nervosa as well as the utilization of treatment and services.

Binge eating and purging are dangerous. In rare cases bingeing can cause esophageal ruptures, and purging can result in life-threatening cardiac (heart) conditions because the body loses vital minerals. The acid in vomit wears down tooth enamel and the lining of the esophagus, throat, and mouth and can cause scarring on the hands when fingers are pushed down the throat to induce vomiting. The esophagus may become inflamed, and glands in the neck may become swollen.

Bulimics often talk of being "hooked" on certain foods and needing to feed their "habits." This addictive behavior carries over into other areas of their life, including

TABLE 3.2

Percentage of high school students engaging in dangerous dieting behaviors, 2009

Category	Did not eat for 24 or more hours to lose weight or to keep from gaining weight			Took diet pills, powders, or liquids to lose weight or to keep from gaining weight		
	Female	Male	Total	Female	Male	Total
	%	%	%	%	%	%
Race/ethnicity						
White*	14.7	6.1	10.1	7.0	3.6	5.2
Black*	12.8	8.0	10.4	3.7	3.8	3.8
Hispanic	15.2	8.8	12.0	6.9	4.6	5.7
Grade						
9	15.7	6.7	10.9	4.7	3.7	4.2
10	14.5	6.5	10.3	6.0	3.0	4.4
11	14.8	7.2	10.9	8.1	4.0	6.0
12	12.6	7.3	9.9	6.6	4.6	5.6
Total	**14.5**	**6.9**	**10.6**	**6.3**	**3.8**	**5.0**

*Non-Hispanic.

Note: Dangerous dieting behaviors include not eating for 24 or more hours to lose weight or to keep from gaining weight during the 30 days before the survey and taking diet pills, powders, or liquids without a doctor's advice.

SOURCE: Adapted from Danice K. Eaton et al., "Table 96. Percentage of Students Who Did Not Eat for 24 or More Hours and Who Took Diet Pills, Powders, or Liquids, by Sex, Race/Ethnicity and Grade—United States, Youth Risk Behavior Survey, 2009," in "Youth Risk Behavior Surveillance—United States, 2009," *Morbidity and Mortality Weekly Report*, vol. 59, no. SS–5, June 4, 2010, http://www.cdc.gov/mmwr/pdf/ss/ss5905.pdf (accessed October 7, 2011)

TABLE 3.3

Percentage of students who vomited or took laxatives to lose or maintain their weight, by sex, race/ethnicity and grade, 2009

Category	Female	Male	Total
	%	%	%
Race/ethnicity			
White*	5.2	1.8	3.4
Black*	3.6	4.6	4.1
Hispanic	6.9	4.0	5.4
Grade			
9	5.6	2.8	4.1
10	5.3	2.2	3.7
11	6.3	2.7	4.5
12	4.2	2.6	3.4
Total	**5.4**	**2.6**	**4.0**

*Non-Hispanic.

Notes: Vomiting and laxatives used in order to lose weight or to keep from gaining weight during the 30 days before the survey.

SOURCE: Adapted from Danice K. Eaton et al., "Table 98. Percentage of High School Students Who Vomited or Took Laxatives, by Sex, Race/Ethnicity, and Grade—United States, Youth Risk Behavior Survey, 2009," in "Youth Risk Behavior Surveillance—United States, 2009," *Morbidity and Mortality Weekly Report*, vol. 59, no. SS-5, June 4, 2010, http://www.cdc.gov/mmwr/pdf/ss/ss5905.pdf (accessed October 7, 2011)

developing anorexia is about one out of 200, but when a family member has the disorder, the risk increases to one out of 30. Twin studies demonstrate that when one twin is affected, there is a 50% chance the other will develop an eating disorder. Cynthia M. Bulik et al. calculated heritability estimates for anorexia nervosa and bulimia nervosa and published the estimates of their genetic correlation in "Understanding the Relation between Anorexia Nervosa and Bulimia Nervosa in a Swedish National Twin Sample" (*Biological Psychiatry*, vol. 67, no. 1, January 1, 2010). Consistent with the findings of other researchers, Bulik et al. find an overlap of genetic and unique environmental factors that influence the development of both eating disorders.

Besides a genetic predisposition, bulimics and anorexics seem to have different temperaments. Bulimics are likely to be impulsive (acting without thought of the consequences) and are more likely to abuse alcohol and drugs. Anorexics tend to be perfectionists, good students, and competitive athletes. They usually keep their feelings to themselves and rarely disobey their parents. However, bulimics and anorexics do share certain traits: they lack self-esteem, have feelings of helplessness, and fear gaining weight. In both disorders the eating problems appear to develop as a way of handling stress and anxiety.

Bulimics consume huge amounts of food (often junk food) in a search for comfort and stress relief. The bingeing, however, brings only guilt and depression. By contrast, anorexics restrict food to gain a sense of control and mastery over some aspect of their lives. Controlling their weight seems to offer two advantages: they can take control of their body, and they can gain approval from others.

the likelihood of alcohol and drug abuse. Many bulimics suffer from coexisting medical or mental health problems, such as severe depression, which increases their risk of committing suicide.

CAUSES OF EATING DISORDERS

As described earlier, research suggests there is a genetic component to susceptibility to eating disorders. For example, in the general population the chance of

FIGURE 3.2

Bulimia prevalence, demographics and treatment

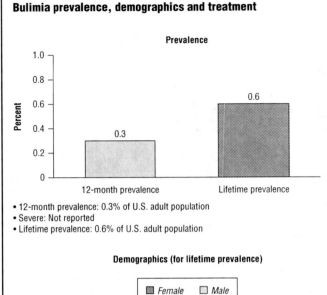

Prevalence

- 12-month prevalence: 0.3% of U.S. adult population
- Severe: Not reported
- Lifetime prevalence: 0.6% of U.S. adult population

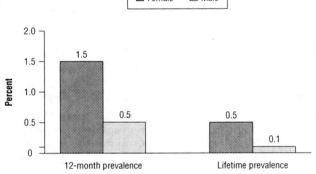

Demographics (for lifetime prevalence)

- Sex:
- Race: Not reported
- Age: People ages 18–29, 30–44, and 45–59 were all significantly more likely than 60+ year olds to suffer from bulimia nervosa

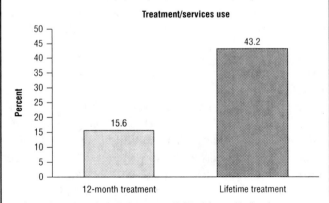

Treatment/services use

- 12-month treatment for bulimia nervosa: 15.6% of those with disorder are receiving treatment
- Lifetime treatment for bulimia nervosa: 43.2% of those with disorder are receiving treatment

Average age-of-onset: 20 years old

SOURCE: "Bulimia Nervosa," in *Eating Disorders among Adults—Bulimia Nervosa*, U.S. Department of Health and Human Services, National Institute of Mental Health, undated, http://www.nimh.nih.gov/statistics/pdf/NCS-R_Bulimia_Nervosa.pdf (accessed October 7, 2011)

Psychological theories that explain the origins of bulimia include conflicted relationships between mothers and daughters, attempts to control one's own body in the face of seemingly uncontrollable family or other interpersonal relationships, or ambivalence about sexual development and attention. The latter theory has also been used to explain overweight and obesity in teenaged girls and young women—as protection from or defense against attention from males who make them fearful or uncomfortable.

In "Childhood Anxiety Associated with Low BMI in Women with Anorexia Nervosa" (*Behaviour Research and Therapy*, vol. 48, no. 1, January 2010), Jocilyn E. Dellava et al. look at risk factors for developing anorexia nervosa and low BMI after they interviewed 326 women and their mothers who participated in the Genetics of Anorexia Nervosa Study. The researchers find that women with anorexia nervosa who had been especially fearful or anxious as children were at greater risk for dangerously low BMI and that childhood anxiety was associated with caloric restriction. Dellava et al. posit that "measures of anxiety and factors associated with anxiety-proneness in childhood may index children at risk for restrictive behaviors and extremely low BMIs in [anorexia nervosa]." In another study, Tamar B. Rubinstein et al. consider risk factors for developing eating disorders and report their findings in "Disordered Eating in Adulthood Is Associated with Reported Weight Loss Attempts in Childhood" (*International Journal of Eating Disorders*, vol. 43, no. 7, November 1, 2009). The researchers indicate that adults who had made efforts to lose weight when they were children (aged 12 years and younger) were at increased risk of unhealthy eating behaviors, especially binge-eating disorder.

OCCURRENCE OF EATING DISORDERS

Sonia A. Swanson et al. of the NIMH analyzed eating disorders using data from the National Comorbidity Survey Replication Adolescent Supplement, a nationally representative sample of adolescents aged 13 to 18 years in the United States. In "Prevalence and Correlates of Eating Disorders in Adolescents: Results from the National Comorbidity Survey Replication Adolescent Supplement" (*Archives of General Psychiatry*, vol. 68, no. 7, July 2011), the researchers note that the lifetime prevalence rates of anorexia nervosa, bulimia nervosa, and binge eating disorder were 0.3%, 0.9%, and 1.6%, respectively, and their 12-month prevalence rates were 0.2%, 0.6%, and 0.9%, respectively. The majority of adolescents with an eating disorder also met criteria for at least one other mental disorder and nearly all adolescents with anorexia nervosa reported social problems. Adolescents with eating disorders were also at increased risk for other self-destructive and suicidal behavior. Swanson et al. conclude that "the prevalence of these disorders is higher than previously expected in this age range, and the patterns of comorbidity, role impairment, and suicidality indicate that eating disorders represent a major public health concern."

The Eating Disorders Coalition for Research, Policy, and Action notes in the fact sheet "Facts about Eating Disorders: What the Research Shows" (May 20, 2009, http://www.eatingdisorderscoalition.org/documents/Talking pointsEatingDisordersFactSheetUpdated5-20-09.pdf) that about 11 million Americans are affected by eating disorders and that anorexia is the third most common illness among adolescents. The coalition observes that the incidence of eating disorders is increasing in younger age groups and is becoming more common in diverse ethnic and sociocultural groups. Eating disorders have been diagnosed in children as young as seven years old, 40% of nine-year-old girls have dieted, and even five-year-old girls express concern about weight. About 40% to 60% of high school–aged girls diet and 13% engage in purging.

According to Swanson et al., the prevalence of eating disorders among adults range from 0.5% to 1% for anorexia nervosa and from 0.5% to 3% for bulimia nervosa. In the *Textbook of Psychiatric Epidemiology* (2011), the editors Ming Tsuang, Mauricio Tohen, and Peter B. Jones observe that the lifetime prevalence of anorexia nervosa across studies from North America, Europe, Australia, and New Zealand ranges from 0.9% to 2.2%; for bulimia nervosa the range is from 1.5% to 4.6%; and for binge eating disorder the range is from 0.6% to 3.5%. Research reveals that males are much less likely to suffer from eating disorders, with their lifetime prevalence of anorexia nervosa ranging from 0.1% to 0.4% and bulimia nervosa of about 0.5%. When all other eating disorders are added, between 8.7% and 15.9% of women will suffer from an eating disorder during their lifetime.

Eating disorders are often associated with various impulsive behaviors. In "Obsessive-Compulsive Disorder, Impulse Control Disorders, and Drug Addiction: Common Features and Potential Treatments" (*Drugs*, vol. 71, no. 7, May 7, 2011), Leonardo F. Fontenelle et al. examine the relationship between compulsive, impulsive, and addictive behaviors. They find a relationship between these behaviors and posit that impulsive or addictive features of eating disorders might be effectively treated with drugs that address the quality of the underlying drives and the involvement of neural systems such as those that act to reduce or prevent relapse of addiction.

According to Jessica H. Baker et al., in "Eating Disorder Symptomatology and Substance Use Disorders: Prevalence and Shared Risk in a Population Based Twin Sample" (*International Journal of Eating Disorders Review*, vol. 43, no. 7, November 1, 2010), there is a significant association between eating disorders and substance use disorders, in that high rates of substance abuse

(alcohol and illicit drugs) are reported by women with eating disorders. The researchers analyzed data from the Virginia Adult Twin Study of Psychiatric and Substance Use Disorders and focused on female-female twin pairs who were born between 1934 and 1968. Baker et al. find comparable prevalence of substance use disorders among women with anorexia nervosa and those with bulimia nervosa. The difference between women suffering from these eating disorders and substance use disorders was the chronology of the onset of substance use. A majority of women with bulimia nervosa reported that their eating disorder preceded their substance use, whereas women with anorexia nervosa were more likely to report substance use before the onset of their eating disorder. One possible explanation for this difference is that women with anorexia nervosa begin experimenting with substances in an effort to lose weight, whereas women with bulimia nervosa begin using substances to suppress or relieve bulimic urges.

TREATMENT OF EATING DISORDERS

Generally, physicians treat the medical complications of the disorder, whereas nutritionists advise the affected individuals about specific diet and eating plans. To help people with eating disorders face their underlying problems and emotional issues, psychotherapy is usually necessary. For people with eating disorders, the initial challenge is to convince them to seek and obtain treatment; after they start treatment, the challenge then becomes helping them to stay in the program. Many anorexics deny their illness, and getting and keeping anorexic patients in treatment can be difficult. Treating bulimia is also difficult. Many bulimics are easily frustrated and want to leave treatment if their symptoms are not quickly relieved.

Several approaches are used to treat eating disorders. Cognitive-behavioral therapy (CBT) teaches people how to monitor their eating and change unhealthy eating habits. It also teaches them how to change the way they respond to stressful situations. CBT is based on the premise that thinking influences emotions and behavior—that feelings and actions originate with thoughts. CBT posits that it is possible to change the way people feel and act even if their circumstances do not change. It teaches the advantages of feeling calm when faced with undesirable situations. CBT clients learn that they will confront undesirable events and circumstances whether they become troubled about them or not. When they are troubled about events or circumstances, they have two problems: the troubling event or circumstance, and the troubling feelings about the event or circumstance. Clients learn that when they do not become troubled about trying events and circumstances, they can reduce the number of problems they face by half.

Interpersonal psychotherapy (IPT) helps people look at their relationships with friends and family and make changes to resolve problems. IPT is short-term therapy that has demonstrated effectiveness for the treatment of depression. According to the International Society for Interpersonal Psychotherapy, IPT emphasizes that mental health and emotional problems occur within an interpersonal context. For this reason the therapy aims to intervene specifically in social functioning to relieve symptoms.

Group therapy has been found helpful for bulimics, who are relieved to find that they are not alone or unique in their eating behavior. A combination of behavioral therapy and family systems therapy is often the most effective with anorexics. Family systems therapy considers the family as the unit of treatment and focuses on relationships and communication patterns within the family rather than on the personality traits or symptoms displayed by individual family members. Problems are addressed by modifying the system rather than by trying to change an individual family member. People with eating disorders who also suffer from depression may benefit from antidepressant and antianxiety medications to help relieve coexisting mental health problems.

Recovery from eating disorders is uneven and the lack of consensus about the criteria for recovery further confounds efforts to assess how people fare as a result of treatment. Greta Noordenbos of Leiden University explains in "When Have Eating Disordered Patients Recovered and What Do the DSM-IV Criteria Tell about Recovery?" (Eating Disorders, vol. 19, no. 3, May 2011) that varying criteria result in a wide range of estimates of recovered patients. Noordenbos laments that "outcome studies not only use different criteria for recovery, but also quite different instruments, rendering their results incomparable. The same problem occurs among studies of predictors for recovery from eating disorders. Without consensus on criteria for recovery, it is not clear which goals of treatment are important to realize full recovery."

In "Facts about Eating Disorders," the Eating Disorders Coalition for Research, Policy, and Action characterizes recovery as a process that frequently entails multiple rehospitalizations, limited ability to work or attend school, and limited capacity for interpersonal relationships. With treatment, which can take months to years, about one-third of people with an eating disorder recover after an initial episode, one-third fluctuates between recovery and relapse, and the remaining third suffer chronic deterioration.

Eating disorders are difficult to treat effectively because many sufferers resist entering treatment and/or fail to complete treatment programs. Because attrition (dropping out of treatment) is a known problem, Karen Farchaus Stein et al. report in "An Eating Disorder Randomized Clinical Trial and Attrition: Profiles and Determinants of Dropout" (International Journal of Eating Disorders, vol. 44, no. 4, May 2011) their efforts to determine whether attrition is related to changes in symptoms during treatment, including participants' perceptions of dissatisfaction with their body. To do this, the researchers compared the perceptions of dropouts to those of participants who remained in treatment for six months.

Farchaus Stein et al. find that both dropouts and those who remained in treatment experienced decreases in the drive for thinness, body dissatisfaction, and bulimia during the treatment phase, but that women who dropped out of treatment had a greater decrease in body dissatisfaction after one month of treatment than those who remained. The researchers theorize that a decrease in symptoms along with changes in self-perception, such as diminished body dissatisfaction, discourage participants from continuing in treatment. Farchaus Stein et al. opine that "attention to treatment response from the earliest phases of intervention through follow-up may help to identify those at greatest risk of dropping and lead to strategies for promoting participant retention."

New Directions in Research and Treatment

According to the NIMH, in "Eating Disorders," the results of its research are aiding both the understanding of eating disorders and their treatment. Research on intervening in the binge-eating cycle demonstrates that initiating structured patterns of eating enables people with eating disorders to experience less hunger, less deprivation, and fewer negative feelings about food and eating. When the two key predictors of bingeing—hunger and negative feelings—are reduced, the frequency of binges declines.

Continued study of the human genome promises the identification of susceptibility genes (genes that indicate an individual's increased risk for developing eating disorders) that will help develop more effective treatments for these disorders. Other research is investigating the relationship between brain functions and emotional and social behavior related to eating disorders and the role of the brain in feeding behavior. Scientists have learned that both appetite and energy expenditure are regulated by a highly complex network of nerve cells and intercellular messengers called neuropeptides. The role of sex hormones, known as gonadal steroids, in the development of eating disorders is suggested by gender and the onset of puberty as a risk for these disorders. These discoveries provide insight into the biochemical mechanisms of eating disorders and offer potential direction for the development of new drugs and treatments for these disorders.

In "Update on Course and Outcome in Eating Disorders" (International Journal of Eating Disorders, vol. 43, no. 3, April 2010), Pamela K. Keel and Tiffany A. Brown review 26 studies that describe inpatient and outpatient treatment of eating disorders and the outcomes (how patients fared) as a result of treatment. The researchers find that inpatient treatment and the co-occurrence of serious psychiatric disorders were significant predictors of poor outcomes. Keel and Brown note that even though treatment may serve to stabilize or reduce the progression of symptoms and minimize the medical consequences and complications of eating disorders for many people, it is not yet known if treatment (or if a specific type of treatment) increases the number of people who fare well long term. Furthermore, little is known about the other factors that predict good or poor results of treatment.

Kelly L. Klump and Kyle L. Gobrogge summarize in "A Review and Primer of Molecular Genetic Studies of Anorexia Nervosa" (International Journal of Eating Disorders, vol. 37, suppl. S43–48, July 2005) the genetic underpinnings of eating disorders. They report that research reveals a role for the chemical serotonin in the development of anorexia nervosa. Serotonin is a neurotransmitter involved in the regulation of mood and certain mental disorders, such as depression and anxiety. Genomic regions on chromosomes 1 and 10 are likely to harbor susceptibility genes for anorexia as well as for other eating disorders. The findings from these genetic studies support those of neurobiologic studies indicating that alterations in serotonin functioning may contribute to the development of eating disorders.

The considerable proportion of people with eating disorders who do not fare well in treatment, along with the high mortality rates that are associated with these disorders, prompts questions about factors that may influence recovery. In view of the genetic component in the genesis and progression of eating disorders, it seems likely that there may be genetic variants that contribute to the prospects for recovery. Identifying these variants may lead to more personalized treatment that includes more effective psychotherapies and/or pharmacological interventions for the most treatment-resistant patients. In "Genetic Association of Recovery from Eating Disorders: The Role of GABA Receptor SNPs" (Neuropsychopharmacology, vol. 36, no. 11, October 2011), Cinnamon S. Bloss et al. tested more than 5,000 single nucleotide polymorphisms (SNPs) in approximately 350 genes to determine whether any of these SNPs were associated with recovery from eating disorders. SNPs associated with g-aminobutyric acid (a neurotransmitter that acts to inhibit the central nervous system, exerting a calming effect) were overrepresented among people with eating disorders. Bloss et al. conclude that their findings "could provide new insights into the development of more effective interventions for the most treatment-resistant patients."

PREVENTING EATING DISORDERS

Conventional public health definitions describe primary prevention as the prevention of new cases and secondary prevention as the prevention of recurrence of a disease or prevention of its progression. Primary prevention measures fall into two categories: actions to protect against disease and disability and actions to promote health such as good nutrition and hygiene, adequate exercise and rest, and avoidance of environmental and health risks. Health promotion also includes education about other interdependent dimensions of health known as wellness. Examples of health promotion programs aimed at preventing eating disorders include programs to enhance self-esteem, nutrition education classes, and programs that support children and teens to resist unhealthy pressures to conform to unrealistic body weight.

Secondary prevention programs are intended to identify and detect disease in its earliest stages, when it is most likely to be successfully treated. With early detection and diagnosis, it may be possible to cure the disease, slow its progression, prevent or minimize complications, and limit disability. Secondary prevention of eating disorders includes efforts to identify affected individuals to intervene early and prevent the development of serious and potentially life-threatening consequences.

Tertiary prevention programs aim to improve the quality of life for people with various diseases by limiting complications and disabilities, reducing the severity and progression of the disease, and providing rehabilitation (therapy to restore function and self-sufficiency). Unlike primary and secondary prevention, tertiary prevention involves actual treatment for the disease, and in the case of eating disorders it is conducted primarily by medical and mental health practitioners rather than by public health or social service agencies. An example of tertiary prevention is a program that monitors people with eating disorders to ensure that they maintain appropriate body weight and adhere to healthy diets and other prescribed medication or treatment. Because the treatment of eating disorders is not always effective or lasting, many health professionals contend that initiatives directed at controlling or eliminating the disorders by treating each affected individual or by training enough professionals as interventionists are ill advised. Instead, they advocate redirecting time, energy, and resources to primary and secondary prevention efforts.

Table 3.4 lists the basic principles for the prevention of eating disorders prepared by the National Eating Disorders Association (NEDA). These principles underscore the complexity of addressing eating disorders and the need for comprehensive, community-wide prevention programs that address the social and cultural issues promoting the rise of these disorders. The NEDA also urges parents to spearhead efforts to prevent eating disorders by

TABLE 3.4

Eating disorders prevention

What is eating disorders prevention?

Prevention is any systematic attempt to change the circumstances that promote, initiate, sustain, or intensify problems like eating disorders.

- **Primary prevention** refers to programs or efforts that are designed to prevent the occurrence of eating disorders before they begin. Primary prevention is intended to help promote healthy development.
- **Secondary prevention** (sometimes called "targeted prevention") refers to programs or efforts that are designed to promote the early identification of an eating disorder—to recognize and treat an eating disorder before it spirals out of control. The earlier an eating disorder is discovered and addressed, the better the chance for recovery.

Basic principles for the prevention of eating disorders

1. Eating disorders are serious and complex problems. We need to be careful to avoid thinking of them in simplistic terms, like "anorexia is just a plea for attention," or "bulimia is just an addiction to food." Eating disorders arise from a variety of physical, emotional, social, and familial issues, all of which need to be addressed for effective prevention and treatment.
2. Eating disorders are not just a "woman's problem" or "something for the girls." Males who are preoccupied with shape and weight can also develop eating disorders as well as dangerous shape control practices like steroid use. In addition, males play an important role in prevention. The objectification and other forms of mistreatment of women by others contribute directly to two underlying features of an eating disorder: obsession with appearance and shame about one's body.
3. Prevention efforts will fail, or worse, inadvertently encourage disordered eating, if they concentrate solely on warning the public about the signs, symptoms, and dangers of eating disorders. Effective prevention programs must also address:
   - Our cultural obsession with slenderness as a physical, psychological, and moral issue.
   - The roles of men and women in our society.
   - The development of people's self-esteem and self-respect in a variety of areas (school, work, community service, hobbies) that transcend physical appearance.
4. Whenever possible, prevention programs for schools, community organizations, etc., should be coordinated with opportunities for participants to speak confidentially with a trained professional with expertise in the field of eating disorders, and, when appropriate, receive referrals to sources of competent, specialized care.

SOURCE: Michael Levine and Margo Maine, "Eating Disorders Can Be Prevented!" National Eating Disorders Association, 2005, http://www .nationaleatingdisorders.org/nedaDir/files/documents/handouts/EDsPrev .pdf (accessed October 10, 2011)

TABLE 3.5

Ten things parents can do to prevent eating disorders

1. Consider your thoughts, attitudes, and behaviors toward your own body and the way that these beliefs have been shaped by the forces of weightism and sexism. Then educate your children
   (a) the genetic basis for the natural diversity of human body shapes and sizes, and
   (b) the nature and ugliness of prejudice.
   - Make an effort to maintain positive, healthy attitudes & behaviors. Children learn from the things you say and do!
2. Examine closely your dreams and goals for your children and other loved ones. Are you overemphasizing beauty and body shape, particularly for girls?
   - Avoid conveying an attitude which says in effect, "I will like you more if you lose weight, don't eat so much, look more like the slender models in ads, fit into smaller clothes, etc."
   - Decide what you can do and what you can stop doing to reduce the teasing, criticism, blaming, staring, etc. that reinforce the idea that larger or fatter is "bad" and smaller or thinner is "good."
3. Learn about and discuss with your sons and daughters (a) the dangers of trying to alter one's body shape through dieting, (b) the value of moderate exercise for health, and (c) the importance of eating a variety of foods in well-balanced meals consumed at least three times a day.
   - Avoid categorizing foods into "good/safe /no-fat or low-fat" vs."bad/dangerous/ fattening."
   - Be a good role model in regard to sensible eating, exercise, and self-acceptance.
4. Make a commitment not to avoid activities (such as swimming, sunbathing, dancing, etc.) simply because they call attention to your weight and shape. Refuse to wear clothes that are uncomfortable or that you don't like but wear simply because they divert attention from your weight or shape.
5. Make a commitment to exercise for the joy of feeling your body move and grow stronger, not to purge fat from your body or to compensate for calories eaten.
6. Practice taking people seriously for what they say, feel, and do, not for how slender or "well put together" they appear.
7. Help children appreciate and resist the ways in which television, magazines, and other media distort the true diversity of human body types and imply that a slender body means power, excitement, popularity, or perfection.
8. Educate boys and girls about various forms of prejudice, including weightism, and help them understand their responsibilities for preventing them.
9. Encourage your children to be active and to enjoy what their bodies can do and feel like. Do not limit their caloric intake unless a physician requests that you do this because of a medical problem.
10. Do whatever you can to promote the self-esteem and self-respect of all of your children in intellectual, athletic, and social endeavors. Give boys and girls the same opportunities and encouragement. Be careful not to suggest that females are less important than males, e.g., by exempting males from housework or child care. A well-rounded sense of self and solid self-esteem are perhaps the best antidotes to dieting and disordered eating.

SOURCE: Michael Levine, "10 Things Parents Can Do to Help Prevent Eating Disorders," National Eating Disorders Association, 2005, http://www .nationaleatingdisorders.org/nedaDir/files/documents/handouts/10Parent.pdf (accessed October 10, 2011)

practicing positive, healthy attitudes and behaviors and encouraging children to resist media stereotypes about body shape and weight. Furthermore, it outlines the philosophies and actions parents can adopt and the behaviors they can model to help their children cultivate healthy attitudes about food, eating, exercise, and body weight. Table 3.5 outlines 10 steps parents can take to help prevent eating disorders.

Changing Social and Cultural Norms

The cultural idealization of thinness as a standard of female beauty and worth and the societal acceptance of dieting as a female ritual have been widely cited as sociocultural causes of eating disorders. The widespread misperception that the body is readily reshaped and that one can, and should, strive to change its size and form to correspond with aesthetic preferences also contributes to distorted perceptions and unrealistic expectations.

Media images that create, reflect, communicate, and reinforce cultural definitions of attractiveness, especially female beauty, are often acknowledged as factors that contribute to the rise of eating disorders. They exert powerful influences on values, attitudes, and practices for body image, diet, and activity. The role of the media, in conjunction with the fashion and entertainment industries, in promoting unrealistic standards of female beauty and unhealthy eating habits has been named as a causative factor for body dissatisfaction, unhealthy dieting behavior, and the rise of eating disorders.

Even though media messages portraying thinness as a desirable attribute do not directly cause eating disorders, they help create the context in which people learn to place a value on the size and shape of their body. To the extent that media advertising defines cultural values about that which is beautiful and desirable, the media have potent power over the development of self-esteem and body image. Even if the media were to present more diverse and realistic images of people, this change would be unlikely to immediately reduce or eliminate eating disorders. Many observers, however, believe it would reduce the pressures to conform to one ideal, lessen feelings of body dissatisfaction, and ultimately decrease the potential for eating disorders.

ADVERTISING CAMPAIGN EMPHASIZING REALISTIC BODIES DRAWS PRAISE AND CRITICISM. In June 2005 Dove, a skin and hair care division of the Unilever company, launched the "Campaign for Real Beauty," which featured a purportedly unretouched photo of six smiling women of various sizes and ethnicities posing in plain white underwear to promote a skin-firming cream. The women, who were not models, ranged from a slim size 6 to a curvy size 14 and graced print advertisements and billboards. The campaign generated considerable discussion and debate in the media.

According to the article "Dove Ads with 'Real' Women Get Attention" (Associated Press, July 29, 2005), Philippe Harousseau, the Dove marketing director, described the campaign as responsive to "our belief that beauty comes in different shapes, sizes and ages. Our mission is to make more women feel beautiful every day by broadening the definition of beauty." Industry observers wondered whether the company was in fact broadening the definition of beauty and improving women's body image and self-esteem or simply launching a provocative advertising campaign. Even though the company did not disclose just how much the advertisements helped promote its products, it conceded that the campaign was beneficial for all Dove products, not just the firming creams.

The article notes that the ads were not, however, universally well received. For example, the *Chicago Sun-Times* columnist Richard Roeper characterized the women as "chunky," which earned him angry letters from about a thousand readers. Some skeptics asserted that even though they endorsed the notion of the ads featuring real women who felt good about their body, they believed the ads sent contradictory messages—promoting a product to reduce the curves the models were flaunting. The most impassioned detractors accused the company of appearing hypocritical because the ads aimed to profit from "improving" the same curves the campaign exhorted women to celebrate.

The Dove advertising campaign ended in early 2011, but its long-running campaign had prompted some attitu-dinal change. The campaign coined the term *Dove beauties*, which referred to attractive women with healthy bodies as opposed to model-thin frames. It also inspired some other advertisers and editors to use more average-sized models instead of relying solely on extremely thin models.

For example, in September 2009 *Glamour* magazine ran an unretouched nearly nude photo of the plus-sized model Lizzi Miller (1989–), in which her rounded belly was clearly visible. The photo touched a nerve with readers who were generally overjoyed to see the photograph of a clearly happy, self-confident young woman who was not extremely thin. Readers and others in the media pleaded for more images of beautiful women of all sizes, and the magazine complied with its November 2009 issue, which featured photos of seven models who were all several sizes larger than the typical thin model.

Among the models was Crystal Renn (1986–), the coauthor (with Marjorie Ingall) of *Hungry: A Young Model's Story of Appetite, Ambition, and the Ultimate Embrace of Curves* (2009), a memoir that describes her as having an eating disorder. When she acknowledged her disorder and began to eat healthily, her career as a fashion model took off. Renn became a healthy, successful plus-sized model and advocate for media recognition and celebration of women of all sizes. However, in September 2011 the poster girl for curvier plus-sized models debuted a new, much thinner look. According to Sarah Bull and Laura Schreffler, in "Plus-Size Past: Former 'Big' Model Crystal Renn Shows Full Extent of Weight Loss in Slinky Gold Dress at Metropolitan Opera" (*Daily Mail*, September 29, 2011), Renn denied that her weight loss was attributable to pressure from the fashion industry. Renn claimed she was happy with her body, opining, "I think the most important thing that we all need to know, whether you're a model, you're a normal person walking around, you're an editor, you're a photographer, you're anybody out in the world—it's about individual health."

In "Waif Goodbye! Average-Size Female Models Promote Positive Body Image and Appeal to Consumers" (*Psychology and Health*, vol. 26, no. 10, October 2011), Phillippa C. Diedrichs and Christina Lee examine the effectiveness of advertising using average-sized models compared with thin models. Among men and women, the average-sized models were associated with a more positive body image than the thin models. Based on their findings, Diedrichs and Lee conclude that "average-size female models can promote positive body image and appeal to consumers."

CHAPTER 4
DIET, NUTRITION, AND WEIGHT ISSUES AMONG CHILDREN AND ADOLESCENTS

Over the last year we've fundamentally changed the conversation about how we eat, how we move and how we get our food. Communities across the country...are implementing creative solutions to ending childhood obesity. Together, we're making a real difference in the lives of children and today there's a real sense of hope that we can end childhood obesity.

—Michelle Obama, "Remarks by the First Lady on the One Year Anniversary of the Let's Move! Campaign" (February 8, 2011)

One of the most disturbing observations about overweight and obesity in the United States is the epidemic of supersized (overweight and obese) kids. Boyd A. Swinberg et al. find in "The Global Obesity Pandemic: Shaped by Global Drivers and Local Environments" (*Lancet*, vol. 378, no. 9793, August 2011) that in 2008 an estimated 170 million children under the age 18 years were considered overweight or obese. More than 25% of children in Australia, Chile, the United Kingdom, and the United States were overweight—twice as many as were overweight during the mid-1970s, when the epidemic began. Swinberg et al. report that the prevalence of overweight and obesity in children appears to be leveling off, or in some instances, decreasing in Australia, France, Sweden, and Switzerland.

The National Center for Health Statistics reports in *Health, United States, 2010* (2011, http://www.cdc.gov/nchs/data/hus/hus10.pdf) that in 2005–08 nearly three times as many American children aged six to 11 years and more than three times as many children aged 12 to 19 years were seriously overweight than were overweight in 1976–80. (See Table 4.1.) In just the last 25 years, from 1988–94 to 2005–08, the prevalence of overweight among children and adolescents increased from 7.2% to 10.7% for children two to five years and from 11.3% to 17.4% for children aged six to 11 years. Among teenagers aged 12 to 19 years the percentage nearly doubled, from 10.5% to 17.9%.

With children and teens as well as with adults, the body mass index (BMI; body weight in kilograms divided by height in meters squared) is used to determine underweight, healthy weight, overweight, and at risk for overweight. Children's body fatness changes over the years as they grow, and girls and boys differ in their body fatness as they mature. In light of these differences, the BMI for children (also referred to as BMI-for-age) is gender and age specific. For example, Figure 4.1 shows BMI percentiles for boys aged two to 20 years and demonstrates how different BMI numbers are interpreted for a 10-year-old boy. Figure 4.2 shows that children of different ages (and genders) may have the same BMI number, but that number will fall into a different percentile for each child, classifying a 10-year-old boy as overweight and a 15-year-old boy as at a healthy weight.

Overweight is defined as at or above the age- and gender-specific 95th percentile on the BMI. (See Table 4.2.) Still, even children at the 85th percentile are considered at risk for overweight- and obesity-induced illnesses and overweight throughout their adult life.

Overweight children are much more likely to become overweight adults, and those children who are likely to become overweight and obese can be identified as toddlers and preschoolers. Laura E. Pryor et al. indicate in "Developmental Trajectories of Body Mass Index in Early Childhood and Their Risk Factors: An 8-Year Longitudinal Study" (*Archives of Pediatric and Adolescent Medicine*, vol. 165, no. 10, October 2011) that by plotting age against BMI an "atypically elevated BMI trajectory" is identifiable at age three and a half. They also find that two maternal risk factors—high maternal BMI and smoking during pregnancy—were associated with the sharply rising trajectory predictive of overweight and obesity.

The prevalence of overweight and obesity among adolescents is of particular concern because overweight and obese adolescents are at even greater risk than overweight children of becoming overweight or obese adults.

TABLE 4.1

Obesity among children and teens, selected years 1963–2008

[Data are based on physical examinations of a sample of the civilian noninstitutionalized population]

Sex, age, race and Hispanic origin[a], and percent of poverty level	1963–1965 1966–1970[b]	1971–1974	1976–1980[c]	1988–1994	1999–2002	2005–2008
			Percent of population			
2–5 years of age						
Both sexes[d]	—	—	—	7.2	10.3	10.7
Not Hispanic or Latino:						
White only	—	—	—	5.2	8.7	9.4
Black or African American only	—	—	—	7.7	8.8	14.0
Mexican	—	—	—	12.3	13.1	14.1
Boys	—	—	—	6.1	10.0	10.2
Not Hispanic or Latino:						
White only	—	—	—	4.5	8.2	7.8
Black or African American only	—	—	—	7.7	8.0	13.8
Mexican	—	—	—	12.4	14.1	17.3
Girls	—	—	—	8.2	10.6	11.1
Not Hispanic or Latina:						
White only	—	—	—	5.9	9.0	11.3
Black or African American only	—	—	—	7.6	9.6	14.2
Mexican	—	—	—	12.3	12.2	10.7
Percent of poverty level:[e]						
Below 100%	—	—	—	9.7	10.9	12.5
100%–199%	—	—	—	7.2	13.8	10.8
200%–399%	—	—	—	5.6	7.6	11.5
400% or more	—	—	—			
6–11 years of age						
Both sexes[d]	4.2	4.0	6.5	11.3	15.9	17.4
Boys	4.0	4.3	6.6	11.6	16.9	18.7
Not Hispanic or Latino:						
White only	—	—	6.1	10.7	14.0	16.5
Black or African American only	—	—	6.8	12.3	17.0	18.7
Mexican	—	—	13.3	17.5	26.5	28.4
Girls	4.5	3.6	6.4	11.0	14.7	16.0
Not Hispanic or Latina:						
White only	—	—	5.2	9.8	13.1	14.5
Black or African American only	—	—	11.2	17.0	22.8	21.3
Mexican	—	—	9.8	15.3	17.1	21.2
Percent of poverty level:[e]						
Below 100%	—	—	—	11.4	19.1	21.5
100%–199%	—	—	—	11.1	16.4	22.2
200%–399%	—	—	—	11.7	15.3	16.8
400% or more	—	—	—	8.3	12.9	9.5
12–19 years of age						
Both sexes[d]	4.6	6.1	5.0	10.5	16.0	17.9
Boys	4.5	6.1	4.8	11.3	16.7	18.7
Not Hispanic or Latino:						
White only	—	—	3.8	11.6	14.6	16.1
Black or African American only	—	—	6.1	10.7	18.8	19.1
Mexican	—	—	7.7	14.1	24.7	26.2
Girls	4.7	6.2	5.3	9.7	15.3	17.0
Not Hispanic or Latina:						
White only	—	—	4.6	8.9	12.6	14.0
Black or African American only	—	—	10.7	16.3	23.5	29.5
Mexican	—	—	8.8	13.4	19.6	21.3

Natalie S. The et al. observe in "Association of Adolescent Obesity with Risk of Severe Obesity in Adulthood" (*Journal of the American Medical Association*, vol. 304, no. 18, November 2010) that previous studies have shown that obesity in childhood continues into adolescence and adulthood. The researchers find that there is strong persistence of severe obesity from adolescence to young adulthood and that obese adolescents are significantly more likely to become severely obese in adulthood. The et al. recommend that "primary prevention efforts should focus on the prevention of obesity prior to adolescence, while secondary prevention efforts should focus on the identification and treatment of high-risk groups in adolescence, including overweight and obese adolescents."

According to Richard Kones of the Texas Medical Center in Houston, Texas, in "Is Prevention a Fantasy, or the Future of Medicine? A Panoramic View of Recent Data, Status, and Direction in Cardiovascular Prevention"

TABLE 4.1

Obesity among children and teens, selected years 1963–2008 [CONTINUED]

[Data are based on physical examinations of a sample of the civilian noninstitutionalized population]

Sex, age, race and Hispanic origin[a], and percent of poverty level	1963–1965 1966–1970[b]	1971–1974	1976–1980[c]	1988–1994	1999–2002	2005–2008
			Percent of population			
Percent of poverty level:[e]						
Below 100%	—	—	—	15.8	19.8	23.1
100%–199%	—	—	—	11.2	15.1	19.8
200%–399%	—	—	—	9.4	15.7	19.8
400% or more	—	—	—	2.7	13.9	14.0

—Data not available.

*Estimates are considered unreliable. Data not shown have an RSE (relative standard error) greater than 30%.

[a]Persons of Mexican origin may be of any race. Starting with 1999 data, race-specific estimates are tabulated according to the 1997 Revisions to the Standards for the Classification of Federal Data on Race and Ethnicity and are not strictly comparable with estimates for earlier years. The two non-Hispanic race categories shown in the table conform to the 1997 Standards. Starting with 1999 data, race-specific estimates are for persons who reported only one racial group. Prior to data year 1999, estimates were tabulated according to the 1977 Standards. Estimates for single-race categories prior to 1999 included persons who reported one race or, if they reported more than one race, identified one race as best representing their race.

[b]Data for 1963–1965 are for children 6–11 years of age; data for 1966–1970 are for adolescents 12–17 years of age, not 12–19 years.

[c]Data for Mexicans are for 1982–1984.

[d]Includes persons of all races and Hispanic origins, not just those shown separately.

[e]Percent of poverty level is based on family income and family size. Persons with unknown percent of poverty level are excluded (5% in 2005–2008).

Notes: Obesity is defined as body mass index (BMI) at or above the sex-and age-specific 95th percentile BMI cutoff points from the 2000 CDC Growth Charts: United States. Kuczmarski RJ, Ogden CL, Guo SS, Grummer-Strawn LM, Flegal KM, Mei Z, Wei R, Curtin LR, Roche AF, Johnson CL. 2000 CDC Growth Charts for the United States: methods and development. Vital Health Stat 11. 2002 May; (246): 1–190. Starting with Health United States, 2010, the terminology describing weight for height among children changed from prior editions. The term "obesity" now refers to children who were formerly labeled as overweight. This is a change in terminology only and not measurement; the previous definition of overweight is now the definition of obesity. Ogden CL, Flegal KM. Changes in terminology for childhood overweight and obesity. National health statistics report; no. 25. Hyattsville, MD: NCHS; 2010. Age is at time of examination at the mobile examination center. Crude rates, not age-adjusted rates, are shown. Excludes pregnant females starting with 1971–1974. Pregnancy status not available for 1963–1965 and 1966–1970.

SOURCE: "Table 72. Obesity among Children and Adolescents 2–19 Years of Age, by Selected Characteristics: United States, Selected Years 1963–1965 through 2005–2008," in *Health, United States, 2010: With Special Feature on Death and Dying*, Centers for Disease Control and Prevention, National Center for Health Statistics, 2011, http://www.cdc.gov/nchs/data/hus/hus10.pdf#listtables (accessed September 30, 2011)

(*Therapeutic Advances in Cardiovascular Disease*, vol. 5, no. 1, December 2010), 32% of children were overweight or obese in 2010, and fewer than 17% got enough exercise. Kones also notes that approximately 20% of adolescents aged 12 to 19 years had abnormal lipid levels, which are associated with an increased risk for heart disease. Type 2 diabetes and hypertension (high blood pressure) also occur with increased frequency among overweight youth. Furthermore, overweight children and teens are at risk for psychosocial problems that range from teasing and ostracism to social isolation and discrimination. The Centers for Disease Control and Prevention (CDC) reports in *Basics about Childhood Obesity* (April 26, 2011, http://www.cdc.gov/obesity/childhood/basics.html) that among five- to 17-year-olds, "70% of obese children had at least one [cardiovascular disease] risk factor, and 39% had two or more."

PREVALENCE OF OVERWEIGHT AND OBESE TEENS BY SEX, GRADE, RACE, AND ETHNICITY

The Youth Risk Behavior Surveillance System (YRBSS) is a national school-based survey conducted by the CDC. It examines health-risk behaviors among youth and young adults, including unhealthy dietary behaviors, physical inactivity, and overweight.

The 2009 YRBSS found that throughout the United States, 15.8% of students were overweight. (See Table 4.3.)

The prevalence of overweight was higher among Hispanic males (19.7%) and non-Hispanic African-American males (18.7%) than among non-Hispanic white males (13.9%). For females, the prevalence of overweight was higher among non-Hispanic African-Americans (23.3%) and Hispanics (19.5%) than among non-Hispanic whites (13.2%). Overall, the prevalence of overweight was higher among non-Hispanic African-Americans (21%) and Hispanics (19.6%) than among non-Hispanic whites (13.6%).

The prevalence of overweight was higher among ninth-grade students (17.2%) than among 12th-grade students (14.7%) and higher among ninth-grade females (17.9%) than among 10th-grade (16.9%), 11th-grade (13.5%), and 12th-grade (15.1%) females. (See Table 4.3.) The prevalence of overweight ranged from 10.5% to 18% across state surveys and from 12.8% to 21.1% across local surveys. (See Table 4.4.)

The 2009 YRBSS found that 12% of high school students were obese. (See Table 4.3.) The prevalence of obesity was higher among male students (15.3%) than among female students (8.3%). It was also higher among non-Hispanic African-American females (12.6%) and Hispanic females (11.1%) than among non-Hispanic white females (6.2%) and higher among non-Hispanic African-American males (17.5%) and Hispanic males (18.9%) than among non-Hispanic white males (13.8%). Overall, there were higher rates of obesity among

FIGURE 4.1

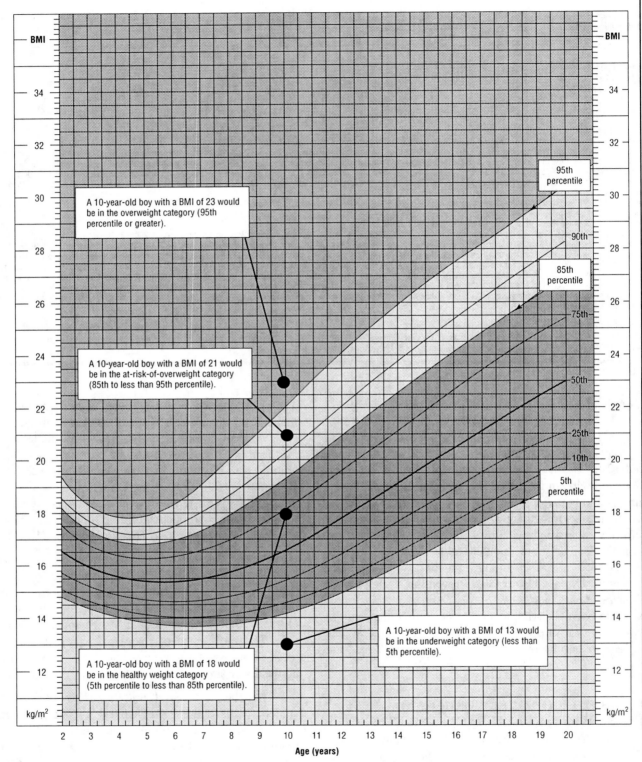

Body mass index (BMI) percentiles for boys, ages 2–20

SOURCE: "Body Mass Index-for-Age Percentiles: Boys, 2 to 20 Years," in *About BMI for Children and Teens*, Centers for Disease Control and Prevention, National Center for Chronic Disease Prevention and Health Promotion, Division of Nutrition, Physical Activity, and Obesity, January 27, 2009, http://cdc.gov/nccdphp/dnpa/bmi/childrens_BMI/about_childrens_BMI.htm (accessed October 15, 2011)

FIGURE 4.2

The interpretation of body mass index (BMI) varies by age

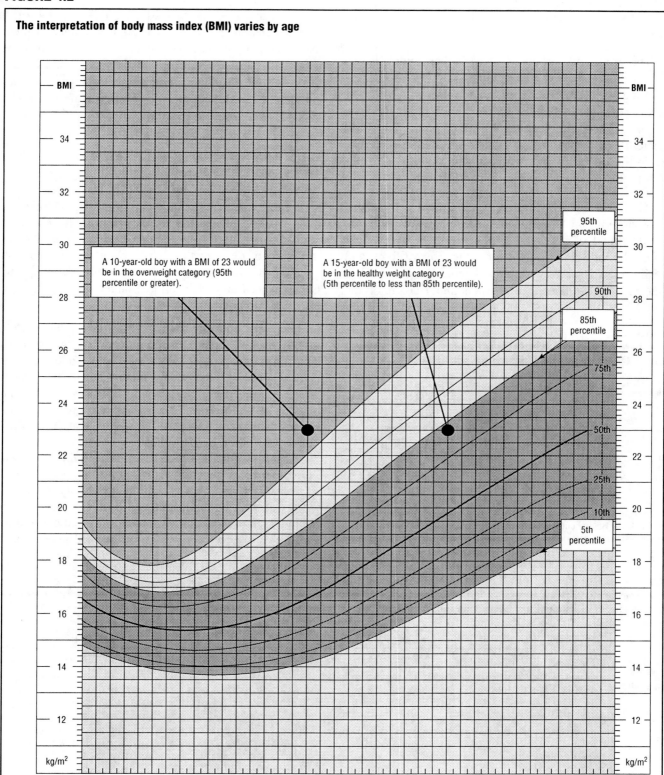

A 10-year-old boy with a BMI of 23 would be in the overweight category (95th percentile or greater).

A 15-year-old boy with a BMI of 23 would be in the healthy weight category (5th percentile to less than 85th percentile).

95th percentile

90th

85th percentile

75th

50th

25th

10th

5th percentile

Age (years)

SOURCE: "Body Mass Index-for-Age Percentiles: Boys, 2 to 20 years," in *About BMI for Children and Teens*, Centers for Disease Control and Prevention, National Center for Chronic Disease Prevention and Health Promotion, Division of Nutrition, Physical Activity, and Obesity, January 27, 2009, http://cdc.gov/nccdphp/dnpa/bmi/childrens_BMI/about_childrens_BMI.htm (accessed October 15, 2011) non-Hispanic African-American (15.1%) and Hispanic (15.1%) students than among non-Hispanic white (10.3%) students.

The prevalence of obesity was higher among ninth-grade males (15.3%), 10th-grade males (13.8%), 11th-grade males (14.5%), and 12th-grade males (17.7%) than among ninth-grade females (7.6%), 10th-grade females (7.7%), 11th-grade females (8.9%), and 12th-grade females (9.1%). (See Table 4.3.) The prevalence of obesity ranged from 6.4% to 18.3% across state surveys and from 8.4% to 20.8% across local surveys. (See Table 4.4.)

The 2009 YRBSS finding of significant percentages of overweight and obese teens in lower grades suggests the likelihood of yet another generation of overweight adults who may be at risk for subsequent overweight- and obesity-related health problems. According to Y. Claire Wang et al., in "Health and Economic Burden of the Projected Obesity Trends in the USA and the UK" (*Lancet*, vol. 378, no. 9793, August 2011), forecasts based on the National Health and Nutrition Examination Surveys predict that if the current trends continue, three out of four Americans will be overweight or obese by 2020 and by 2030 there will be 65 million more obese American adults. In children, at the current rate, the prevalence of overweight is likely to nearly double by 2030.

WHY ARE SO MANY CHILDREN AND TEENS OVERWEIGHT?

Most children are overweight for the same reason as their adult counterparts: they consume more calories than they expend. Infants and toddlers appear to be effective regulators of caloric consumption, taking in only the calories needed for growth and development. By the time children are school age, this self-regulatory mechanism has weakened and when offered larger portions, they will eat them.

Heredity and environment play key roles in determining a child's risk of becoming overweight or obese. The American Academy of Child and Adolescent Psychiatry notes in "Obesity in Children and Teens" (March 2008, http://www.aacap.org/cs/root/facts_for_families/obesity_in_children_and_teens) that if one parent is obese, then there is a 50% chance that a child will be obese, and when both parents are obese, a child has an 80% chance of being obese. Even though there is mounting evidence of genetic predisposition and susceptibility to overweight and obesity, childhood obesity is still considered largely an environmental problem—the result of behaviors, attitudes, and preferences learned early in life. Children's relationships with food develop in response to

TABLE 4.2

Weight status categories by BMI-for-age percentiles

Weight status category	Percentile range
Underweight	Less than the 5th percentile
Healthy weight	5th percentile to less than the 85th percentile
At risk of overweight	85th to less than the 95th percentile
Overweight	Equal to or greater than the 95th percentile

BMI = Body mass index.

SOURCE: "Weight Status Category," in *About BMI for Children and Teens*, Centers for Disease Control and Prevention, National Center for Chronic Disease Prevention and Health Promotion, Division of Nutrition, Physical Activity, and Obesity, January 27, 2009, http://www.cdc.gov/nccdphp/dnpa/bmi/childrens_BMI/about_childrens_BMI.htm (accessed October 15, 2011)

TABLE 4.3

Percentages of overweight and obese high school students, by sex, race, ethnicity, and grade, 2009

	Obese			Overweight		
	Female	Male	Total	Female	Male	Total
Category	%	%	%	%	%	%
Race/ethnicity						
White*	6.2	13.8	10.3	13.2	13.9	13.6
Black*	12.6	17.5	15.1	23.3	18.7	21.0
Hispanic	11.1	18.9	15.1	19.5	19.7	19.6
Grade						
9	7.6	15.3	11.8	17.9	16.7	17.2
10	7.7	13.8	11.0	16.9	16.9	16.9
11	8.9	14.5	11.8	13.5	14.4	14.0
12	9.1	17.7	13.5	15.1	14.4	14.7
Total	**8.3**	**15.3**	**12.0**	**15.9**	**15.7**	**15.8**

*Non-Hispanic.
Notes: Overweight references students who were ≥85th percentile buy <95th percentile for body mass index, by age and sex, based on reference data. Obese references student who were ≥95th percentile for body mass index, by age and sex, based on reference data.

SOURCE: Adapted from Danice K. Eaton et al., "Table 90. Percentage of High School Students Who Were Obese and Who Were Overweight, by Sex, Race/Ethnicity, and Grade—United States, Youth Risk Behavior Survey, 2009," in "Youth Risk Behavior Surveillance—United States, 2009," *Morbidity and Mortality Weekly Report*, vol. 59, no. SS-5, June 4, 2010, http://www.cdc.gov/mmwr/pdf/ss/ss5905.pdf (accessed October 7, 2011)

TABLE 4.4

Percentages of overweight and obese high school students by sex and selected U.S. sites, 2009

	Obese			Overweight		
	Female	Male	Total	Female	Male	Total
Site	%	%	%	%	%	%
State surveys						
Alabama	9.9	17.0	13.5	19.9	15.1	17.5
Alaska	10.0	13.5	11.8	14.9	13.9	14.4
Arizona	8.9	16.9	13.1	15.2	14.0	14.6
Arkansas	10.1	18.5	14.4	15.4	16.1	15.7
Colorado	5.4	8.6	7.1	10.4	11.7	11.1
Connecticut	6.7	13.8	10.4	12.2	16.6	14.5
Delaware	11.8	15.3	13.7	16.8	14.8	15.8
Florida	7.3	13.2	10.3	13.3	16.1	14.7
Georgia	10.5	14.3	12.4	16.0	13.8	14.8
Hawaii	11.7	17.0	14.5	14.8	13.2	14.0
Idaho	4.9	12.3	8.8	11.5	12.4	12.0
Illinois	9.0	14.7	11.9	14.1	16.8	15.5
Indiana	9.7	15.7	12.8	17.9	14.0	15.9
Kansas	9.5	15.0	12.4	13.0	13.2	13.1
Kentucky	14.4	20.5	17.6	16.4	14.9	15.6
Louisiana	11.3	18.1	14.7	21.0	14.8	18.0
Maine	8.0	16.7	12.5	13.5	16.7	15.1
Maryland	8.8	15.5	12.2	15.4	15.9	15.6
Massachusetts	7.2	14.3	10.9	14.8	13.8	14.3
Michigan	8.0	15.7	11.9	13.2	15.2	14.2
Mississippi	16.6	20.0	18.3	16.8	16.2	16.5
Missouri	10.5	18.3	14.4	13.9	14.8	14.4
Montana	7.5	13.1	10.4	9.4	14.3	11.9
Nevada	6.7	15.1	11.0	13.5	13.4	13.4
New Hampshire	7.7	16.4	12.4	12.9	13.6	13.3
New Jersey	6.7	13.8	10.3	13.6	14.9	14.2
New Mexico	8.5	18.3	13.5	14.5	14.6	14.6
New York	7.4	14.6	11.0	14.0	17.2	15.6
North Carolina	10.1	16.8	13.4	15.2	13.9	14.6
North Dakota	7.2	14.6	11.0	12.4	14.6	13.5
Oklahoma	13.6	14.7	14.1	16.5	16.4	16.4
Pennsylvania	10.1	13.5	11.8	16.2	15.6	15.9
Rhode Island	8.2	12.4	10.4	16.9	16.5	16.7
South Carolina	14.4	18.9	16.7	16.1	14.0	15.0
South Dakota	6.0	13.1	9.6	12.0	13.1	12.6
Tennessee	13.0	18.6	15.8	17.5	14.8	16.1
Texas	11.0	15.9	13.6	15.7	15.5	15.6
Utah	4.4	8.3	6.4	10.9	10.2	10.5
Vermont	8.1	16.1	12.2	12.5	14.7	13.6
West Virginia	7.7	20.3	14.2	15.8	13.1	14.4
Wisconsin	6.8	11.7	9.3	13.7	14.2	14.0
Wyoming	8.4	11.1	9.8	11.9	13.2	12.6
Median	8.6	15.2	12.3	14.6	14.6	14.6
Range	4.4–16.6	8.3–20.5	6.4–18.3	9.4–21.0	10.2–17.2	10.5–18.0
Local surveys						
Boston, MA	12.2	17.7	15.0	19.1	17.3	18.2
Broward County, FL	6.1	13.1	9.7	14.9	16.3	15.6
Charlotte-Mecklenburg, NC	9.7	13.3	11.5	16.9	16.1	16.5
Chicago, IL	11.7	18.1	15.1	22.4	19.9	21.1
Clark County, NV	7.7	16.7	12.3	12.9	13.0	12.9
Dallas, TX	12.7	21.0	16.9	20.0	18.5	19.2
Detroit, MI	18.9	22.8	20.8	21.4	17.9	19.6
Duval County, FL	10.5	15.4	12.9	18.4	14.8	16.6
Los Angeles, CA	7.1	20.3	14.1	21.7	16.7	19.1
Memphis, TN	15.5	18.2	16.8	21.2	16.1	18.7
Miami-Dade County, FL	7.2	13.3	10.3	15.0	17.1	16.1
Milwaukee, WI	15.1	18.1	16.6	19.7	14.5	17.1
New York City, NY	8.5	13.1	10.7	16.9	16.3	16.6
Orange County, FL	8.9	14.3	11.6	15.8	15.6	15.7
Palm Beach County, FL	6.3	13.3	9.8	13.8	12.9	13.3
Philadelphia, PA	15.2	19.6	17.4	22.5	16.3	19.4

family and cultural values and practices as well as to the influences of school, peers, and the media.

The question remains: Which environmental factors have given rise to the increasing prevalence of overweight children and teens during the past three decades? Many observers point to a reliance on fat-laden convenience and fast foods, along with time spent watching television, playing video games, and surfing the Internet, instead of being outdoors and getting physical activity. The Federal

TABLE 4.4

Percentages of overweight and obese high school students by sex and selected U.S. sites, 2009 [CONTINUED]

Site	Obese			Overweight		
	Female	Male	Total	Female	Male	Total
	%	%	%	%	%	%
San Bernardino, CA	13.4	21.2	17.4	20.2	14.9	17.5
San Diego, CA	7.9	14.9	11.5	14.4	13.6	14.0
San Francisco, CA	5.5	11.1	8.4	13.2	12.4	12.8
Seattle, WA	6.8	13.2	10.2	12.5	13.5	13.0
Median	9.3	16.0	12.6	17.6	16.1	16.6
Range	5.5–18.9	11.1–22.8	8.4–20.8	12.5–22.5	12.4–19.9	12.8–21.1

Notes: Overweight references students who were ≥85th percentile buy <95th percentile for body mass index, by age and sex, based on reference data. Obese references student who were ≥95th percentile for body mass index, by age and sex, based on reference data.

SOURCE: Adapted from Danice K. Eaton et al., "Table 91. Percentage of High School Students Who Were Obese and Who Were Overweight, by Sex—Selected U.S. Sites, Youth Risk Behavior Survey 2009," in "Youth Risk Behavior Surveillance—United States, 2009," *Morbidity and Mortality Weekly Report*, vol. 59, no. SS-5, June 4, 2010, http://www.cdc.gov/mmwr/pdf/ss/ss5905.pdf (accessed October 7, 2011)

TABLE 4.5

Percentages of high school students who used computers, played video games or watched television for 3 or more hours/day, by sex, race/ethnicity and grade, 2009

Category	Used computers 3 or more hours/day			Watched television 3 or more hours/day		
	Female	Male	Total	Female	Male	Total
	%	%	%	%	%	%
Race/ethnicity						
White*	17.8	25.9	22.1	22.7	26.6	24.8
Black*	27.5	33.2	30.4	57.4	53.7	55.5
Hispanic	23.0	28.4	25.7	41.5	42.4	41.9
Grade						
9	24.6	32.2	28.7	33.9	36.3	35.2
10	22.5	28.2	25.5	33.6	35.7	34.7
11	19.3	27.2	23.4	29.6	31.8	30.8
12	17.7	24.5	21.2	31.0	28.4	29.7
Total	**21.2**	**28.3**	**24.9**	**32.1**	**33.5**	**32.8**

*Non-Hispanic.
Notes: Use of computer would not include school work. Three or more hours would be on an average school day.

SOURCE: Adapted from Danice K. Eaton et al., "Table 84. Percentage of High School Students Who Played Video or Computer Games or Used a Computer for 3 or More Hours/Day and Who Watched 3 or More Hours/Day of Television, by Sex, Race/Ethnicity, and Grade—United States, Youth Risk Behavior Survey 2009," in "Youth Risk Behavior Surveillance—United States, 2009," *Morbidity and Mortality Weekly Report*, vol. 59, no. SS-5, June 4, 2010, http://www.cdc.gov/mmwr/pdf/ss/ss5905.pdf (accessed October 7, 2011)

Interagency Forum on Child and Family Statistics reports in *America's Children: Key National Indicators of Well-Being, 2011* (2011, http://www.childstats.gov/pdf/ac2011/ac_11.pdf) that only 18% of adolescents get the recommended one hour of physical activity per day and only one out of five eat five or more servings of fruits and vegetables per day. Television viewing, media advertising, dwindling school physical education programs, neighborhoods where it is unsafe for children to play outdoors, and even working parents have been implicated. The 2009 YRBSS found that 24.9% of high school students used computers or played video games for three or more hours per day and that 32.8% watched television for three or more hours per day. (See Table 4.5.)

Eating alone, in front of a television or computer, kids are more likely to overeat because they are lonely, bored, or susceptible to advertising cues. Overcome with guilt because they are not home to prepare meals, some working parents may intensify the problem by indulging their children with too many food treats. However, stay-at-home parents do not necessarily convey healthier attitudes about food, eating, and nutrition than parents who work outside the home. Both groups may use food, especially sweets, to reward good behavior or may pressure children to clean their plates. Even though these suppositions remain unproven, it is known that parents with eating disorders, obsessive dieters, and those with unhealthy eating habits are powerful, negative role models for children.

HOW HIGH SCHOOL STUDENTS EAT AND DIET

The 2009 YRBSS found that only 13.8% of students had eaten vegetables at least three times per day during the seven days preceding the survey. (See Table 4,6.) About one-third (33.9%) of students reported eating fruits or drinking fruit juice two or more times per day. Less than one-quarter (22.3%) of students ate fruits and vegetables five or more times per day. (See Table 4.7.)

Even fewer students (14.5%) had drunk at least three glasses of milk per day than had eaten the recommended servings of fruits and vegetables during the seven days preceding the survey. (See Table 4.7.) The prevalence of having consumed at least three glasses of milk per day was more than two times higher among male (19.8%) than among female (8.7%) students.

TABLE 4.6

Percentages of high school students who ate fruit or drank fruit juice 2 or more times/day and who ate vegetables 3 or more times/day, by sex, race/ethnicity and grade, 2009

	Ate fruit or drank 100% fruit juices two or more times/day			Ate vegetables three or more times/day		
	Female	Male	Total	Female	Male	Total
Category	%	%	%	%	%	%
Race/ethnicity						
White*	31.2	33.1	32.2	12.8	12.8	12.8
Black*	35.0	39.6	37.3	13.1	15.4	14.3
Hispanic	32.4	35.9	34.1	11.5	15.9	13.7
Grade						
9	33.9	36.5	35.3	13.3	15.7	14.6
10	30.3	37.6	34.1	12.9	14.5	13.8
11	32.8	33.9	33.4	13.6	13.0	13.3
12	31.4	32.5	32.0	12.2	14.0	13.2
Total	**32.2**	**35.3**	**33.9**	**13.0**	**14.5**	**13.8**

*Non-Hispanic.

Notes: The timeframe is during the 7 days prior to the survey. Vegetables include green salad, potatoes (excluding French fries, fried potatoes, or potato chips), carrots, or other vegetables.

SOURCE: Adapted from Danice K. Eaton et al., "Table 74. Percentage of High School Students Who Ate Fruit or Drank 100% Fruit Juices Two or More Times/Day and Who Ate Vegetables Three or More Times/Day, by Sex, Race/Ethnicity, and Grade—United States, Youth Risk Behavior Survey 2009," in "Youth Risk Behavior Surveillance—United States, 2009," *Morbidity and Mortality Weekly Report*, vol. 59, no. SS-5, June 4, 2010, http://www.cdc.gov/mmwr/pdf/ss/ss5905.pdf (accessed October 7, 2011)

TABLE 4.7

Percentage of students who ate 5 or more servings per day of fruits and vegetables and who drank 3 glasses of milk per day, by sex, race/ethnicity and grade, 2009

	Ate fruits and vegetables five or more times/day			Drank three or more glasses/day of milk		
	Female	Male	Total	Female	Male	Total
Category	%	%	%	%	%	%
Race/ethnicity						
White*	19.6	21.3	20.5	10.4	22.7	17.0
Black*	25.2	28.0	26.6	4.4	13.9	9.1
Hispanic	18.6	25.3	22.0	7.2	15.9	11.6
Grade						
9	21.1	24.6	23.0	10.3	20.1	15.6
10	19.7	25.2	22.6	9.7	23.3	16.9
11	21.4	23.1	22.3	6.7	17.5	12.2
12	19.6	21.9	20.8	7.9	17.9	13.0
Total	**20.5**	**23.9**	**22.3**	**8.7**	**19.8**	**14.5**

*Non-Hispanic.

Notes: Fruits and vegetables include 100% fruit juice, fruit, green salad, potatoes (excluding French fries, fried potatoes, or potato chips), carrots or other vegetables. The timeframe is the 7 days prior to the survey.

SOURCE: Adapted from Danice K. Eaton et al., "Table 76. Percentage of High School Students Who Ate Fruits and Vegetables Five or More Times/Day and Who Drank Three or More Glasses/Day of Milk, by Sex, Race/Ethnicity, and Grade—United States, Youth Risk Behavior Survey 2009," in "Youth Risk Behavior Surveillance—United States, 2009," *Morbidity and Mortality Weekly Report*, vol. 59, no. SS-5, June 4, 2010, http://www.cdc.gov/mmwr/pdf/ss/ss5905.pdf (accessed October 7, 2011)

TABLE 4.8

Percentage of students who described themselves as overweight and percentage trying to lose weight, by sex, race, ethnicity, and grade, 2009

	Described themselves as overweight			Were trying to lose weight		
	Female	Male	Total	Female	Male	Total
Category	%	%	%	%	%	%
Race/ethnicity						
White*	32.3	21.3	26.4	61.3	28.4	43.7
Black*	28.7	17.2	22.9	47.3	26.3	36.8
Hispanic	37.6	28.8	33.3	62.4	41.8	52.1
Grade						
9	32.2	22.7	27.1	57.0	31.8	43.5
10	31.1	21.2	25.9	59.4	29.5	43.6
11	33.5	21.8	27.5	60.8	28.0	44.0
12	36.0	25.5	30.6	60.3	32.8	46.4
Total	**33.1**	**22.7**	**27.7**	**59.3**	**30.5**	**44.4**

*Non-Hispanic.

SOURCE: Adapted from Danice K. Eaton et al., "Table 92. Percentage of High School Students Who Described Themselves As Slightly or Very Overweight and Who Were Trying to Lose Weight, by Sex, Race/Ethnicity, and Grade—United States, Youth Risk Behavior Survey, 2009," in "Youth Risk Behavior Surveillance—United States, 2009," *Morbidity and Mortality Weekly Report*, vol. 59, no. SS-5, June 4, 2010, http://www.cdc.gov/mmwr/pdf/ss/ss5905.pdf (accessed October 7, 2011)

TABLE 4.9

Percentage of students who exercised and ate less, counted calories, or chose foods low in fat to lose or keep from gaining weight, 2009

	Ate less food, fewer calories, or low-fat foods to lose weight or to keep from gaining weight			Exercised to lose weight or to keep from gaining weight		
	Female	Male	Total	Female	Male	Total
Category	%	%	%	%	%	%
Race/ethnicity						
White*	56.5	28.4	41.4	72.2	53.8	62.3
Black*	35.0	23.2	29.2	54.2	51.1	52.6
Hispanic	48.0	32.8	40.4	66.3	64.8	65.6
Grade						
9	49.1	27.5	37.5	67.4	57.6	62.2
10	52.6	26.7	38.9	69.6	53.6	61.1
11	52.7	27.8	39.9	67.5	53.6	60.3
12	52.0	32.4	42.1	66.7	58.0	62.3
Total	**51.6**	**28.4**	**39.5**	**67.9**	**55.7**	**61.5**

*Non-Hispanic.
Notes: Timeframe is 30 days before the survey.

SOURCE: Adapted from Danice K. Eaton et al., "Table 94. Percentage of High School Students Who Ate Less Food, Fewer Calories, or Low-fat Foods and Who Exercised, by Sex, Race/Ethnicity, and Grade—United States, Youth Risk Behavior Survey, 2009," in "Youth Risk Behavior Surveillance—United States, 2009," *Morbidity and Mortality Weekly Report*, vol. 59, no. SS-5, June 4, 2010, http://www.cdc.gov/mmwr/pdf/ss/ss5905.pdf (accessed October 7, 2011)

Table 4.8 reveals that less than one-third (27.7%) of high school students described themselves as "slightly" or "very" overweight. More teenaged girls (33.1%) than teenaged boys (22.7%) considered themselves overweight. Almost half (44.4%) of the students said they were trying to lose weight, but nearly twice as many female teens (59.3%) as male teens (30.5%) reported making an effort to lose weight.

Strategies for losing weight varied. Table 4.9 shows that more than two-thirds (67.9%) of teenaged girls and more than half (55.7%) of teenaged boys exercised to lose or maintain their weight. More than half (51.6%) of female teens and over a quarter (28.4%) of male teens said they had tried to lose or control their weight by eating less, counting calories, or choosing foods low in fat during the month preceding the survey. However, 14.5% of teenaged girls and 6.9% of teenaged boys said they had gone without eating for 24 hours or more, and 6.3% of teenaged girls and 3.8% of teenaged boys had taken diet pills, powders, or liquids without a doctor's advice in an effort to lose weight. (See Table 3.2 in Chapter 3.)

Is Fast Food to Blame?

In "Trends in Energy Intake among US Children by Eating Location and Food Source, 1977–2006" (*Journal of the American Dietetic Association*, vol. 111, no. 8, August 2011), Jennifer M. Poti and Barry M. Popkin indicate that children's increased food consumption between 1977 and 2006 was associated with a major increase in food that was eaten away from home. The researchers analyzed data from 29,217 children aged two to 18 years from the 1977–78 Nationwide Food Consumption Survey, the 1989–91 and 1994–98 Continuing Survey of Food Intakes by Individuals, and the 2003–06 National Health and Nutrition Examination Surveys. They find that the percentage of daily energy (as measured in calories) children ate away from home increased from 23.4% to 33.9% between 1977 and 2006. During the same period there were significant increases in children's consumption of fast food eaten at home and store-bought food eaten away from home. Poti and Popkin conclude that "foods prepared away from home, including fast food eaten at home and store-prepared food eaten away from home, are fueling the increase in total energy intake."

Echoing the sentiments of many health professionals, the Committee on Nutrition of the European Society for Paediatric Gastroenterology, Hepatology, and Nutrition named fast-food consumption as a contributing factor to childhood obesity. In "Role of Dietary Factors and Food Habits in the Development of Childhood Obesity: A Commentary by the ESPGHAN Committee on Nutrition" (*Journal of Pediatric Gastroenterology and Nutrition*, vol. 52, no. 6, June 2011), Carlo Agostino et al. observe that fast foods offer large portions of high-energy-dense foods that are low in fiber and high in saturated and trans fats, glycemic load (a ranking system for carbohydrate content in food based on its glycemic index [a measure of a food's ability to raise blood glucose] and the portion size), and tastiness, which may promote not only a lifelong preference for foods high in fat, salt, and sugar but also excessive weight gain. Agostino et al. reviewed the relevant literature and conclude that increasing consumption of fast food is associated with excess weight gain and recommend that "regular consumption of fast food with large portion sizes and high energy density should be avoided."

Because high intake of sugar-sweetened beverages in childhood is linked to an increased risk of obesity, Gentry Lasater, Carmen Piernas, and Barry M. Popkin of the University of North Carolina, Chapel Hill, looked at beverage consumption patterns and trends among school-aged children in the United States between 1989–91 and 2007–08 and reported their findings in "Beverage Patterns and Trends among School-Aged Children in the US, 1989–2008" (*Nutrition Journal*,

vol. 10, October 2, 2011). The researchers analyzed the dietary records of 3,583 children aged six to 11 years to determine the amounts of sugar-sweetened beverages (SSBs; e.g., soda, fruit drinks, sweetened coffee and tea, and sports drinks), caloric nutritional beverages (CNBs; e.g., 100% fruit and vegetable juice and high-fat low-sugar milk), and low-calorie beverages (LCBs; e.g., skim milk, unsweetened coffee and tea, and diet drinks) that were consumed per child. Over the course of the two-decade study period the researchers find that the total caloric contribution from beverages remained constant, but that the types of beverages consumed changed. The consumption of SSBs increased and CNBs decreased in similar magnitude. A substantial increase in the consumption of certain SSBs, such as fruit drinks and soda, high-fat high-sugar milk, and sports drinks, coupled with a decrease in the consumption of high-fat low-sugar milk, was responsible for this shift. The percentage consuming SSBs as well as the amount per child (both portion size and the number of portions) increased significantly over time. Lasater, Piernas, and Popkin also observe that milk was displaced in children's diets by soda. The researchers applaud efforts to limit SSB consumption at schools made by the American Beverage Association with the support of the William J. Clinton Foundation and the American Heart Association, but believe that "further interventions to reduce SSB consumption within this age group should be considered."

The 2009 YRBSS confirmed that soda remains popular with high school students. Almost one-third (29.2%) of students reported drinking at least one soda per day. (See Table 4.10.) More males (34.6%) than females (23.3%) drank one or more sodas per day.

TABLE 4.10

Percentage of students who drank soda at least once a day, 2009

Category	Female %	Male %	Total %
Race/ethnicity			
White*	21.5	35.6	29.0
Black*	32.3	35.0	33.7
Hispanic	24.0	32.2	28.1
Grade			
9	24.6	35.6	30.5
10	23.2	34.6	29.2
11	21.3	35.2	28.5
12	23.8	32.7	28.3
Total	**23.3**	**34.6**	**29.2**

*Non-Hispanic.
Notes: Soda or pop does not include diet soda or diet pop. The timeframe is 7 days before the survey.

SOURCE: Adapted from Danice K. Eaton et al., "Table 78. Percentage of High School Students Who Drank a Can, Bottle, or Glass of Soda or Pop, At Least One Time/Day—United States, Youth Risk Behavior Survey, 2009," in "Youth Risk Behavior Surveillance—United States, 2009," *Morbidity and Mortality Weekly Report*, vol. 59, no. SS-5, June 4, 2010, http://www.cdc.gov/mmwr/pdf/ss/ss5905.pdf (accessed October 7, 2011)

The Role of the Media

Despite television and print media antiobesity campaigns, many industry observers condemn corporate marketing efforts and media for continuing to assault children with unhealthy messages that encourage them to eat junk foods. The CDC defines junk foods as those that provide calories primarily through fats or added sugars and have minimal amounts of vitamins and minerals.

The Interagency Working Group on Food Marketed to Children with representation from the Federal Trade Commission, the CDC, the U.S. Food and Drug Administration, and the U.S. Department of Agriculture (USDA) was formed in 2009 and tasked with recommending principles for the marketing of food to children to help the food industry self-regulate its marketing and advertising practices. In April 2011 the Interagency Working Group released the fact sheet "Food for Thought: Interagency Working Group Proposal on Food Marketing to Children" (http://www.ftc.gov/os/2011/04/110428foodmarketfactsheet.pdf) to discuss its principles for food marketing to children aged two to 16 years. The first principle is that the foods "make a meaningful contribution to a healthful diet" and contain fruit, vegetable, whole grain, fat-free or low-fat (1%) milk products, fish, extra lean meat or poultry, eggs, nuts and seeds, or beans. The second principle is that the foods should "contain limited amounts of nutrients that have a negative impact on health or weight," which is defined as a saturated fat content of 1 gram or less per serving or less than 15% of calories, 0 grams of trans-fat per serving, no more than 13 grams of added sugars per serving, and no more than 210 milligrams of sodium per serving. The principles are simply guidelines and even though they become effective in 2016, adherence to them is entirely voluntary.

According to Mark Bittman, in the editorial "Junk Food 'Guidelines' Won't Help" (*New York Times*, May 3, 2011), food marketing "to children needs to be reined in" and requesting voluntary compliance from the food industry is highly unlikely to achieve this objective. Bittman describes many of the food products marketed to children as being composed of "multiple forms of sugar, highly refined carbohydrates, chemically extracted fats and mystery ingredients only a food scientist or profiteer could love."

Other researchers and industry observers concur that the obesity epidemic cannot be effectively combatted without dramatic changes in food marketing that is aimed at children. In "Protecting Children from Harmful Food Marketing: Options for local Government to Make a Difference" (*Preventing Chronic Diseases*, vol. 8, no. 5, September 2011), Jennifer L. Harris and Samantha K. Graff note that even though much of the marketing of calorie-dense, nutrient-poor foods to children is via nationwide media such as the Internet and television, it is also conducted using local venues such as billboards, restaurants, and schools. The researchers assert that "although the federal government has jurisdiction to regulate national media and the First Amendment to the US Constitution limits what government at any level can do to restrict advertising, municipalities do have constitutionally viable options to protect children from the harmful food marketing that permeates their communities."

According to Harris and Graff, local food marketing efforts include product packaging, signs, and promotions in stores that are designed and placed at eye level for children, and school and local child-focused activities and product tie-ins that appeal to children by associating foods with popular movies, cartoon characters, and sports and entertainment celebrities. School-based promotions include food company incentives such as rewarding children for reading with coupons for free pizza; fund-raising programs that entail submitting proof of purchase of food items; branded food items that are served in school cafeterias, stores, and vending machines; corporate logos on scoreboards, book covers, and team jerseys; and sponsored books, workbooks, and materials with corporate logos and prominent mention of food products. Harris and Graff observe that logo placement, associations with celebrities, and video and Internet games are "designed to create lifelong customers by imprinting brand meaning into the minds of young children. Before children know better, they have learned to love the products they encounter most frequently and associate with positive experiences."

Harris and Graff suggest that local policies should restrict or limit the marketing of unhealthful food to children. For example, supermarkets and other retailers may opt to:

- Impose excise taxes or fees on sugar-sweetened beverages, and earmark a portion or all of the revenue to fund obesity prevention programs

- Limit sales of unhealthy food and beverages near schools before, during, and immediately after the school day

- Prohibit food sales in other retail venues that are frequented by children, such as toy stores

Restaurants and other food service providers may choose to:

- Eliminate use of trans fats

- Prohibit fast-food restaurants from opening near schools

- Establish nutritional standards for children's meals that include toys or other incentives

Schools can reduce children's exposure to food marketing by:

- Banning the sale and advertising of unhealthful foods on school property

- Requiring vendors to sharply restrict or eliminate the sale of unhealthful food and beverages

- Eliminating food company sponsorships, fund-raisers, and materials that are imprinted with corporate logos

In "With 'Healthy' Foods Like These, Who Needs Junk?" (*Huffington Post*, September 29, 2011), Michael F. Jacobson, the executive director of the Center for Science in the Public Interest (a nonprofit advocacy group for nutrition, food safety, health, and other issues), asserts that even though the Interagency Working Group principles for marketing to children are entirely voluntary, the food industry is agitating to "get the government to withdraw their marketing recommendations." Jacobson observes that the food industry considers products such as Kool-Aid, popsicles, and Cookie Crisp cereal to be healthy choices for children. He contends that such food products "aren't the worst of the worst foods in the food supply, mind you. But are these healthy foods that should be aggressively promoted to young children as they grow and form lifelong eating habits?"

The Role of Schools Schools

In many parts of the country students are beginning to have some healthier beverage and food options in school. Nancy D. Brener et al. of the CDC find in *School Health Profiles 2010: Characteristics of Health Programs among Secondary Schools in Selected U.S. Sites* (2011, http://www.cdc.gov/healthyyouth/profiles/2010/profiles_report.pdf) that fewer secondary schools in the United States sold less nutritious foods and beverages in vending machines, school stores, and snack bars in 2010 than in 2008. For example, in 2008, 58.8% of schools sold sports drinks and 37.2% sold soda; in 2010 the percentages were 50.7% and 29.8%, respectively.

Even though there is widespread agreement that removing soda from schools is a healthy move, some nutritionists feel the proposed beverages that will replace soda, which include sports drinks and vitamin-enhanced water, still favor beverage company interests rather than students' health. Brener et al. confirm that in 2010 many schools still offered less nutritious food and beverages that students could purchase. (See Figure 4.3.)

FIGURE 4.3

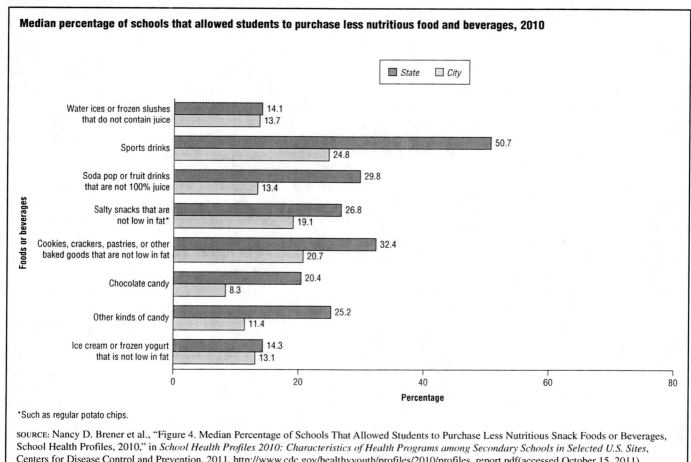

Median percentage of schools that allowed students to purchase less nutritious food and beverages, 2010

*Such as regular potato chips.

SOURCE: Nancy D. Brener et al., "Figure 4. Median Percentage of Schools That Allowed Students to Purchase Less Nutritious Snack Foods or Beverages, School Health Profiles, 2010," in *School Health Profiles 2010: Characteristics of Health Programs among Secondary Schools in Selected U.S. Sites*, Centers for Disease Control and Prevention, 2011, http://www.cdc.gov/healthyyouth/profiles/2010/profiles_report.pdf(accessed October 15, 2011)

Many Schools Offer and Promote Unhealthy Food Choices

Food manufacturers and marketers know that schools are ideal sites to promote their products to children and teens. Nearly all youth attend school and spend many of their waking hours at school. Furthermore, the presence of foods in schools allows food companies to benefit from the implied endorsement of the schools and teachers. According to Brener et al., in 2010 many schools had vending machines, stores, or snack bars on campus that sold "competitive foods [which] are any foods or beverages sold or served at school separately from the USDA school meal programs." Competitive foods are usually low in nutrients and high in fat, sugar, and calories. Brener et al. state that "while foods and beverages sold through the school meal programs must meet federal nutrition requirements, competitive foods are not subject to any federal nutrition standards unless they are sold inside the food service area during mealtimes." The nutritional value of competitive foods is essentially unregulated, and students often purchase these foods instead of, or in addition to, school meals. In December 2011 the USDA issued federal nutrition standards for competitive foods that are sold on school grounds. These standards are consistent with the *Dietary Guidelines for Americans* and aim to increase the proportion of schools that offer other nutritious food and beverage choices, in addition to school meals.

Besides selling food in schools, food manufacturers advertise on vending machines, posters, book covers, scoreboards, and banners and offer schools educational materials, contests in which children receive prizes or food rewards for achievement, and fund-raising opportunities. Some critics, including the Center for Science in the Public Interest, assert that the manufacturers are taking unfair advantage of cash-strapped school districts.

Food for Thought Has New Meaning at Many Schools

In December 2010 President Barack Obama (1961–; http://www.whitehouse.gov/sites/default/files/Child _Nutrition_Fact_Sheet_12_10_10.pdf) signed the Healthy, Hunger-Free Kids Act, which reauthorizes funding for federal school meal and child nutrition programs and increases access to healthy food for low-income children. The act not only grants the USDA the authority to establish nutritional standards for all foods that are regularly sold in schools during the school day, including vending machines, the à la carte lunch lines, and school stores, but also provides additional funding to schools that meet updated nutritional standards for federally subsidized lunches. This additional funding represents the first increase in the reimbursement rate in more than 30 years. Additional improvements in food and beverage offerings in schools are anticipated in response to the USDA nutrition standards for competitive foods that were issued at the close of 2011. However, even before these legislation-mandated changes and revised nutrition standards were put into place, and certainly afterward, many school districts were in the process of replacing some of the food and beverages that were available in their schools.

For example, New Jersey schools have adopted what may be the most ambitious statewide school nutrition policy in the nation. Since 2007 all the state's public schools adhere to a policy stipulating that soda, any food item listing sugar as its first ingredient, all forms of candy, and foods of minimal nutritional value (per the USDA definition) cannot be served, sold, or given for free anytime during the school day. Snacks and drinks sold anywhere on a school campus must have no more than 8 grams of fat and 2 grams of saturated fat per serving, and drinks cannot exceed more than 12 ounces (355 mL), except bottled water. This policy applies to vending machines, cafeterias, à la carte items, school stores, school fund-raisers, and the after-school snack program. The policy also makes nutrition education a requirement in school curricula.

Another example is a school initiative to improve nutrition, which is described in the article "Gold Medal School Has Taken on a Hefty Task—Reversing Obesity" (October 17, 2011, http://latino.foxnews.com/latino/health/ 2011/10/17/gold-medal-school-has-taken-on-hefty-task-reversing-obesity/). Northeast Elementary Magnet School in Danville, Illinois, is the first elementary school to earn a gold medal from the Alliance for a Healthier Generation, a joint venture between the American Heart Association and the William J. Clinton Foundation that aims to eliminate childhood obesity. The school earned the award by establishing nutrition and physical activity policies, including daily gym classes for all students and eliminating soda, fried foods, and gooey desserts from the cafeteria in favor of fresh fruits and vegetables. Birthdays are celebrated without sweets, students learn to be critical food shoppers, teachers wear pedometers to track their steps, and parents must sign on endorsing the program.

The Media Can Deliver Powerful Nutrition and Health Education

Greater emphasis on children's diets has inspired the media to offer nutrition education. In 2008 *Sesame Street* launched the "Healthy Habits for Life" program. Rather than subsisting on a diet of cookies alone, *Sesame Street*'s Cookie Monster now champions healthful food choices. The beloved character also sings a new tune, "A Cookie Is a Sometimes Food." Bonnie Rochman reports in "More Muppets? The New 'Superfoods' Want Kids to Eat Healthy" (*Time*, December 1, 2010) that in December 2010 *Sesame Street* introduced new Muppet characters: the Superfoods—an animated broccoli stalk, a wedge of low-fat cheese, a banana, and a whole-wheat bun. These new characters are aimed at encouraging healthy eating, especially among the 17 million children in the United States who do not have food that meets their nutritional needs, due to financial instability.

Children's television programming such as Disney's *Little Einsteins* and *Phineas and Ferb* aim to inspire young viewers to be physically active. Blending fitness and entertainment, video game makers have developed a genre of active rhythm games including *Dance Dance Revolution*, which features a workout mode that can track how many calories the user burns while playing. *In the Groove* and *Pump It Up: Exceed* are video games in which players try to match the onscreen action by stepping on different sections of a floor pad, and *Yourself!Fitness* and *Kinetic* offer teens exercise routines in video game formats. Nintendo's *Wii Fit* instructs and coaches users in yoga, balance games, strength training, aerobics, and simulated sports. As part of its antiobesity efforts, the National Institutes of Health (NIH) is funding video game research projects in the United States.

In 2011 the Ad Council collaborated with McCann, a global marketing communications company, and HUSH Studios to produce public service announcements and the Action Hero Alliance website (http://www.ActionHero Alliance.com/#content3). Both the public service announcements and the website encourage children to eat like action heroes—a balanced diet that contains fruit, vegetables, protein, dairy, and whole grains. More specifically, the website encourages children to "fuel up" with foods such as "berry boosters," to enhance immune system function, and "bone builders," which are dairy products that contain calcium.

FOOD AND BEVERAGE MARKETING PRACTICES IMPROVE. In 2005 the Institute of Medicine (IOM) published the report *Food Marketing to Children and Youth: Threat or Opportunity?* (http://www.iom.edu/Reports/2005/Food-Marketing-to-Children-and-Youth-Threat-or-Opportunity.aspx) to evaluate the influence of food marketing on the health of American children and teens. The IOM found that marketing practices, particularly television advertising, did not support a healthful diet and called on food and beverage companies as well as restaurants, trade associations, and the media to promote programs and practices to support healthful eating. The IOM report offered 10 recommendations for promoting healthful diets to children and teens. In 2006 the IOM Committee on Progress in Preventing Childhood Obesity followed up with the publications *Food Marketing and the Diets of Children and Youth* (http://www.iom.edu/Activities/Children/KidsFoodMarketing.aspx), which included a framework to guide the development of marketing and advertising strategies to foster healthy food choices among children and teens, and *Progress in Preventing Childhood Obesity: How Do We Measure Up?* (http://books.nap.edu/

openbook.php?record_id=11722), which addressed the competing interests of stakeholders and the challenges of balancing corporate goals with promoting children's health.

Vivica I. Kraak et al. conducted a literature review and a review of government, food company, entertainment industry, and media websites between December 1, 2005, and January 31, 2011, to assess progress made by each sector toward the 2005 IOM recommendations and published their findings in "Industry Progress to Market a Healthful Diet to American Children and Adolescents" (*American Journal of Preventive Medicine*, vol. 41, no. 3, September 2011). The researchers indicate that food and beverage companies made "moderate progress" in reformulating and improving the nutritional content of some products, reducing television advertising of sweets and sugar-sweetened beverages, developing package labels to identify healthful products, and establishing partnerships to promote healthy diets and lifestyles. Kraak et al. also determine that moderate progress had been achieved in the improvement and enforcement of marketing practice standards. By 2010, 17 companies, which were responsible for two-thirds of the industry marketing expenditures for children and adolescents, reported progress in "revising, applying, and evaluating their advertising standards."

By contrast, Kraak et al. note that restaurants, industry trade associations, and media and entertainment companies made only "limited progress." For example, the 2005 IOM report exhorted restaurants to expand healthier options, reduce portion sizes, and promote menu labeling. According to two studies that were conducted in 2008 and 2009, less than 10% of children's meals met the nutritional criteria of the *Dietary Guidelines for Americans*. Similarly, Kraak et al. note that a study performed in 2010 found that just one-quarter of entertainment companies had "a clear policy on food marketing to children" and that the percentage of advertisements for unhealthful food products "decreased only slightly between 2005 and 2009 (before and after the [Children's Food and Beverage Advertising Initiative] was implemented) from about nine in ten (88%) to eight in ten (79%) food advertisements." Kraak et al. report that in July 2011 the Council of the Better Business Bureaus Inc. and the Children's Food and Beverage Advertising Initiative established an agreement to adhere to uniform nutrition criteria for foods advertised to children. The agreement prompts companies to reformulate their products so they contain less sodium, saturated fat, and sugars and fewer calories. Furthermore, the companies agreed not to advertise older, less healthful food products after December 31, 2013.

School Physical Education Programs

School physical education (PE) programs, especially at the high school level, have been found lacking.

FIGURE 4.4

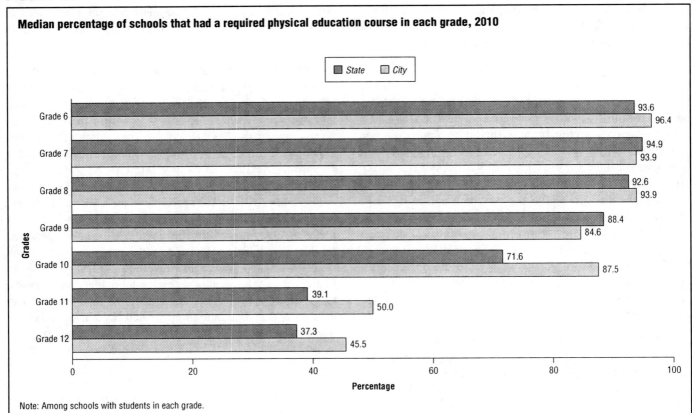

Median percentage of schools that had a required physical education course in each grade, 2010

Note: Among schools with students in each grade.

SOURCE: Nancy D. Brener et al., "Figure 3. Median Percentage of Schools That Taught a Required Physical Education Course in Each Grade, School Health Profiles, 2010," in *School Health Profiles 2010: Characteristics of Health Programs among Secondary Schools in Selected U.S. Sites*, Centers for Disease Control and Prevention, 2011, http://www.cdc.gov/healthyyouth/profiles/2010/profiles_report.pdf(accessed October 15, 2011)

According to Brener et al., the percentage of schools that required PE for students in grades six through 12 ranged from 61.1% to 100% in 2010. Figure 4.4 shows the median (average) percentage of schools that had a required PE course in each grade in 2010. The state percentages ranged from 93.6% in grade six to just 37.3% in grade 12. Danice K. Eaton et al. of the CDC note in "Youth Risk Behavior Surveillance—United States, 2009" (*Morbidity and Mortality Weekly Report*, vol. 59, no. SS-5, June 4, 2010) that in 2009 nearly two-thirds of students did not meet the recommended levels of physical activity (they were not physically active enough to increase their heart rate and cause them to breathe hard some of the time for a total of at least 60 minutes per day on five or more days during the seven days before the survey). (See Table 4.11.)

The importance of school PE programs cannot be underestimated, especially in view of the 2009 YRBSS finding that only a little more than one-third (37%) of high school students had participated in sufficient physical activity during the week preceding the survey. (See Table 4.11.) Many more male teens (45.6%) than female teens (27.7%) said they had been active for 60 minutes or more on at least five of the past seven days.

HEALTH RISKS AND CONSEQUENCES

The harmful health consequences of overweight and obesity can begin during childhood and adolescence. According to Gerald S. Berenson et al., in "Glycemic Status, Metabolic Syndrome, and Cardiovascular Risk in Children" (*Medical Clinics of North America*, vol. 95, no. 2, March 2011), approximately 40% of the U.S. population is overweight or obese by adolescence and "obesity in childhood is the most consistent predictor of adult heart disease." Berenson et al. also assert that the risk for cardiovascular disease increases at the 85th percentile of body weight, which is considerably below the 95th percentile considered to be dangerous by the CDC.

The most frequently occurring medical consequences of overweight among children and adolescents are:

• Elevated blood lipids—overweight children and adolescents display the same elevated levels of cholesterol, triglycerides (a fatty substance found in the blood), and/or low-density lipoproteins as overweight adults. These hyperlipidemias are linked to an increased risk for cardiovascular disease and premature mortality (death) in adulthood.

TABLE 4.11

Percentages of high school students who met recommended levels of physical activity by sex, race, ethnicity, and grade, 2009

Category	Physically active at least 60 minutes/day on all 7 days			Physically active at least 60 minutes/day on 5 or more days		
	Female	Male	Total	Female	Male	Total
	%	%	%	%	%	%
Race/ethnicity						
White*	12.4	26.2	19.7	31.3	47.3	39.9
Black*	10.0	24.4	17.2	21.9	43.3	32.6
Hispanic	10.5	20.7	15.6	24.9	41.3	33.1
Grade						
9	13.6	28.0	21.3	30.8	47.5	39.7
10	12.7	25.3	19.3	30.5	47.4	39.3
11	10.3	23.3	17.0	26.0	46.2	36.4
12	8.6	21.9	15.3	22.4	40.4	31.6
Total	**11.4**	**24.8**	**18.4**	**27.7**	**45.6**	**37.0**

* Non-Hispanic.

Notes: Physical activity refers to any that increased the student's heart rate and made him or her breathe hard some of the time. Timeframe is 7 days before the survey.

SOURCE: Adapted from Danice K. Eaton et al., "Table 80. Percentage of High School Students Who Were Physically Active, by Sex, Race/Ethnicity, and Grade—United States, Youth Risk Behavior Survey, 2009," in "Youth Risk Behavior Surveillance—United States, 2009," *Morbidity and Mortality Weekly Report*, vol. 59, no. SS-5, June 4, 2010, http://www.cdc.gov/mmwr/pdf/ss/ss5905.pdf (accessed October 7, 2011)

- Glucose intolerance and type 2 diabetes—glucose intolerance, a carbohydrate intolerance that varies in severity, is a forerunner of diabetes. The incidence of type 2 diabetes among adolescents is increasing in response to the national rise of overweight teens. A skin condition known as acanthosis nigricans (velvety thickening and darkening of skinfold areas at the neck, elbow, and behind the knee) often coexists with glucose intolerance in youth.

- Fatty liver disease—high concentrations of liver enzymes are associated with fatty degeneration of the liver (also called hepatic steatosis) and have been found in overweight children and adolescents. Excessively high blood insulin levels (hyperinsulinemia) may contribute to the genesis of this disease.

- Gallstones—even though gallstones occur less frequently among children and adolescents who are overweight than in obese adults, nearly half of the cases of inflammation of the gallbladder (also called cholecystitis) in adolescents may be associated with overweight. Like adults, the risk for cholecystitis and gallstones in adolescents may decrease with weight reduction.

Another common health consequence of overweight is early maturation, a condition in which the skeletal age is more than three months greater than the chronological age. Early maturation is linked to overweight in adulthood and is also associated with the distribution of fat—it predicts that the fat will be predominantly located on the abdomen and trunk, which is in turn predictive of increased disease risk.

Less frequently occurring health consequences include hypertension, a condition that is nine times more frequent among children who are overweight, compared with children who have a healthy weight; obstructive sleep apnea (breathing becomes shallow or stops completely for short periods during sleep), a condition that afflicts an estimated 7% of overweight children; and orthopedic problems resulting from excessive stress on the feet, legs, and hips. Hypertension for children and adolescents aged one to 17 years is defined as average blood pressure readings at or above the 95th percentile (based on age, sex, and height) on at least three separate occasions. (See Table 4.12 and Table 4.13 for blood pressures by age and gender that are considered indicative of hypertension or at risk for hypertension; children and adolescents between the 90th and 95th percentiles for their age, sex, and height are at risk for developing hypertension.)

Several studies confirm that blood pressure and change in BMI during childhood are the two most powerful predictors of adult blood pressure across all ages and both genders. Sudhir K. Mehta et al. opine in "Abdominal Obesity, Waist Circumference, Body Mass Index, and Echocardiographic Measures in Children and Adolescents" (*Congenital Heart Diseases*, vol. 4, no. 5, September–October 2009) that waist circumference in children and teens may better predict future risk of cardiovascular disease than BMI alone because waist circumference assesses abdominal obesity, which is associated with an increased risk of heart disease in youth as well as in adults.

Metabolic Syndrome

The metabolic syndrome is a group of risk factors for atherosclerotic cardiovascular disease and type 2 diabetes mellitus in adults that include insulin resistance, obesity,

TABLE 4.12

Blood pressure levels for the 90th and 95th percentiles of blood pressure for boys ages 1 to 17 years

Age	BP percentile*	Systolic BP (mm Hg), by height percentile from standard growth curves							Diastolic BP (mm Hg), by height percentile from standard growth curves						
		5%	10%	25%	50%	75%	90%	95%	5%	10%	25%	50%	75%	90%	95%
1	90th	94	95	97	98	100	102	102	50	51	52	53	54	54	55
	95th	98	99	101	102	104	106	106	55	55	56	57	58	59	59
2	90th	98	99	100	102	104	105	106	55	55	56	57	58	59	59
	95th	101	102	104	106	108	109	110	59	59	60	61	62	63	63
3	90th	100	101	103	105	107	108	109	59	59	60	61	62	63	63
	95th	104	105	107	109	111	112	113	63	63	64	65	66	67	67
4	90th	102	103	105	107	109	110	111	62	62	63	64	65	66	66
	95th	106	107	109	111	113	114	115	66	67	67	68	69	70	71
5	90th	104	105	106	108	110	111	112	65	65	66	67	68	69	69
	95th	108	109	110	112	114	115	116	69	70	70	71	72	73	74
6	90th	105	106	108	110	111	113	114	67	68	69	70	70	71	72
	95th	109	110	112	114	115	117	117	72	72	73	74	75	76	76
7	90th	106	107	109	111	113	114	115	69	70	71	72	72	73	74
	95th	110	111	113	115	116	118	119	74	74	75	76	77	78	78
8	90th	107	108	110	112	114	115	116	71	71	72	73	74	75	75
	95th	111	112	114	116	118	119	120	75	76	76	77	78	79	80
9	90th	109	110	112	113	115	117	117	72	73	73	74	75	76	77
	95th	113	114	116	117	119	121	121	76	77	78	79	80	81	81
10	90th	110	112	113	115	117	118	119	73	74	74	75	76	77	78
	95th	114	115	117	119	121	122	123	77	78	79	80	80	81	82
11	90th	112	113	115	117	119	120	121	74	74	75	76	77	78	78
	95th	116	117	119	121	123	124	125	78	79	79	80	81	82	83
12	90th	115	116	117	119	121	123	123	75	75	76	77	78	78	79
	95th	119	120	121	123	125	126	127	79	79	80	81	82	83	83
13	90th	117	118	120	122	124	125	126	75	76	76	77	78	79	80
	95th	121	122	124	126	128	129	130	79	79	80	81	82	83	84
14	90th	120	121	123	125	126	128	128	76	76	77	78	79	80	80
	95th	124	125	127	128	130	132	132	80	81	81	82	83	84	85
15	90th	123	124	125	127	129	131	131	77	77	78	79	80	81	81
	95th	127	128	129	131	133	134	135	81	82	83	83	84	85	86
16	90th	125	126	128	130	132	133	134	79	79	80	81	82	82	83
	95th	129	130	132	134	136	137	138	83	83	84	85	86	87	87
17	90th	128	129	131	133	134	136	136	81	81	82	83	84	85	85
	95th	132	133	135	136	138	140	140	85	85	86	87	88	89	89

*Blood pressure percentile determined by a single measurement.

BP = blood pressure. mm Hg = millimeters of mercury.

SOURCE: "Table 16. Blood Pressure Levels for the 90th and 95th Percentiles of Blood Pressure for Boys Ages 1 to 17 Years," in *Overweight Children and Adolescents: Screen, Access, and Manage,* Centers for Disease Control and Prevention, National Center for Chronic Disease Prevention and Promotion, Division of Nutrition, Physical Activity and Obesity, May 2000, http://www.cdc.gov/nccdphp/dnpa/growthcharts/training/modules/module3/text/hypertension_tables.htm (accessed October 18, 2011)

TABLE 4.13

Blood pressure levels for the 90th and 95th percentiles of blood pressure for girls ages 1 to 17 years

Age	BP percentile*	Systolic BP (mm Hg), by height percentile from standard growth curves							Diastolic BP (mm Hg), by height percentile from standard growth curves						
		5%	10%	25%	50%	75%	90%	95%	5%	10%	25%	50%	75%	90%	95%
1	90th	97	98	99	100	102	103	104	53	53	53	54	55	56	56
	95th	101	102	103	104	105	107	107	57	57	57	58	59	60	60
2	90th	99	99	100	102	103	104	105	57	57	58	58	59	60	61
	95th	102	103	104	105	107	108	109	61	61	62	62	63	65	65
3	90th	100	100	102	103	104	105	106	61	61	61	62	63	63	64
	95th	104	104	105	107	108	109	110	65	65	65	66	67	68	68
4	90th	101	102	103	104	106	107	108	63	63	64	65	65	66	67
	95th	105	106	107	108	109	111	111	67	67	68	69	69	70	71
5	90th	103	103	104	106	107	108	109	65	66	66	67	68	68	69
	95th	107	107	108	110	111	112	113	69	70	70	71	72	73	73
6	90th	104	105	106	107	109	110	111	67	67	68	69	69	70	71
	95th	108	109	110	111	112	114	114	71	71	72	73	73	74	75
7	90th	106	107	108	109	110	112	112	69	69	69	70	71	72	72
	95th	110	110	112	113	114	115	116	73	73	73	74	75	76	76
8	90th	108	109	110	111	112	113	114	70	70	71	71	72	73	74
	95th	112	112	113	115	116	117	118	74	74	75	75	76	77	78
9	90th	110	110	112	113	114	115	116	71	72	72	73	74	74	75
	95th	114	114	115	117	118	119	120	75	76	76	77	78	78	79
10	90th	112	112	114	115	116	117	118	73	73	73	74	75	76	76
	95th	116	116	117	119	120	121	122	77	77	77	78	79	80	80
11	90th	114	114	116	117	118	119	120	74	74	75	75	76	77	77
	95th	118	118	119	121	122	123	124	78	78	79	79	80	81	81
12	90th	116	116	118	119	120	121	122	75	75	76	76	77	78	78
	95th	120	120	121	123	124	125	126	79	79	80	80	81	82	82
13	90th	118	118	119	121	122	123	124	76	76	77	78	78	79	80
	95th	121	122	123	125	126	127	128	80	80	81	82	82	83	84
14	90th	119	120	121	122	124	125	126	77	77	78	79	79	80	81
	95th	123	124	125	126	128	129	130	81	81	82	83	83	84	85
15	90th	121	121	122	124	125	126	127	78	78	79	79	80	81	82
	95th	124	125	126	128	129	130	131	82	82	83	83	84	85	86
16	90th	122	122	123	125	126	127	128	79	79	79	80	81	82	82
	95th	125	126	127	128	130	131	132	83	83	83	84	85	86	86
17	90th	122	123	124	125	126	128	128	79	79	79	80	81	82	82
	95th	126	126	127	129	130	131	132	83	83	83	84	85	86	86

*Blood pressure percentile determined by a single measurement.

BP = blood pressure. mm Hg = millimeters of mercury.

SOURCE: "Table 17. Blood Pressure Levels for the 90th and 95th Percentiles of Blood Pressure for Girls Ages 1 to 17 Years," in *Overweight Children and Adolescents: Screen, Access, and Manage*, Centers for Disease Control and Prevention, National Center for Chronic Disease Prevention and Promotion, Division of Nutrition, Physical Activity and Obesity, May 2000, http://www.cdc.gov/nccdphp/dnpa/growthcharts/training/modules/module3/text/hypertension_tables.htm (accessed October 18, 2011) hypertension, and hyperlipidemia. (Atherosclerosis is a hardening of the walls of the arteries caused by the buildup of fatty deposits on the inner walls of the arteries that interferes with blood flow.) Atherosclerotic cardiovascular disease is the leading cause of death among adults, but it rarely occurs in young people. Recently, however, the risk factors—high blood pressure, elevated triglycerides, obesity, and low levels of the "good" high-density lipoprotein (HDL) cholesterol—that are associated with the development of metabolic syndrome have been appearing during childhood. Berenson et al. indicate that in the United States more than 17% of children with a BMI greater than the 95th percentile are considered to have all the conditions that are associated with metabolic syndrome.

Mental Health Consequences

One of the most immediate, distressing, and widespread consequences of being overweight as described by children themselves is social discrimination and low self-esteem. Overweight and obese children and adolescents are at risk for psychological and social adjustment problems, such as considering themselves less competent than normal-weight youth in social, athletic, and appearance arenas, and for suffering from overall diminished self-worth.

In "Modelling the Relationship between Obesity and Mental Health in Children and Adolescents: Findings from the Health Survey for England 2007" (*Child and Adolescent Psychiatry and Mental Health*, vol. 5, October 7, 2011), Paul A. Tiffin et al. report the results of a study of 3,898 children aged five to 16 years that looked at the relationship between mental health, overweight, and obesity. The researchers find no relationship between overweight and mental health problems but do find a relationship between obesity and poor mental health. They also find that the psychological impact of obesity was independent of reported physical activity and did not differ between boys and girls. Tiffin et al. conclude that "given our current knowledge of the long-term outcomes of both childhood mental health problems as well as the recognised complications of chronic obesity this has implications for the long-term health and social care burdens in the developed world."

Lana M. Bell et al. analyze in "High Incidence of Obesity Co-morbidities in Young Children: A Cross-Sectional Study" (*Journal of Paediatrics and Child Health*, vol. 47, no. 12, December 2011) the medical and psychological problems of overweight, obese, and normal-weight children aged six to 13 years. The researchers find that in addition to more abnormal laboratory test results such as impaired glucose tolerance, hyperinsulinemia, and hyperlipidemia, overweight and obese children were more likely to complain of musculoskeletal pain, depression, anxiety, and bullying than their normal-weight peers.

SCREENING AND ASSESSMENT OF OVERWEIGHT CHILDREN AND ADOLESCENTS

In view of the rising prevalence of overweight youth, screening children and adolescents for overweight and risk for overweight has assumed a prominent place in pediatric practice (the medical specialty devoted to the diagnosis and treatment of children) and public health programs. The Recommendations for Preventive Pediatric Health Care by the American Academy of Pediatrics advise a frequent schedule of accurate weight and height measurements to determine whether children require further assessment or treatment for overweight. Screening distinguishes between youths who are not at risk of overweight, at risk of overweight, and overweight. Those deemed to be overweight receive an in-depth medical assessment; those considered at risk are assessed for changes in BMI, blood pressure, and cholesterol levels; and annual screening is advised for those who are not at risk of being overweight.

The comprehensive assessment that is performed on overweight children and adolescents generally includes obtaining a detailed medical history to identify any underlying medical conditions that may contribute to overweight and analyzing family history for the presence of familial risks for overweight or obesity. Relevant familial factors include the occurrence of obesity, eating disorders, type 2 diabetes, heart disease, high blood pressure, and abnormal lipid profiles such as high cholesterol among immediate family members. The assessment may also involve:

- A dietary evaluation to consider the quantity, quality, and timing of food consumed to identify foods and patterns of eating that may lead to excessive calorie intake. A food record or food diary may be used to assess eating habits.

- An evaluation of daily activities. This assessment involves an estimate of time that is devoted to exercise and activity as well as time spent on sedentary behaviors such as television, video games, and computer use.

- A physical examination to provide information about the extent of overweight and any complications of overweight, including high blood pressure. Children and adolescents with a BMI-for-age at or above the 95th percentile and who are athletic and muscular may be further assessed using the triceps skinfold measurement to assess body fat. A measurement of greater than the 95th percentile indicates that the child has excess fat rather than increased lean body mass or a large frame.

TABLE 4.14

Classification of cholesterol levels in high-risk children and adolescents

	Total cholesterol, ng/dL	LDL cholesterol, ng/dL
Acceptable	<170	<110
Borderline	170–199	110–129
High	Greater than or equal to 200	Greater than or equal to 130

Note: High-risk children are defined as those from families with hypercholesterolemia or premature cardiovascular disease.
LDL = low density lipoprotein. ng/dL = nanograms per deciliter.

SOURCE: "Table 15. Classification of Cholesterol Levels in High-Risk Children and Adolescents," in *Overweight Children and Adolescents: Screen, Assess, and Manage,* Centers for Disease Control and Prevention, National Center for Chronic Disease Prevention and Promotion, Division of Nutrition, Physical Activity and Obesity, 2001, http://www.cdc.gov/nccdphp/dnpa/growthcharts/training/modules/module3/text/cholesterol.htm (accessed October 18, 2011)

- Laboratory tests, such as cholesterol screening, that are dictated by the degree of overweight, family history, and the results of the physical examination. Table 4.14 shows the range of values for total blood cholesterol and low-density lipoprotein cholesterol that are considered acceptable, borderline, and high.

- A mental health evaluation to determine the readiness of children and adolescents to change behaviors and to identify a history of eating disorders or depression that may require treatment. An assessment of the family's ability to support a child's weight-loss or weight-management efforts may also be performed.

INTERVENTION AND TREATMENT OF OVERWEIGHT AND OBESITY

In the absence of acute medical necessity, such as with children who are dangerously obese, most health professionals concur that drastic caloric restriction is an inappropriate weight-loss strategy for children who are still growing. Instead, they advise efforts to stabilize body weight with a healthy, balanced diet, increased physical activity, and education about nutrition, food choices, and preparation. This approach is especially effective for children who are just slightly overweight, because maintaining body weight often allows them to outgrow overweight and become normal-weight adults.

When active weight loss is indicated, it is generally for children with a BMI greater than the 95th percentile or those experiencing complications of overweight or obesity. Among children aged two to seven, gradual weight loss of about 1 pound (0.5 kg) per month is advised. Older children with serious health risks who are severely overweight (BMI greater than 35) may be advised to lose between 1 and 2 pounds (0.5 and 0.9 kg) per week.

In "Pediatric Obesity: Etiology and Treatment" (*Pediatric Clinics of North America*, vol. 58, no. 5, October 2011), Melissa K. Crocker and Jack A. Yanovski observe that pediatric childhood obesity has been shown to have a tremendous impact on later health, even independent of adult weight. The researchers consider lifestyle modification and restricting energy intake to be the foundation of successful treatment of obesity in children. They explain that interventions for overweight and obese children range from basic diets and lifestyle interventions to more intensive very-low-energy diets, medications, and surgery. These methods achieve varying levels of success and all are optimally successful when the child and family are motivated and educated. Crocker and Yanovski assert that "the participation and cooperation of the entire family is critical regardless of the mode of therapy employed."

Crocker and Yanovski observe that dietary changes alone may benefit children who are overweight but are relatively ineffective for children and adolescents with severe obesity. Similarly, exercise without dietary intervention is relatively ineffective. Comprehensive approaches to weight loss that involve behavior modification to reduce screen time, increase physical activity, motivate children to improve their eating behavior, and engage the school system and family to support weight-loss goals appear to be more effective than diet alone.

Pharmacotherapy (drug treatment to support weight loss) has shown limited success when combined with diet and exercise. As of 2011, only one weight-loss drug, orlistat (a drug that induces weight loss by blocking the absorption of about one-third of the fat contained in a meal), was approved for use in children aged 16 years and younger. However, many physicians believe that in view of orlistat's limited effectiveness and potential side effects, it should be limited to children and adolescents with a BMI over the 95th percentile who also have significant obesity-related medical complications.

Some adolescents who are obese may be treated with weight-loss surgery. The NIH criteria for adolescents aged 13 to 17 years are the same as those applied to adults: a BMI greater than or equal to 40 or a BMI greater than or equal to 35 with at least one comorbidity (a coexisting serious medical condition) such as type 2 diabetes, hypertension, or obstructive sleep apnea. Evan P. Nadler et al. compare in "Morbidity in Obese Adolescents Who Meet the Adult National Institutes of Health Criteria for Bariatric Surgery" (*Journal of Pediatric Surgery*, vol. 44, no. 10, October 2009) the medical records of 134 adolescents who met the NIH criteria for weight-loss surgery to the records of 4,736 adolescents who did not meet the criteria to determine the differences between these populations and whether stricter criteria should be adopted for teens. The researchers find that "adolescents who meet NIH consensus criteria for weight loss surgery in adults require specialized health services and have functional impairment. Thus, we advocate the use of the standard adult criteria defined by the NIH as the initial screening requirements so that enhanced access to weight loss surgery for morbidly obese adolescents may be achieved."

Meghan L. Butryn et al. examine in "Maintenance of Weight Loss in Adolescents: Current Status and Future Directions" (*Journal of Obesity*, January 2011) how different approaches—lifestyle modification, dietary and physical activity interventions, use of Internet, and medication—assist adolescents to maintain their weight loss. Butryn et al. find that lifestyle modification programs, especially those that involve parents, are likely to be more successful than other approaches because parents can exert a strong impact on the adolescent's behavior by supporting healthy eating and physical activity. Even though definitive data are lacking, Internet-based interventions that maximize and prolong engagement and participation also appear promising, especially for adolescents without access to in-person treatment. Medication used as a component of a lifestyle modification program appears to offer some weight-maintenance benefits; however, adolescents must adhere to a low-fat diet when taking the medication.

Educating Parents

Researchers agree that primary prevention is the strategy with the greatest potential for reversing the alarming rise in overweight and obesity among children and teens. Public health educators recommend counseling parents and caregivers about healthy eating habits for children. They advise offering children a variety of healthful foods, in reasonable quantities, to assist children to make wise food choices. Children should be encouraged, but not forced, to sample new foods and should not be pressured to clean their plates. No foods or food groups should be entirely off-limits, or children may become fixated on obtaining the forbidden foods.

Even though it is difficult to impress on children the future health risks that are associated with excess weight, parents should be informed that obese children are more likely to suffer from diabetes, heart, and joint diseases such as osteoarthritis, as well as breast and colon cancer. Adults should model healthy habits by consuming no more than 30% of calories from fat, exercising regularly, and limiting time spent in front of the television. Health educators are especially eager to reduce children's television viewing, with its destructive blend of junk-food advertising and enforced inactivity. Finally, health professionals caution that food should not be used to punish or reward behavior or as a way to comfort or console children. The undivided attention of a parent or caregiver or an expression of sympathy, reassurance, or encouragement may satisfy a child's need better than an ice cream cone or an order of french fries.

Launching of Let's Move! by First Lady Michelle Obama

In February 2010 First Lady Michelle Obama (1964–) launched Let's Move! (http://www.letsmove.gov/), a comprehensive set of strategies that are aimed at combatting childhood obesity. The antiobesity initiative involves private- and public-sector resources in alliances with states, local communities, athletic organizations, and schools. The ambitious program aims to:

- Inform parents to enable them to make healthy choices for their family

- Assist retailers and manufacturers to implement new nutritionally sound and user-friendly front-of-package labeling

- Educate health professionals about obesity to ensure they regularly monitor children's BMI, provide counseling for healthy eating, and write prescriptions for parents detailing the steps they can take to increase healthy eating and physical activity

- Use the media to enhance public awareness of the need to combat obesity through public service announcements, special programming, and marketing

- Promote the USDA interactive database—the Food Environment Atlas—that helps identify communities with diet and obesity-related problems such as high incidences of diabetes; this information should prove useful for parents, educators, government, and businesses

- Improve food choices in schools by doubling the number of schools that participate in the Healthier U.S. School Challenge, which sets rigorous standards for schools' food quality, participation in meal programs, and physical activity and nutrition education

- Encourage food suppliers to decrease the amount of sugar, fat, and salt in school meals; increase whole grains; and double the amount of produce they serve within 10 years

- Improve Americans' access to healthy affordable foods by bringing grocery stores to underserved areas, helping places such as convenience stores and bodegas to carry healthier food options, and investing in farmers' markets

- Increase physical activity by challenging children and adults to commit to physical activity five days per week for six weeks and supporting efforts to get children physically active in and outside of school

Let's Move! celebrated its first anniversary in February 2011. Its website offers success stories involving children, chefs, faith-based and community organizations, mayors and municipal officials, parents, teachers, and schools. Nikki Sutton reports in "The White House Kitchen Garden Fall Harvest and Grilled Garden Pizza" (http://www.letsmove.gov/blog/2011/10/05/white-house-kitchen-garden-fall-harvest-and-grilled-garden-pizza) that in October 2011 the first lady invited local school children to help harvest fresh produce from the White House kitchen garden and then sample some of the vegetables they picked on grilled garden pizzas.

EATING DISORDERS

Overweight and obesity are among the most stigmatizing and least socially acceptable conditions in childhood and adolescence. Society, culture, and the media send children powerful messages about body weight and shape ideals. For girls these messages include the "thin ideal" and encouragement to diet and exercise. Messages to boys emphasize a muscular body and pressure to body build and even use potentially harmful dietary supplements and steroids. Gender has not been identified as a specific risk factor for obesity in children, but the pressure placed on girls to be thin may put them at a greater risk for developing eating-disordered behaviors. Even though society presents boys with a wider range of acceptable body images, they are also at risk for developing disordered eating and body image disturbances.

Adolescence is a developmental period marked by great physical change, and it is a time when many teens subject themselves to painful scrutiny. Uneven growth, puberty, and sexual maturation may make teens feel awkward and self-conscious about their bodies. Teenaged girls are especially susceptible to developing negative body images—ignoring other qualities and focusing exclusively on appearance to measure their self-worth. This single-minded, and often distorted, destructive focus can result in lowered self-esteem and increased risk for mental health problems, including eating disorders. The 2009 YRBSS found that 5.4% of female high school students engaged in dangerous dieting behaviors (vomiting or taking laxatives). (See Table 3.3 in Chapter 3.)

Who Is at Risk?

Even though there are biological, genetic, and familial factors that predispose certain people to eating disorders such as anorexia nervosa (intense fear of becoming fat even when dangerously underweight) and bulimia nervosa (recurrent episodes of binge eating followed by purging to prevent weight gain), the emergence of these disorders is triggered by environmental factors. Chief among the environmental triggers is body image. Many researchers and health professionals believe that teenaged girls who identify with the idealized body images projected throughout U.S. culture are at an increased risk for eating disorders.

Other risk factors are peer group pressures and sociocultural forces such as the fashion and entertainment industries and the media. The National Eating Disorders Association identifies media definitions of attractiveness, beauty, and health as among the myriad factors that contribute to the rise of eating disorders.

Historically, most adolescents with eating disorders have been first- or second-born white females from middle- to upper-class families. Girls who suffer from anorexia are often academically successful, with athletic prowess or training in dance. They tend to be perfectionists, well behaved, emotionally dependent, socially anxious, and intent on receiving approval from others. Adolescent girls with bulimia are generally more extroverted and socially involved. According to the Eating Disorders Coalition for Research, Policy, and Action, in the fact sheet "Facts about Eating Disorders: What the Research Shows" (May 20, 2009, http://www.eating disorderscoalition.org/documents/TalkingpointsEatingDis ordersFactSheetUpdated5-20-09.pdf), in the early 21st century the occurrence of eating disorders is increasing among younger children and throughout diverse ethnic and sociocultural groups.

Research reveals that the incidence of eating disorders in young children is relatively high. In "Incidence and Age-Specific Presentation of Restrictive Eating Disorders in Children" (*Archives of Pediatric and Adolescent Medicine*, vol. 165, no. 10, October 2011), Leora Pinhas et al. analyze data from 2,453 pediatricians in Canada about the children they care for. The researchers find that the incidence of restrictive eating disorders (intentional limitation or avoidance of nutrition) among children aged five to 12 years is 2.6 per 100,000 children, with girls outnumbering boys by a ratio of 6:1. Pinhas et al. also note delayed growth in about half of children with eating disorders and that more than one-third had unstable blood pressure and heart rates. Nearly half of the children with eating disorders had been hospitalized as a result of the disorder.

Which Variables Are Associated with Dieting, Overweight, and Eating Disorders?

Dianne Neumark-Sztainer and Peter J. Hannan of the University of Minnesota, Minneapolis, analyzed a representative sample of 6,728 adolescents in grades five through 12 who completed the Commonwealth Fund surveys about the health of adolescent girls and boys. The results of the research were detailed in the landmark study "Weight-Related Behaviors among Adolescent Girls and Boys: Results from a National Survey" (*Archives of Pediatrics and Adolescent Medicine*, vol. 154, no. 6, June 2000). The research aimed to assess the prevalence of dieting and disordered eating among adolescents; the sociodemographic, psychosocial, and behavioral variables that were associated with dieting and disordered eating; and whether adolescents report having discussed weight-related issues with their health care providers. (Neumark-Sztainer and Hannan defined disordered eating as weight-related behaviors such as anorexia and bulimia, self-induced vomiting, binge eating, inappropriate or extreme dieting, and obesity.)

Subjects were assessed by calculating their BMI and eliciting weight-related attitudes and behaviors. For example, dieting was assessed by asking questions such as "Have you ever been on a diet?" and "Why were you dieting?" Behaviors were assessed by posing a question such as "Have you ever binged and purged (which is when you eat a lot of food and then make yourself throw up, vomit, or take something that makes you have diarrhea) or not?" Subjects were also asked "Right now, how would you describe yourself?" to gain an understanding of their perceptions of their weight. Psychosocial and behavioral variables including self-esteem, stress, depression, substance use (of tobacco, alcohol, or illegal drugs), and level of physical activity were also measured and scored using standardized questionnaires and inventories.

Alcohol and drug use were directly associated with dieting and disordered eating among girls and boys; however, the association between substance use and disordered eating was stronger than the association between substance use and dieting. Tobacco use was associated with dieting and disordered eating among girls, but not among boys.

Neumark-Sztainer and Hannan noted that "about half of the youth reported that a health care provider had discussed nutrition and weight issues with them" and observed that even though the content of such discussions was unclear, "at least the youth remembered that these issues had been discussed." They concluded that "the high rates of dieting and disordered eating behaviors, coupled with the high prevalence of obesity found in this and previous studies, indicate a clear need for interventions aimed at the primary and secondary prevention of weight-related disorders. The large scope of the problem and the complexity of the issues at hand indicate that there is a need for multiple interventions at the individual and familial level (e.g., within clinical practices), at the group level (e.g., within school settings), and at the community or larger societal level (e.g., changes in the physical and social environment)."

Alison E. Field et al. confirm in "Family, Peer, and Media Predictors of Becoming Eating Disordered" (*Archives of Pediatric and Adolescent Medicine*, vol. 162, no. 6, June 2008), a study to identify the predictors of eating disorders in adolescents, some of the findings that were reported by Neumark-Sztainer and Hannan and discover other risk factors. The researchers looked at whether various suspected risk factors for eating disorders were independently associated with starting to binge, purge, or both binge and purge over the course of seven years in 12,534 subjects in the Growing up Today Study, who were nine to 15 years old at the beginning of the study.

Field et al. find that the rates and risk factors varied by sex and age. Girls younger than 14 years whose mothers had a history of an eating disorder were nearly three times more likely than their peers to start purging at least weekly, but a maternal history of an eating disorder was unrelated to the risk of starting to binge or purge in girls older than the age of 14 years. Frequent dieting and striving to look like people in the media were independent predictors of binge eating in females of all ages. In males, negative comments about weight by fathers predicted starting to binge at least weekly.

In "Characteristics Measured by the Eating Disorder Inventory for Children at Risk and Protective Factors for Disordered Eating in Adolescent Girls" (*International Journal of Women's Health*, October 28, 2010), Sanna Aila Gustafsson et al. seek to identify risk factors for eating disorders and factors that protect against the development of disordered eating. Like other investigators, Gustafsson et al. find that an excessive drive for thinness and body dissatisfaction are risk factors. Not surprisingly, teenaged girls with healthy attitudes about eating and acceptance of a range of health body sizes in early adolescence are less likely to develop disordered eating.

CHAPTER 5
DIETARY TREATMENT FOR OVERWEIGHT AND OBESITY

We rarely repent of having eaten too little.

—Thomas Jefferson

Americans have long been consumed with losing weight, seemingly willing to suffer deprivation and to embrace each new diet that debuts—even if the "new diet" is simply a twist on a previous weight-loss plan. The fixation with weight loss is so long-standing that even the word *diet* has assumed a new meaning. As a verb, diet means to eat and drink a prescribed selection of foods; however, since the latter part of the 20th century dieting became synonymous with an effort to lose weight.

During the 19th century fashionable body shapes and sizes varied from decade to decade, but most periods celebrated plumpness as a sign of health and prosperity and considered being thin a sign of poverty and ill health. At the start of the 20th century rising interest in dieting seemingly coincided with some of the social and cultural changes that would make it necessary: food became increasingly plentiful, and sedentary work and public transportation reduced Americans' level of physical activity. In *Fat History: Bodies and Beauty in the Modern West* (1997), Peter N. Stearns explains how fat became "a turn-of-the-century target" with anti-fat sentiments intensifying from the 1920s to the 21st century.

Stearns asserts that the contemporary obsession with fat arose in tandem with the dramatic growth in consumer culture, women's increasing equality, and changes in women's sexual and maternal roles. Dieting, with its emphasis on deprivation, self-control, and moral discipline, seemed the perfect antidote to the indulgence of consumer culture, and Stearns contends that "weight morality bore disproportionately on women precisely because of their growing independence, or seeming independence, from other standards."

Fashion trends fueled anti-fat sentiments as women shed the corsets that had created the illusion of narrow waists and aspired to duplicate the wasp-waisted silhouettes by becoming slimmer. The shorter, close-fitting "flapper" dresses of the 1920s revealed women's legs and rekindled their desire to be slender. The emergence of the first actuarial tables (data compiled to assess insurance risk and formulate life insurance premiums), which showed the relationship between overweight and premature mortality (death), reinforced the growing sentiment that thinness was the key to health and longevity. Capitalizing on the increasing interest in monitoring and reducing body weight, the new Detecto and Health-o-Meter bathroom scales enabled people to weigh themselves regularly in the privacy of their own home, as opposed to relying on periodic visits to the physician's office or the pharmacy to use the balance scale.

SELECTED MILESTONES IN THE HISTORY OF DIETING

Not unlike fashion trends, the history of dieting reveals the emergence and popularity of specific diets, which over time are cast aside in favor of different approaches but then are recycled and resurface as "new and miraculous." The first low-carbohydrate diet to earn popular acclaim was described by William Banting (1797–1878) during the 1860s. In *Letter on Corpulence, Addressed to the Public* (1863), Banting, then 66 years old, claimed that by adhering to his low-carbohydrate regimen he was never hungry and had lost 46 pounds (20.9 kg) of his initial 202 pounds (91.6 kg) in one year.

The early 1900s marked the beginning of diets that restricted calories. *Diet and Health, with Key to the Calories* (1918) by Lulu Hunt Peters (1873–1930) advised readers to think in terms of consuming calories rather than food items and remained in print for 20 years. Peters wrote, "You should know and use the word calorie as frequently, or more frequently, than you use the foot, yard, quart, gallon and so forth...hereafter you are going to eat calories of food. Instead of saying one slice of bread, or a piece of pie, you will say 100 calories of bread, 350 calories of pie." The 1920s saw the rise of very-low-calorie diets to promote weight loss. For example, the Hollywood 18-day diet advised just 585 calories per day, which required the dieter to eat mostly citrus fruit.

Throughout the 1920s and 1930s the low-calorie diet remained a popular weight-loss strategy. Other approaches, however, such as food-limiting plans that restricted dieters to just one or two foods (e.g., lamb chops, pineapples, grapefruits, or cabbage), were introduced, as were diets that prescribed combinations of certain foods and forbid others. For example, some diets prohibited eating protein and carbohydrates together; others were more specific, advising which vegetables could be served together. The 1930s also saw the first condemnations of carbohydrates as causes of overweight. A high-fat, low-fiber diet consisting primarily of milk and meat was thought to be protective against disease. The Italian poet Filippo Tommaso Marinetti (1876–1944) exhorted Italians to forgo their pasta because he claimed it made them sluggish, pessimistic, and fat.

In 1943 the U.S. Department of Agriculture (USDA) released the "Basic Seven" food guide in the *National Wartime Nutrition Guide*. It emphasized a patriotic wartime austerity diet that included between two and four servings of protein-rich meat and milk products, three servings of fruits or vegetables, and the rather vague recommendation of "bread, flour, and cereals every day and butter, fortified margarine—some daily."

In 1948 Esther Manz (1908–1996), a 208-pound (94.3-kg) homemaker, established Take Off Pounds Sensibly (TOPS; http://www.tops.org/), the first support-group program for weight loss. Manz was inspired to start the program after she attended childbirth preparation classes, where women benefited from mutual support and encouragement. As of January 2012, the annual membership of $26 supported the international nonprofit organization, which is based in Milwaukee, Wisconsin. Along with weekly meetings and private weigh-ins, TOPS participants are encouraged to adhere to a calorie-counting meal plan that is based on a program developed by the Academy of Nutrition and Dietetics. In "TOPS Quick Facts" (March 10, 2010, http://www.tops.org/MediaKit/ PI-009BTopsQuickFactsflyer.pdf), TOPS indicates that in 2009 it had about 170,000 members in nearly 10,000 chapters worldwide. Members who achieve their weight goals become KOPS (Keep Off Pounds Sensibly) and often keep attending meetings to maintain their weight and serve as role models for others.

In 1950 the physician and biophysicist John W. Gofman (1918–2007) hypothesized that blood cholesterol was involved in the rise in coronary heart disease.

Gofman found not only that heart attacks correlated with elevated levels of cholesterol but also that the cholesterol was contained in one lipoprotein particle: low-density lipoprotein (LDL). Early reports of the connection between overweight and elevated blood cholesterol intensified interest in weight loss, which was now promoted as a strategy for preventing heart disease. During the late 1950s injections of human chorionic gonadotropin, which was derived from the urine of pregnant women or animals, enjoyed fleeting popularity as a weight-loss agent; however, it was quickly proven entirely ineffective. Fad diets, such as a diet advocating the consumption of several bananas to satisfy sugar cravings and another that involved ingesting a blend of oils to boost metabolism, continued to lure Americans seeking quick weight loss. In 1959 the American Medical Association called dieting a "national neurosis."

In 1960 Metrecal, the first high-protein beverage, was widely advertised by the Mead Johnson Company as a weight-reducing aid. It was originally sold as a powder, which when mixed with 1 quart (0.9 L) of water yielded four 8-ounce (237-mL) glasses intended to serve as four meals per day, totaling 900 calories. The powder was made from milk, soy flour, starch, corn oil, yeast, vitamins, coconut oil, and vanilla, chocolate, or butterscotch flavoring. The low-calorie regimen enabled a dieter to lose 10 pounds (4.5 kg) in a few weeks, without the trouble of meal preparation or counting calories. Later, Metrecal was sold in a premixed, liquid form that could be consumed right from the can. Mead Johnson made over $10 million selling Metrecal in the first two years. It was the forerunner of liquid diet products such as Slim-Fast.

The 1960s also witnessed the birth of Overeaters Anonymous (OA) and Weight Watchers. OA began as a support group modeled on the 12-step emotional, physical, and spiritual recovery program used by Alcoholics Anonymous. In "About OA" (2012, http://www.oa.org/ new-to-oa/about-oa.php), the OA notes that about 6,500 OA groups meet each week in more than 75 countries. In 1961 Jean Nidetch (1923–), an overweight housewife in New York City, invited a few friends to her home to gain support for her efforts to diet and overcome an "obsession for cookies." From this first meeting, the friends gathered weekly, offering one another encouragement and sharing advice and ideas. The weekly support meetings proved successful, providing motivation and encouragement for long-term weight loss. In 1963 Nidetch incorporated Weight Watchers, and hundreds of people turned out for its first meeting. Weight Watchers grew in both size and popularity by developing nutritious and convenient eating plans and promoting exercise, cookbooks, healthful prepared food, and a magazine. The company became so successful that it was acquired by the H. J. Heinz Company in 1978. Weight Watchers states in "About Us: History and Philosophy" (2012, http://www.weightwatchers.com/about/his/hello.aspx) that approximately 50,000 Weight Watcher groups meet every week.

Two best-selling diet books also debuted during the 1960s. The first was Herman Taller's *Calories Don't Count* (1961), which told dieters to avoid carbohydrates and refined sugars and to eat a high-protein diet that included large quantities of unsaturated fat. The second was Irwin Maxwell Stillman and Samm Sinclair Baker's *The Doctor's Quick Weight Loss Diet* (1967), which instructed dieters to avoid carbohydrates altogether and to consume just meat, poultry, fish, cheese, eggs, and water. Even though Taller and Stillman and Baker were not the first to tout low-carbohydrate diets, they introduced the first modern high-protein weight-loss diets. Taller's career as a diet guru ended abruptly in 1967, when he was convicted of mail fraud for the sale of safflower capsules as weight-loss aids. Stillman and Baker, however, followed up their wildly successful first book with several other additional weight-loss titles, including *The Doctor's Quick Teenage Diet* (1971), one of the first diet books to address the needs of overweight adolescents. High-protein, low-carbohydrate diets washed down by liberal amounts of alcohol were also advocated by other books from the 1960s, including Gardener Jameson's *The Drinking Man's Diet* (1965) and Sidney Petrie's *Martinis and Whipped Cream: The New Carbo-Cal Way to Lose Weight and Stay Slim* (1966) and *The Lazy Lady's Easy Diet: A Fast-Action Plan to Lose Weight Quickly for Sustained Slenderness and Youthful Attractiveness* (1969).

During this same decade chemically processed, nonnutritive sweeteners were marketed as calorie- and guilt-free substitutes that enabled dieters to enjoy many of their favorite sweet treats. Saccharin, which is 300 times sweeter than sugar, was the first artificial sweetener to be widely used in diet foods and beverages. Other chemically processed, artificial, and nonnutritive sweeteners followed, including cyclamate, which was withdrawn from the U.S. market in 1969 because research findings in animals suggested that it might increase the risk of bladder cancer in humans. According to the National Cancer Institute, in "Artificial Sweeteners and Cancer" (August 5, 2009, http://www.cancer.gov/cancertopics/factsheet/Risk/artificial-sweeteners), recent animal studies have failed to demonstrate that cyclamate is a carcinogen (a substance known to cause cancer) or a cocarcinogen (a substance that enhances the effect of a cancer-causing substance); regardless, cyclamate is not approved for commercial use as a food additive in the United States.

Aspartame and acesulfame potassium were approved by the U.S. Food and Drug Administration (FDA) in

1981 and 1988, respectively. In 1999 the FDA approved the noncaloric sweetener sucralose for general use. Sucralose has gained popularity because it is derived from and tastes like sugar, has no aftertaste, does not promote tooth decay, and is deemed safe for use by pregnant women and diabetics, as well as by those in the general population who are trying to cut down on their sugar intake.

In 2002 the FDA approved neotame, another nonnutritive sweetener, for use as a general-purpose sweetener. Neotame is approximately 7,000 to 13,000 times sweeter than sugar and has been approved for use in food products including baked goods, nonalcoholic beverages (including soft drinks), chewing gum, confections and frostings, frozen desserts, gelatins and puddings, jams and jellies, processed fruits and fruit juices, toppings, and syrups.

In 2008 the FDA approved the sale of stevia, a naturally occurring, zero-calorie sweetener, as a sugar substitute. Stevia is sold in various forms: in combination with other naturally occurring flavors and sweeteners, such as the sugar alcohol erythritol, as well as on its own. Because it has a negligible effect on blood glucose, it is an attractive sugar alternative for people on low-carbohydrate diets.

However, some researchers think sugar substitutes may sabotage dieters by interfering with the body's own innate ability to monitor calorie consumption based on a food's flavor: sweet or savory. Susan E. Swithers, Ashley A. Martin, and Terry L. Davidson of Purdue University report in "High-Intensity Sweeteners and Energy Balance" (*Physiology and Behavior*, vol. 100, no.1, April 26, 2010) the results of additional research confirming that nonnutritive sweeteners promote food intake, body weight gain, and metabolic disorders. The researchers suggest that the consumption of nonnutritive sweeteners may result in sweet tastes no longer serving as consistent predictors of energy consumption and physiological consequences. This disconnect between the sweet taste cues and the caloric consequences may lead to a decrease in the ability of sweet tastes to stimulate the bodily responses that regulate energy balance.

In 1972 the cardiologist Robert Atkins (1930–2003) published *Dr. Atkins' Diet Revolution: The High Calorie Way to Stay Thin Forever*, which provided a new explanation about how an extremely low-carbohydrate diet targets insulin to promote weight loss. Atkins called insulin, the hormone that regulates blood sugar levels, a "fat-producing hormone." He asserted that most overeaters are continually in a state of hyperinsulinism, in that they are primed and ever-ready to convert excess carbohydrates to fat. As a result, they have excess circulating insulin, which primes the body to store fat. Atkins contended that when people with hyperinsulinism dieted to lose weight—especially when they reduced their fat intake and increased carbohydrate consumption—their efforts were doomed to fail. He claimed that dieters could alter their metabolism and burn fat by inducing a state of ketosis (the accumulation of ketones from partly digested fats due to inadequate carbohydrate intake) that they monitored by testing their urine for the presence of ketones. Dieters who were tired of limiting portion size, weighing and measuring their foods, counting calories, and assiduously avoiding fatty foods such as steak, bacon, butter, cheese, and heavy cream embraced the low-carbohydrate diet with religious fervor.

The high-protein, low-carbohydrate diet not only was satisfying but also produced the immediate benefit of weight loss through water loss because the body flushes the waste products of protein digestion in the form of urine. Especially during the early weeks of dieting this additional weight loss delivered a psychological boost to dieters and provided the motivation to continue. Many researchers and health professionals agreed with Atkins's premise that sharply limiting carbohydrate intake can help curb the appetite by maintaining even levels of insulin and preventing the insulin surges and blood sugar drops that may trigger hunger. For example, in "A High-Protein Diet Induces Sustained Reductions in Appetite, Ad Libitum Caloric Intake, and Body Weight Despite Compensatory Changes in Diurnal Plasma Leptin and Ghrelin Concentrations" (*American Journal of Clinical Nutrition*, vol. 82, no. 1, July 2005), David S. Weigle et al. observe that there is considerable evidence that high-protein diets, such as the Atkins regimen, increase satiety (the feeling of fullness or satisfaction after eating). The researchers posit that the increased satiety produced by high-protein diets may help explain the weight loss produced by low-carbohydrate diets.

Atkins and his devotees were celebrating weight loss, good health, and improved mood as a result of the low-carbohydrate diet, but nutritionists and health professionals were countering by trumpeting the benefits of low-fat diets that were high in complex carbohydrates and fiber. Fat was demonized, and nutritionists pointed dieters to the USDA Food Guide Pyramid, which advised using fats sparingly. (The updated 2005 USDA Food Guide Pyramid continued to promote a low-fat diet and minimal use of fats and oils.) Critics of the low-carbohydrate regimen were concerned about the long-term health consequences of the high-fat diet and wondered if it might elevate cholesterol and triglyceride levels in people who by virtue of being overweight were already at increased risk for heart disease. There were also concerns that high-protein diets might cause kidney damage or bone loss over time. Rigorous research to compare the effectiveness and assess the health outcomes of low-carbohydrate and low-fat diets

was not conducted until the late 1990s. Even though Atkins enjoyed tremendous popularity, published a series of weight-loss books, and oversaw the sale of food products bearing his name, his contributions to the scientific understanding of nutrition and weight loss were not fully appreciated until the year preceding his death in 2003.

The 1970s also witnessed several fad diets. Robert Linn's *The Last Chance Diet—When Everything Else Has Failed* (1976) advised a protein-sparing fast, which was so dangerously deficient in essential nutrients that several deaths were attributed to it. In *The Complete Scarsdale Medical Diet Plus Dr. Tarnower's Lifetime Keep-Slim Program* (1978), Herman Tarnower advocated a fat-free, high-protein diet that allowed 700 calories per day.

At the close of the 1970s Nathan Pritikin's (1915–1985) *The Pritikin Program for Diet and Exercise* (1979) championed a nearly fat-free diet that consisted of fresh and cooked fruits and vegetables, whole grains, breads and pasta, and small amounts of lean meat, fish, and poultry, in concert with daily aerobic exercise. Advocating heart health and fitness, in 1975 Pritikin opened the Pritikin Longevity Center, where people could learn to modify not only their diet but also their lifestyle. Even though Pritikin's plan, which essentially eliminated fat from the diet, was considered by many health professionals too extreme to gain long-term adherents, Pritikin enjoyed as loyal a following as did Atkins.

During the 1980s Judy Mazel (1943–2007) resurrected the notion of specific food combinations as central to weight loss in *The Beverly Hills Diet* (1981). Mazel asserted that eating foods together, such as protein and carbohydrates, destroyed digestive enzymes and caused weight gain and poor digestion. Her diet featured an abundance of fruit, and some observers speculated that weight loss attributable to the diet resulted from the combined effects of caloric restriction and fluid loss resulting from diarrhea. Celebrity endorsements and Mazel's frequent media interviews stimulated interest in the diet.

In 1983 Jenny Craig (1932–) launched a weight-loss program that would become one of the world's two largest diet companies (the other being Weight Watchers). With over 725 centers in Australia, Guam, New Zealand, North America, and Puerto Rico, the company (2012, http://www.jennycraig.com/corporate/company-profile/) that bears her name sells prepared foods, along with other weight-loss materials. The company offers telephone and online support and home delivery of food and support materials. In 2002 the company founders Jenny Craig and Sid Craig sold their majority stake in the company to ACI Capital Co. and MidOcean Capital Partners Inc., but retained 20% interest in the company.

Celebrity endorsements, including paid spokespeople such as Carrie Fisher (1956–) and Valerie Bertinelli (1960–), have helped promote the program.

The 1990s served up so-called new and revised versions of high-protein, high-fat, and low-carbohydrate diets and the low-fat diet as well as an update of Mazel's Beverly Hills diet. The cardiologist Dean Ornish (1953–) rekindled enthusiasm for low-fat eating with *Eat More, Weigh Less: Dr. Dean Ornish's Life Choice Program for Losing Weight Safely While Eating Abundantly* (1993). Atkins's 1999 update of *Dr. Atkins' New Diet Revolution*, which offered advice about how to achieve total wellness and weight loss, spent more than four years on the *New York Times* best-seller list and won over a new generation of dieters. Ornish's approach was directly opposed to Atkins's—he espoused the health benefits of vegetarianism and limiting dietary fat to just 10% of the total daily calories. However, both physicians took a holistic approach to health and weight loss by encouraging readers to engage in moderate exercise, foster social support, and reconnect with themselves to support their physical and emotional well-being.

The diet that generated the most fanfare during the 1990s was by the biochemist Barry Sears (1947–), who published *The Zone: A Dietary Road Map* (1995). Sears's high-protein, low-carbohydrate plan promised that by eating the correct ratio of protein, fat, and carbohydrates dieters would lose weight permanently, avoid disease, enhance mental productivity, achieve maximum physical performance, balance and control insulin levels, and enter "that mysterious but very real state in which your body and mind work together at their ultimate best."

Since the start of the 21st century the fiery debate about the merits of low-carbohydrate and low-fat diets has intensified, with both sides citing scientific evidence to support the supremacy of one diet as the healthier and more effective weight-loss strategy. The cardiologist Arthur Agatston (1947–) offered a kind of compromise between the two regimens in *The South Beach Diet: The Delicious, Doctor-Designed, Foolproof Plan for Fast and Healthy Weight Loss* (2003). Agatston condemned simple carbohydrates, such as white flour and white sugar, citing them as the source of the continuous cravings that sabotage dieters, but did not eliminate complex carbohydrates from the diet. (Carbohydrates are classified as simple or complex. The classification depends on the chemical structure of the particular food source and reflects how quickly the sugar is digested and absorbed. Simple carbohydrates have one or two sugars, whereas complex carbohydrates have three or more.) Agatston's diet program was a modified carbohydrate plan that recommended plenty of high-fiber foods, lean proteins, and healthful fats, while cutting back on, but not entirely banishing, bread, rice, pastas, and fruits.

Americans' enthusiasm for low-carbohydrate diets cooled during 2004, and Atkins Nutritionals Inc., the company that catapulted low-carbohydrate diets into a national obsession, filed for bankruptcy court protection in August 2005. Many dieters abandoned low-carbohydrate diets in favor of regimens that focused on the glycemic index—a ranking system for carbohydrates according to their immediate effect on blood glucose levels, in which a numerical value is assigned to a carbohydrate-rich food based on its average increase in blood glucose.

In 2004 diet books that extolled the virtues of the low glycemic index diet—including Michel Montignac's *Eat Yourself Slim* (1999), Rick Gallop's *The G.I. Diet: The Easy, Healthy Way to Permanent Weight Loss* (2002), and H. Leighton Steward et al.'s *The New Sugar Busters!: Cut Sugar to Trim Fat* (2003)—became quite popular. Proponents of low glycemic index diets observed that the regimen not only produced weight loss but also improved overall health by reducing the risk for both type 2 diabetes and cardiovascular disease.

Even though diet industry observers cannot predict the next craze, they are certain that a replacement for the low-carbohydrate diet will emerge. Contenders among the diets and diet books that debuted since 2006 include:

- *The Diet Code: Revolutionary Weight Loss Secrets from Da Vinci and the Golden Ratio* (2006) by Stephen Lanzalotta promotes Mediterranean-style eating and emphasizes bread, fish, cheese, vegetables, meat, nuts, and wine.

- *The Total Wellbeing Diet* (2006) by Manny Noakes details a low-carbohydrate, high-protein diet that was developed by the Commonwealth Scientific and Industrial Research Organization to help Australians lose weight.

- *The Rice Diet Cookbook: 150 Easy, Everyday Recipes and Inspirational Success Stories from the Rice Diet Program Community* (2007) by Kitty Gurkin Rosati counters the low-carbohydrate diet trend with a low-salt diet that features rice, vegetables, and fruit. This diet was developed in 1939 by Walter Kempner (1903–1997) at Duke University.

- *I Can Make You Thin* (2007) by Paul McKenna encourages mindful eating and exhorts people to savor every mouthful of food. McKenna suggests eliminating food cravings by tapping 10 times on various parts of one's body and humming "Happy Birthday" until cravings subside.

- *The End of Overeating: Taking Control of the Insatiable American Appetite* (2009) by David A. Kessler details why we overeat and how to focus on choosing sensible portions of healthful foods.

- *Food Rules: An Eater's Manual* (2009) by Michael Pollan offers advice such as "eat mostly plants, especially leaves," "eat your colors," "limit your snacks to unprocessed plant food," "don't eat anything your great-grandmother wouldn't recognize as food," "avoid food products that contain more than five ingredients," and "avoid foods that contain high-fructose corn syrup."

- *The Eat This, Not That! No Diet! Diet: The World's Easiest Weight-Loss Plan* (2011) by David Zinczenko describes how to navigate the supermarket to select healthful foods.

- *The Amen Solution: The Brain Healthy Way to Lose Weight and Keep It Off* (2011) by Daniel G. Amen describes how to determine an individual's type of overeating, such as compulsive overeater or emotional eater, and then tailor weight-loss and nutritional strategies for each type of overeater.

- *Why We Get Fat and What to Do about It* (2011) by Gary Taubes asserts that certain types of carbohydrates have fueled the obesity epidemic and offers explanations of why are some people thin and others fat, the roles that exercise and genetics play in determining and managing weight, and the foods to eat and avoid.

AMERICANS' DIETS

Hazel A. B. Hiza and Lisa Bente of the Center for Nutrition Policy and Promotion offer in *Nutrient Content of the U.S. Food Supply: Developments between 2000 and 2006* (July 2011, http://www.cnpp.usda.gov/Publications/FoodSupply/Final_FoodSupplyReport_2006.pdf) historical data about the nutrients in the U.S. food supply and trends in Americans' diets. Table 5.1 shows the consumption of macronutrients (nutrients that the body uses in relatively large amounts: carbohydrates, fats, and proteins) in selected years between 1909 and 2006. Trends include:

- An increase of 800 calories per day between 1960–69 and 2006

- An increase of 3.3 ounces (93 g) of carbohydrate per day between 1960–69 and 2006

- An increase of 1.3 ounces (38 g) of fat per day between 1960–69 and 2006

Table 5.2 shows Americans' decreased consumption of whole milk in favor of low-fat milk; increased consumption of cheese and legumes, nuts, and soy; and decreased consumption of grain products. It also documents the shift from butter to margarine use, a decline in total consumption of vegetables, and a dramatic increase in consumption of salad, cooking, and other edible oils.

Dietary Guidelines for Americans

Every five years the *Dietary Guidelines for Americans* are updated and revised to translate the most current scientific knowledge about individual nutrients and food components into dietary recommendations that may be adopted by the public. The recommendations are based on the preponderance of scientific evidence for reducing the risk of chronic disease and promoting health.

According to the U.S. Department of Health and Human Services and the USDA, in *Dietary Guidelines for Americans, 2010* (December 2010, http://health.gov/dietaryguidelines/dga2010/DietaryGuidelines2010.pdf), a

TABLE 5.1

Food energy and macronutrients per capita per day, selected years 1909–2006

Year	Food energy (kilocalories)	Carbohydrate (grams)	Fiber (grams)	Protein (grams)	Fat (grams)	Saturated fatty acids (grams)	Monounsaturated fatty acids (grams)	Polyunsaturated fatty acids (grams)	Cholesterol (milligrams)
1909–19	3,300	484	28	96	117	48	45	13	430
1920–29	3,300	476	26	92	124	52	47	14	460
1930–39	3,200	449	25	89	127	53	48	15	440
1940–49	3,300	428	24	97	135	54	52	17	490
1950–59	3,100	389	20	92	135	52	52	19	490
1960–69	3,100	381	19	93	140	52	54	22	460
1970–79	3,200	395	20	96	143	49	57	27	430
1980–89	3,400	421	22	100	151	50	61	30	420
1990–99	3,600	478	24	108	150	48	64	31	400
2000	3,900	495	24	111	169	52	75	35	410
2001	3,800	490	24	109	169	52	76	35	410
2002	3,900	484	24	110	173	53	78	36	420
2003	3,900	481	24	110	181	55	79	39	420
2004	3,900	481	24	111	181	55	79	38	420
2005	3,900	478	24	109	177	53	77	39	410
2006	3,900	474	25	111	178	54	77	39	420

SOURCE: Hazel A. B. Hiza and Lisa Bente, "Table 1. Food Energy and Macronutrients per Capita per Day in the U.S. Food Supply, Selected Years," in *Nutrient Content of the U.S. Food Supply: Developments between 2000 and 2006*, U.S. Department of Agriculture, Center for Nutrition Policy and Promotion, July 2011, http://www.cnpp.usda.gov/Publications/FoodSupply/Final_FoodSupplyReport_2006.pdf (accessed October 21, 2011).

TABLE 5.2

Food energy contributed from major food groups, selected years 1909–2006

| Year | Meat, poultry, and fish | | | | Dairy products | | | | | Eggs | Legumes nuts, & soy | Grain products |
	Meat	Poultry	Fish	Total	Whole milk	Lowfat milk	Cheese	Other	Total			
							Percent					
1909–19	12.8	0.9	0.6	14.3	5.1	0.8	0.6	2.1	8.6	1.7	2.4	37.9
1920–29	12.4	0.9	0.6	13.9	5.7	0.7	0.7	2.8	9.8	1.8	2.4	32.4
1930–39	12.0	0.9	0.5	13.4	6.0	0.6	0.8	3.3	10.7	1.8	2.8	29.6
1940–49	14.1	1.2	0.5	15.8	7.3	0.6	1.0	3.7	12.5	2.1	3.1	26.7
1950–59	14.9	1.5	0.6	16.9	7.2	0.5	1.3	3.6	12.6	2.4	3.0	22.8
1960–69	15.7	2.2	0.5	18.4	6.2	0.7	1.6	3.2	11.7	2.0	3.1	21.3
1970–79	13.9	2.8	0.6	17.3	4.7	1.4	2.2	2.8	11.0	1.8	3.2	20.3
1980–89	11.8	3.4	0.6	15.8	2.9	1.9	3.0	2.7	10.4	1.5	3.2	22.2
1990–99	8.8	4.2	0.6	13.6	1.7	2.1	3.3	2.7	9.8	1.3	3.1	24.8
2000	8.1	4.5	0.6	13.2	1.4	1.9	3.4	2.2	8.9	1.3	3.0	24.2
2001	8.0	4.4	0.6	13.0	1.4	1.8	3.4	2.2	8.9	1.3	3.0	24.3
2002	8.2	4.5	0.5	13.3	1.3	1.8	3.5	2.2	8.8	1.3	3.1	23.8
2003	8.5	4.5	0.6	13.6	1.3	1.8	3.4	2.2	8.7	1.3	3.1	23.6
2004	8.5	4.6	0.6	13.8	1.2	1.8	3.5	2.3	8.8	1.3	3.1	23.4
2005	8.5	4.8	0.6	13.8	1.2	1.8	3.6	1.4	8.0	1.3	3.1	23.8
2006	8.1	4.8	0.6	13.6	1.2	1.8	3.7	2.0	8.7	1.3	3.2	23.8

| Year | Fruits | | | Vegetables | | | | | Fats and oils | | | | | | Sugars & sweeteners | Misc-laneous |
	Citrus	Non-citrus	Total	White potatoes	Dark green/deep yellow	Tomatoes	Other	Total	Butter	Marg-arine	Short-ening	Lard & beef tallow	Salad, cooking, & other edible oils	Total		
1909–19	0.2	2.6	2.8	3.9	0.7	0.3	1.3	6.3	4.5	0.6	3.1	3.8	0.7	12.7	13.0	0.3
1920–29	0.3	2.7	3.0	3.4	0.7	0.3	1.5	5.9	4.6	0.7	2.7	4.3	1.4	13.7	16.6	0.5
1930–39	0.5	2.6	3.0	3.1	0.8	0.4	1.6	5.8	4.8	0.7	3.5	4.2	2.0	15.2	17.0	0.6
1940–49	0.8	2.4	3.1	2.8	0.7	0.4	1.7	5.6	3.4	1.1	3.2	4.3	2.4	14.5	15.9	0.6
1950–59	0.8	2.3	3.1	2.6	0.5	0.5	1.5	5.1	2.5	2.3	3.9	3.8	3.4	16.0	17.5	0.6
1960–69	0.8	2.0	2.8	2.7	0.4	0.4	1.4	5.0	1.9	2.9	5.2	2.2	4.8	17.0	18.0	0.7
1970–79	1.3	2.0	3.3	2.7	0.4	0.6	1.6	5.2	1.3	3.1	6.0	1.1	6.9	18.5	18.5	0.8
1980–89	1.2	2.3	3.5	2.5	0.3	0.5	1.4	4.9	1.2	2.8	6.6	1.0	8.1	19.9	17.8	0.9
1990–99	1.0	2.3	3.3	2.5	0.3	0.6	1.4	4.8	1.1	2.4	6.8	0.9	8.2	19.4	18.9	1.0
2000	1.0	2.1	3.1	2.4	0.4	0.5	1.2	4.5	1.0	1.7	8.8	1.4	9.3	22.3	18.5	1.0
2001	1.0	2.1	3.1	2.4	0.3	0.5	1.2	4.5	1.0	1.6	9.3	1.2	9.4	22.6	18.4	1.0
2002	0.9	2.1	3.0	2.3	0.3	0.5	1.2	4.3	1.0	1.5	9.5	1.4	9.9	23.3	18.2	1.0
2003	0.9	2.1	3.0	2.4	0.3	0.5	1.2	4.4	1.0	1.2	9.0	1.5	11.3	23.9	17.3	1.0
2004	0.9	2.2	3.0	2.3	0.3	0.5	1.2	4.4	1.0	1.2	8.9	1.4	11.2	23.7	17.4	1.1
2005	0.9	2.2	3.0	2.2	0.3	0.5	1.2	4.3	1.0	0.9	8.2	1.6	12.2	23.9	17.7	1.1
2006	0.8	2.2	3.0	2.2	0.3	0.5	1.2	4.2	1.1	1.1	8.1	1.6	11.9	23.8	17.3	1.1

SOURCE: Hazel A. B. Hiza and Lisa Bente, "Table 4. Food Energy Contributed from Major Food Groups to the U.S. Food Supply, Selected Years," in *Nutrient Content of the U.S. Food Supply: Developments between 2000 and 2006*, U.S. Department of Agriculture, Center for Nutrition Policy and Promotion, July 2011, http://www.cnpp.usda.gov/Publications/FoodSupply/Final_FoodSupplyReport_2006.pdf (accessed October 21, 2011)

healthy diet includes plenty of fruits, vegetables, whole grains, and fat-free or low-fat milk and milk products, as well as lean meats, poultry, fish, beans, eggs, and nuts. A healthy diet is also low in saturated fats, trans fats (artificial fats created through the hydrogenation of oils, which solidifies the oil and limits the body's ability to regulate cholesterol), cholesterol, salt, and added sugars. Table 5.3 shows the recommended proportions of carbohydrate, protein, and fat for children, adolescents, and adults. Specific recommendations stipulate that fewer than 10% of calories should come from saturated fatty acids, and trans fatty acids, which are considered to be the most harmful to health, should be avoided. Cholesterol intake should be less than 300 milligrams per day. Total fat intake should not exceed 20% to 35% of calories. Preferred fat sources are fish, nuts, and vegetable oils containing polyunsaturated and monounsaturated

TABLE 5.3

Recommended proportions of carbohydrate, protein, and fat, by age group, 2010

	Carbohydrate	Protein	Fat
Young children (1–3 years)	45–65%	5–20%	30–40%
Older children and adolescents (4–18 years)	45–65%	10–30%	25–35%
Adults (19 years and older)	45–65%	10–35%	20–35%

SOURCE: "Table 2-4. Recommended Macronutrient Proportions by Age," in *Dietary Guidelines for Americans, 2010*, 7th ed., U.S. Department of Health and Human Services and U.S. Department of Agriculture, December 2010, http://health.gov/dietaryguidelines/dga2010/dietaryguidelines2010.pdf (accessed October 21, 2011)

fatty acids. Lean, low-fat, or fat-free meats, poultry, dry beans, and milk or milk products are preferable to full-fat foods. Daily sodium intake should be 2,300 milligrams or less for people to age 51 and 1,500 milligrams or less for older adults, African-Americans, and people with diabetes, hypertension, or chronic kidney disease.

In general, the guidelines encourage most Americans to eat fewer calories, increase their physical activity, and choose nutrient-dense foods. They advocate increased consumption of fruits, vegetables, whole grains, and fat-free or low-fat milk and milk products. For example, two cups of fruit and two and a half cups of vegetables per day are recommended for a 2,000-calorie diet, along with three or more servings of whole-grain products per day and three cups per day of fat-free or low-fat milk or equivalent milk products. The guidelines also advise consuming at least half of all grains as whole grains and increasing seafood consumption by replacing some meat and poultry with seafood. Figure 5.1 shows three ways to ensure that at least half of all grains consumed are whole grains.

Table 5.4 compares four eating patterns: the typical American adult diet, the Mediterranean diet, the USDA Dietary Approaches to Stop Hypertension eating plan, and the USDA-recommended food pattern. Compared with the typical American adult diet, the other eating patterns contain greater quantities of vegetables, fruits, beans and peas, whole grains, fat-free and low-fat milk and milk products, and oils and smaller amounts of solid fats, added sugars, and sodium. The other eating patterns also emphasize less red and processed meat and more seafood than the typical American adult diet. Table 5.5 shows the amounts of various food groups that are recommended each day or each week at calorie levels ranging from 1,000 to 3,200.

The guidelines specifically address weight management by advising Americans to "maintain calorie balance over time to achieve and sustain a healthy weight" and to "focus on consuming nutrient-dense foods and beverages." For people who are overweight, the guidelines advise gradual, steady weight loss by decreasing caloric consumption while maintaining sufficient nutrients and increasing physical activity. Parents of overweight children are counseled to reduce the rate of weight gain while children grow and develop and to consult a health care provider before placing children on weight-reduction diets. Women are encouraged to achieve and maintain a healthy weight before becoming pregnant.

In an effort to expand on the guidelines and improve their utility, in 2011 the USDA debuted a new, simple graphic food icon called MyPlate to offer Americans a simple representation of how to construct a healthful meal and diet. (See Figure 5.2.) A full discussion of MyPlate, along with the opinions of supporters and critics of the new icon, is presented in Chapter 10.

FIGURE 5.1

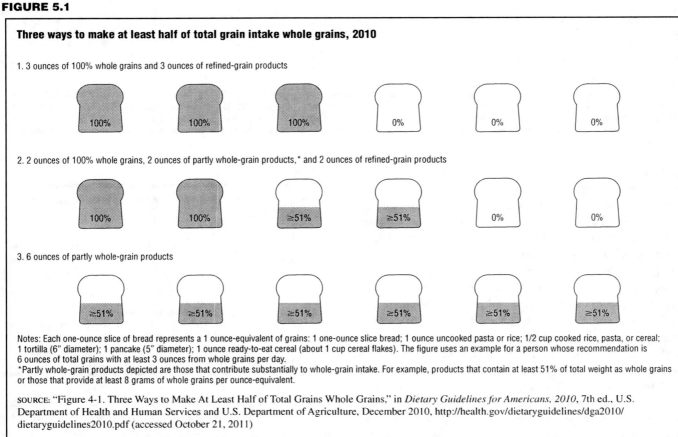

Three ways to make at least half of total grain intake whole grains, 2010

1. 3 ounces of 100% whole grains and 3 ounces of refined-grain products

2. 2 ounces of 100% whole grains, 2 ounces of partly whole-grain products,* and 2 ounces of refined-grain products

3. 6 ounces of partly whole-grain products

Notes: Each one-ounce slice of bread represents a 1 ounce-equivalent of grains: 1 one-ounce slice bread; 1 ounce uncooked pasta or rice; 1/2 cup cooked rice, pasta, or cereal; 1 tortilla (6" diameter); 1 pancake (5" diameter); 1 ounce ready-to-eat cereal (about 1 cup cereal flakes). The figure uses an example for a person whose recommendation is 6 ounces of total grains with at least 3 ounces from whole grains per day.
*Partly whole-grain products depicted are those that contribute substantially to whole-grain intake. For example, products that contain at least 51% of total weight as whole grains or those that provide at least 8 grams of whole grains per ounce-equivalent.

SOURCE: "Figure 4-1. Three Ways to Make At Least Half of Total Grains Whole Grains," in *Dietary Guidelines for Americans, 2010*, 7th ed., U.S. Department of Health and Human Services and U.S. Department of Agriculture, December 2010, http://health.gov/dietaryguidelines/dga2010/dietaryguidelines2010.pdf (accessed October 21, 2011)

TABLE 5.4

Comparison of typical U.S. intake, Mediterranean diet, DASH diet and USDA recommended food intake, 2010

Pattern	Usual U.S. intake adults[a]	Mediterranean patterns Greece (G) Spain (S)	DASH	USDA food pattern
Food groups				
Vegetables: total (c)	1.6	1.2 (S)–4.1 (G)	2.1	2.5
Dark-green (c)	0.1	nd[b]	nd	0.2
Beans and peas (c)	0.1	<0.1 (G)–0.4 (S)	See protein foods	0.2
Red and orange (c)	0.4	nd	nd	0.8
Other (c)	0.5	nd	nd	0.6
Starchy (c)	0.5	nd–0.6 (G)	nd	0.7
Fruit and juices (c)	1.0	1.4 (S)–2.5 (G) (including nuts)	2.5	2.0
Grains: total (oz)	6.4	2.0 (S)–5.4 (G)	7.3	6.0
Whole grains (oz)	0.6	nd	3.9	≥3.0
Milk and milk products (Dairy products) (c)	1.5	1.0 (G)–2.1 (S)	2.6	3.0
Protein foods:				
Meat (oz)	2.5	3.5 (G)–3.6 (S) (including poultry)	1.4	1.8
Poultry (oz)	1.2	nd	1.7	1.5
Eggs (oz)	0.4	nd–1.9 (S)	nd	0.4
Fish/seafood (oz)	0.5	0.8 (G)–2.4 (S)	1.4	1.2
Beans and peas (oz)	See vegetables	See vegetables	0.4 (0.1 c)	See vegetables
Nuts, seeds, and soy products (oz)	0.5	See fruits	0.9	0.6
Oils (g)	18.0	19 (S)–40 (G)	25	27
Solid fats (g)	43.0	nd	nd	16[c]
Added sugars (g)	79.0	nd–24 (G)	12	32[c]
Alcohol (g)	9.9	7.1 (S)–7.9 (G)	nd	nd[d]

[a]1 day mean intakes for adult males and females, adjusted to 2,000 calories and averaged.
[b]nd = Not determined.
[c]Amounts of solid fats and added sugars are examples only of how calories from solid fats and added sugars in the USDA Food Patterns could be divided.
[d]In the USDA Food Patterns, some of the calories assigned to limits for solid fats and added sugars may be used for alcohol consumption instead.
DASH = Dietary Approaches to Stop Hypertension. USDA = United States Department of Agriculture.

SOURCE: "Table 5-1. Eating Pattern Comparison: Usual U.S.. Intake, Mediterranean, DASH, and USDA Food Patterns, Average Daily Intake at or Adjusted to a 2,000 Calorie Level," in *Dietary Guidelines for Americans, 2010*, 7th ed., U.S. Department of Health and Human Services and U.S. Department of Agriculture, December 2010, http://health.gov/dietaryguidelines/dga2010/dietaryguidelines2010.pdf (accessed October 21, 2011)

HOW WEIGHT-LOSS DIETS WORK

Research demonstrates that weight loss is associated with the length of the diet, the pre-diet weight (people who are more overweight tend to lose more weight, more quickly than those who are only mildly overweight), and the number of calories consumed. Any diet that restricts caloric intake such that calories consumed are less than those expended will promote short-term weight loss. The key to weight loss through diet is adherence—if people do not stick to their diet, then they will not lose weight. More than a century ago, Banting, in describing the benefits of his low-carbohydrate diet, wrote that "the great charms and comfort of this system are that its effects are palpable within a week of trial and creates a natural stimulus to persevere for a few weeks more."

The successes achieved using regimens that restrict dieters to a single food or food group such as grapefruit, pineapple, or cabbage are probably in part attributable to the human hankering for variety. When limited to just one food, most dieters experience boredom—there is just no appeal to eating the same food at every meal, for days on end, so naturally less food is consumed. In addition, these diets generally rely on low-calorie foods, so that even if dieters were inspired to consume 15 grapefruits per day, their total daily caloric consumption would be about 1,200 calories, which is sufficient to produce weight loss for most overweight people. Similarly, diets that involve stringent portion control effectively reduce calories to produce weight loss.

Low-Calorie Diets

Traditional dietary therapy for weight loss generally seeks to create a deficit of 500 to 1,000 calories per day with the intent of promoting weight loss of between 1 to 2 pounds (0.5 to 0.9 kg) per week. Low-calorie diets for men usually range from 1,200 to 1,600 calories per day; for women, low-calorie diets contain between 1,000 and 1,200 calories per day. (See Table 5.5 for examples of the recommended percentages of nutrients in low-calorie diets.)

The most successful low-calorie diets take individual food preferences into account to custom-tailor the diet. Table 5.6 and Table 5.7 show examples of how traditional American cuisine may be used to create a low-calorie diet containing 1,200 and 1,600 calories per day, respectively. Table 5.8 incorporates regional southern cuisine into a reduced-calorie diet. Table 5.9 illustrates how Asian-American cuisine may be adapted to 1,200- and 1,600-calorie-per-day diets, and Table 5.10 shows how Mexican-American cuisine may be adapted for low-calorie diets. Table 5.11 is a sample of a reduced-calorie

TABLE 5.5

Recommended intake amounts at various calorie levels

For each food group or subgroup[a], recommended average daily intake amounts[b] at all calorie levels. Recommended intakes from vegetable and protein foods subgroups are per week.

Calorie level of pattern[c]	1,000	1,200	1,400	1,600	1,800	2,000	2,200	2,400	2,600	2,800	3,000	3,200
Fruits	1 c	1 c	1 1/2 c	1 1/2 c	1 1/2 c	2 c	2 c	2 c	2 c	2 1/2 c	2 1/2 c	2 1/2 c
Vegetables[d]	1 c	1 1/2 c	1 1/2 c	2 c	2 1/2 c	2 1/2 c	3 c	3 c	31/2 c	31/2 c	4 c	4 c
Dark-green vegetables	1/2 c/wk	1 c/wk	1 c/wk	1 1/2 c/wk	1 1/2 c/wk	1 1/2 c/wk	2 c/wk	2 c/wk	2 1/2 c/wk	2 1/2 c/wk	2 1/2 c/wk	2 1/2 c/wk
Red and orange vegetables	2 1/2 c/wk	3 c/wk	3 c/wk	4 c/wk	5 1/2 c/wk	5 1/2 c/wk	6 c/wk	6 c/wk	7 c/wk	7 c/wk	7 1/2 c/wk	7 1/2 c/wk
Beans and peas (legumes)	1/2 c/wk	1/2 c/wk	1/2 c/wk	1 c/wk	1 1/2 c/wk	1 1/2 c/wk	2 c/wk	2 c/wk	2 1/2 c/wk	2 1/2 c/wk	3 c/wk	3 c/wk
Starchy vegetables	2 c/wk	3 1/2 c/wk	3 1/2 c/wk	4 c/wk	5 c/wk	5 c/wk	5 c/wk	5 c/wk	7 c/wk	7 c/wk	8 c/wk	8 c/wk
Other vegetables[e]	1 1/2 c/wk	2 1/2 c/wk	2 1/2 c/wk	3 1/2 c/wk	4 c/wk	4 c/wk	5 c/wk	5 c/wk	5 1/2 c/wk	5 1/2 c/wk	7 c/wk	7 c/wk
Grains	3 oz-eq	4 oz-eq	5 oz-eq	5 oz-eq	6 oz-eq	6 oz-eq	7 oz-eq	8 oz-eq	9 oz-eq	10 oz-eq	10 oz-eq	10 oz-eq
Whole grains	1 1/2 oz-eq	2 oz-eq	2 1/2 oz-eq	3 oz-eq	3 oz-eq	3 oz-eq	3 1/2 oz-eq	4 oz-eq	4 1/2 oz-eq	5 oz-eq	5 oz-eq	5 oz-eq
Enriched grains	1 1/2 oz-eq	2 oz-eq	2 1/2 oz-eq	2 oz-eq	3 oz-eq	3 oz-eq	3 1/2 oz-eq	4 oz-eq	4 1/2 oz-eq	5 oz-eq	5 oz-eq	5 oz-eq
Protein foods[d]	2 oz-eq	3 oz-eq	4 oz-eq	5 oz-eq	5 oz-eq	5 1/2 oz-eq	6 oz-eq	6 1/2 oz-eq	6 1/2 oz-eq	7 oz-eq	7 oz-eq	7 oz-eq
Seafood	3 oz/wk	5 oz/wk	6 oz/wk	8 oz/wk	8 oz/wk	8 oz/wk	9 oz/wk	10 oz/wk	10 oz/wk	11 oz/wk	11 oz/wk	11 oz/wk
Meat, poultry, eggs	10 oz/wk	14 oz/wk	19 oz/wk	24 oz/wk	24 oz/wk	26 oz/wk	29 oz/wk	31 oz/wk	31 oz/wk	34 oz/wk	34 oz/wk	34 oz/wk
Nuts, seeds, soy products	1 oz/wk	2 oz/wk	3 oz/wk	4 oz/wk	4 oz/wk	4 oz/wk	4 oz/wk	5 oz/wk	5 oz/wk	5 oz/wk	5 oz/wk	5 oz/wk
Dairy[f]	2 c	2 1/2 c	2 1/2 c	3 c	3 c	3 c	3 c	3 c	3 c	3 c	3 c	3 c
Oils[g]	15 g	17 g	17 g	22 g	24 g	27 g	29 g	31 g	34 g	36 g	44 g	51 g
Maximum SoFAS[h] limit, Calories (% of calories)	137 (14%)	121 (10%)	121 (9%)	121 (8%)	161 (9%)	258 (13%)	266 (12%)	330 (14%)	362 (14%)	395 (14%)	459 (15%)	596 (19%)

[a] All foods are assumed to be in nutrient-dense forms, lean or low-fat and prepared without added fats, sugars, or salt. Solid fats and added sugars may be included up to the daily maximum limit identified in the table. Food items in each group and subgroup are:

Fruits — All fresh, frozen, canned, and dried fruits and fruit juices: for example, oranges and orange juice, apples and apple juice, bananas, grapes, melons, berries, raisins.

Vegetables
- Dark-green vegetables — All fresh, frozen, and canned dark-green leafy vegetables and broccoli, cooked or raw: for example, broccoli; spinach; romaine; collard, turnip, and mustard greens.
- Red and orange vegetables — All fresh, frozen, and canned red and orange vegetables, cooked or raw: for example, tomatoes, red peppers, carrots, sweet potatoes, winter squash, and pumpkin.
- Beans and peas (legumes) — All cooked beans and peas: for example, kidney beans, lentils, chickpeas, and pinto beans. Does not include green beans or green peas. (See additional comment under protein foods group.)
- Starchy vegetables — All fresh, frozen, and canned starchy vegetables: for example, white potatoes, corn, green peas.
- Other vegetables — All fresh, frozen, and canned other vegetables, cooked or raw: for example, iceberg lettuce, green beans, and onions.

Grains
- Whole grains — All whole-grain products and whole grains used as ingredients: for example, whole-wheat bread, whole-grain cereals and crackers, oatmeal, and brown rice.
- Enriched grains — All enriched refined-grain products and enriched refined grains used as ingredients: for example, white breads, enriched grain cereals and crackers, enriched pasta, white rice.

Protein foods — All meat, poultry, seafood, eggs, nuts, seeds, and processed soy products. Meat and poultry should be lean or low-fat and nuts should be unsalted. Beans and peas are considered part of this group as well as the vegetable group, but should be counted in one group only.

Dairy — All milks, including lactose-free and lactose-reduced products and fortiied soy beverages, yogurts, frozen yogurts, dairy desserts, and cheeses. Most choices should be fat-free or low-fat. Cream, sour cream, and cream cheese are not included due to their low calcium content.

[b] Food group amounts are shown in cup (c) or ounce-equivalents (oz-eq). Oils are shown in grams (g). Quantity equivalents for each food group are:
- Grains, 1 ounce-equivalent is: 1 one-ounce slice bread; 1 ounce uncooked pasta or rice 1/2 cup cooked rice, pasta, or cereal; 1 tortilla (6" diameter); 1 pancake (5" diameter); 1 ounce ready-to-eat cereal (about 1 cup cereal flakes).
- Vegetables and fruits, 1 cup equivalent is: 1 cup raw or cooked vegetable or fruit 1/2 cup dried vegetable or fruit; 1 cup vegetable or fruit juice; 2 cups leafy salad greens.
- Protein foods, 1 ounce-equivalent is: 1 ounce lean meat, poultry, seafood; 1 egg; 1 Tbsp peanut butter 1/2 ounce nuts or seeds. Also, 1/4 cup cooked beans or peas may also be counted as 1 ounce-equivalent
- Dairy, 1 cup equivalent is: 1 cup milk, fortified soy beverage, or yogurt; 1/2 ounces natural cheese (e.g., cheddar); 2 ounces of processed cheese (e.g., American).

[c] Food intake patterns at 1,000, 1,200, and 1,400 calories meet the nutritional needs of children ages 2 to 8 years. Patterns from 1,600 to 3,200 calories meet the nutritional needs of children ages 9 years and older and adults. If a child ages 4 to 8 years needs more calories and, therefore, is following a pattern at 1,600 calories or more, the recommended amount from the dairy group can be 2 1/2 cups per day. Children ages 9 years and older and adults should not use the 1,000, 1,200, or 1,400 calorie patterns.

[d] Vegetable and protein foods subgroup amounts are shown in this table as weekly amounts, because it would be dificult for consumers to select foods from all subgroups daily.

[e] Whole-grain subgroup amounts shown in this table are minimums. More whole grains up to all of the grains recommended may be selected, with offsetting decreases in the amounts of enriched refined grains.

[f] The amount of dairy foods in the 1,200 and 1,400 calorie patterns have increased to relect new RDAs for calcium that are higher than previous recommendations for children ages 4 to 8 years.

[g] Oils and soft margarines include vegetable, nut, and fish oils and soft vegetable oil table spreads that have notrans fats.

[h] SoFAS are calories from solid fats and added sugars. The limit for SoFAS is the remaining amount of calories in each food pattern after selecting the speciied amounts in each food group in nutrient-dense forms (forms that are fat-free or low-fat and with no added sugars). The number of SoFAS is lower in the 1,200, 1,400, and 1,600 calorie patterns than in the 1,000 calorie pattern. The nutrient goals for the 1,200 to 1,600 calorie patterns are higher and require that more calories be used for nutrient-dense foods from the food groups.

SOURCE: "Appendix 7. USDA Food Patterns," in *Dietary Guidelines for Americans, 2010*, 7th ed., U.S. Department of Health and Human Services and U.S. Department of Agriculture, December 2010, http://health.gov/dietaryguidelines/dga2010/dietaryguidelines2010.pdf (accessed October 21, 2011)

FIGURE 5.2

MyPlate aims to help consumers plan healthful meals

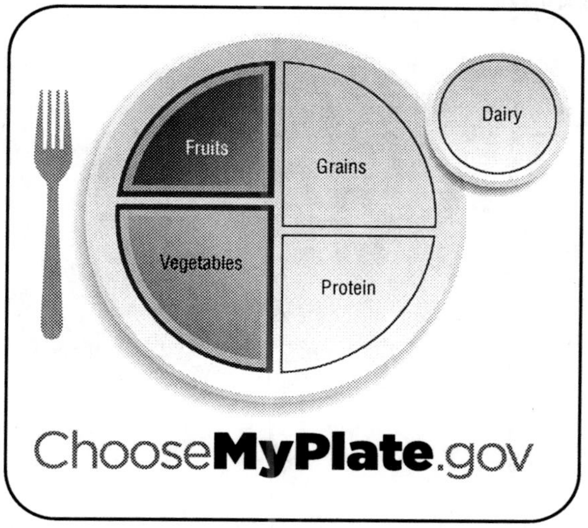

Fruits

Grains

Dairy

Vegetables

Protein

ChooseMyPlate.gov

SOURCE: "MyPlate," in *News and Media* U.S. Department of Agriculture, September 19, 2011, http://www.choosemyplate.gov/images/MyPlateImages/halfplate/PDF/myplate_grayscale_half.pdf (accessed October 21, 2011)

diet that vegetarians who eat milk and eggs but no meat or fish can use to lose weight. Food exchanges, such as those shown in Table 5.12, enable dieters to enjoy a variety of foods in their reduced-calorie meals, which can prevent boredom and the tendency to abandon the diet.

Research reveals that reducing fat in the diet is an effective way to reduce calories and that when low-calorie diets are combined with low-fat diets, better weight loss is achieved than through calorie reduction alone. Furthermore, even though very-low-calorie diets that provide about 500 calories per day have been demonstrated to produce greater initial weight loss than low-calorie diets, the long-term weight loss is not different between the two regimens.

Low-Carbohydrate Diets

During the first decade of the 21st century several rigorous research studies reported that low-carbohydrate diets were as effective, or even more effective, in producing short-term weight loss than low-fat diets. The low-carbohydrate diets owed much of their success to adherence—dieters were better able to stick with their diets, and as a result achieved better results. Another hypothesis about the success of low-carbohydrate regimens is that dieters do not feel as hungry as they do on other diets because protein is the most satisfying of the three macronutrients: carbohydrates, fats, and proteins.

The scientific premise of low-carbohydrate diets is that consuming certain carbohydrates can cause surges in blood sugar and insulin that not only stimulate appetite and weight gain but may also increase the risk for diabetes and heart disease. At first, low-carbohydrate diets viewed all carbohydrates as equally harmful. Increasingly, however, low-carbohydrate diets distinguished between simple and complex carbohydrates, which contain simple (single or double) or complex (three or more) sugars.

Examples of single sugars from foods include fructose, which is found in fruits, and galactose, which is found in milk products. Double sugars include lactose in dairy products; maltose, which is found in certain vegetables and in beer; and sucrose (table sugar). Examples of complex carbohydrates, which are often referred to as starches, include breads, cereals, legumes, brown rice, and pastas. Simple carbohydrates occur naturally in fruits, milk products, and vegetables and, like complex carbohydrates, contain vitamins and minerals, which distinguishes them from the refined simple sugars many nutritionists advise against (or at least recommend limiting in the diet). The simple carbohydrates most nutritionists call "empty calories" are the processed and refined sugars found in candy, table sugar, and sodas, as well as in foods such as white flour and polished white rice.

Besides distinguishing between simple and complex carbohydrates, low-carbohydrate regimens rely on a measure known as the glycemic index (GI), which ranks foods based on how rapidly their consumption raises blood glucose levels. The GI measures how much blood sugar increases over a period of two or three hours after a meal. Carbohydrate foods that break down quickly during digestion have the highest GI. The GI may be used to determine if a particular food will trigger the problematical "carbohydrate–blood sugar–insulin cascade." High-GI foods are those that are rapidly digested and absorbed or transformed metabolically into glucose.

Examples of foods with GI scores of 70 or above are cake, cookies, doughnuts, honey, french fries, rice, baked potato, and white bread. In contrast, lentils have a GI of 29, whereas broccoli, peanuts, and spinach have GIs of less than 15. Carbohydrates that break down slowly, such as whole-grain breads and cereals, beans, leafy greens, or cruciferous vegetables (which include mustard greens, cabbage, broccoli, cauliflower, kale, and brussels sprouts), generate slower glucose release into the bloodstream and lower GI scores—50 or less. Eating low-GI foods supports weight loss by enhancing satiety and thereby decreasing total food consumption.

The measurement of GI is a relatively recent practice. It began during the 1990s, following the discovery that specific carbohydrates such as potatoes and cornflakes raised blood sugar faster than others such as brown rice and oatmeal. Harvard University School of Public Health researchers used GI to calculate glycemic load—a measure that considers the food's GI and the amount of

TABLE 5.6

Sample reduced calorie menus, traditional American cuisine—1,200 calories

	Calories	Fat (grams)	% Fat	Exchange for
Breakfast				
• Whole wheat bread, 1 medium slice	70	1.2	15	(1 bread/starch)
• Jelly, regular, 2 tsp	30	0	0	(1/2 fruit)
• Cereal, shredded wheat, 1/2 cup	104	1	4	(1 bread/starch)
• Milk, 1%, 1 cup	102	3	23	(1 milk)
• Orange juice, 3/4 cup	78	0	0	(1 1/2 fruit)
• Coffee, regular, 1 cup	5	0	0	(free)
Breakfast total	**389**	**5.2**	**10**	
Lunch				
• Roast beef sandwich:				
Whole wheat bread, 2 medium slices	139	2.4	15	(2 bread/starch)
Lean roast beef, unseasoned, 2 oz	60	1.5	23	(2 lean protein)
Lettuce, 1 leaf	1	0	0	(1 vegetable)
Tomato, 3 medium slices	10	0	0	
Mayonnaise, low calorie, 1 tsp	15	1.7	96	(1/3 fat)
• Apple, 1 medium	80	0	0	(1 fruit)
• Water, 1 cup	0	0	0	(free)
Lunch total	**305**	**5.6**	**16**	
Dinner				
• Salmon, 2 ounces edible	103	5	44	(2 lean protein)
• Vegetable oil, 1 1/2 tsp	60	7	100	(1 1/2 fat)
• Baked potato, 3/4 medium	100	0	0	(1 bread/starch)
• Margarine, 1 tsp	34	4	100	(1 fat)
• Green beans, seasoned, with margarine, 1/2 cup	52	2	4	(1 vegetable) (1/2 fat)
• Carrots, seasoned	35	0	0	(1 vegetable)
• White dinner roll, 1 small	70	2	28	(1 bread/starch)
• Iced tea, unsweetened, 1 cup	0	0	0	(free)
• Water, 2 cups	0	0	0	(free)
Dinner total	**454**	**20**	**39**	
Snack				
• Popcorn, 2 1/2 cups	69	0	0	(1 bread/starch)
• Margarine, 3/4 tsp	30	3	100	(3/4 fat)
Total	**1,247**	**34–36**	**24–26**	

Calories	1,247	Saturated fat, % kcals	7	
Total carbohydrate, % kcals	58	Cholesterol, mg	96	
Total fat, % kcals	26	Protein, % kcals	19	
*Sodium, mg	1,043			

Note: Calories have been rounded. Kcal = kilo calorie.
1,200: 100% RDA met for all nutrients except vitamin E 80%, vitamin B$_2$ 96%, vitamin B$_6$ 94%, calcium 68%, iron 63%, and zinc 73%.
*No salt added in recipe preparation or as seasoning. Consume at least 32 ounces of water.

SOURCE: "Appendix D. Traditional American Cuisine—1,200 Calories," in *The Practical Guide: Identification, Evaluation, and Treatment of Overweight and Obesity in Adults*, National Institutes of Health, National Heart, Lung, and Blood Institute, North American Association for the Study of Obesity, October 2000, http://www.nhlbi.nih.gov/guidelines/obesity/prctgd_b.pdf (accessed October 21, 2011).

carbohydrates contained in a single serving. For example, many whole fruits, vegetables, and grains have low glycemic loads, which when consumed prompt a moderate rise in blood glucose and insulin. When the same fruits, vegetables, and grains are squeezed or pulverized into juice or flour, their glycemic load increases—effectively rendering them with the same high glycemic load of sugar water.

After consuming a meal with a high glycemic load, blood sugar rises higher and faster than it does after eating a meal with a low glycemic load. In an effort to recover from the resulting peaks and plummets, the brain transmits a hunger signal long before the next meal is due. Wildly fluctuating blood sugar and insulin may result in overeating, which in turn causes overweight.

For people who are overweight or physically inactive, another potential danger of consuming foods with high glycemic loads is that they may already be insulin resistant, and the overexertion of insulin-producing cells in the pancreas that is required to metabolize the high glycemic loads may ultimately exhaust their insulin-producing cells, leading to diabetes.

Weight-loss diets based on the GI emphasize sharply restricting high-index foods and consuming primarily low-index foods. The proponents of low-carbohydrate, low-GI food diets observe that consuming foods with low glycemic loads stabilizes blood sugar and insulin to prevent the fluctuations that can cause overeating and may increase the risk for diabetes. They also assert that reliance on low-fat diets inadvertently led to diets that

TABLE 5.7

Sample reduced calorie menus, traditional American cuisine—1,600 calories

	Calories	Fat (grams)	% Fat	Exchange for
Breakfast				
• Whole wheat bread, 1 medium slice	70	1.2	15.4	(1 bread/starch)
• Jelly, regular, 2 tsp	30	0	0	(1/2 fruit)
• Cereal, shredded wheat, 1 cup	207	2	8	(2 bread/starch)
• Milk, 1%, 1 cup	102	3	23	(1 milk)
• Orange juice, 3/4 cup	18	0	0	(1 1/2 fruit)
• Coffee, regular, 1 cup	5	0	0	(free)
• Milk, 1%, 1 oz	10	0.3	27	(1/8 milk)
Breakfast total	**502**	**6.5**	**10**	
Lunch				
• Roast beef sandwich:				
Whole wheat bread, 2 medium slices	139	2.4	15	(2 bread/starch)
Lean roast beef, unseasoned, 2 oz	60	1.5	23	(2 lean protein)
American cheese, low fat and low sodium, 1 slice, 3/4 oz	46	1.8	36	(1 lean protein)
Lettuce, 1 leaf	1	1	0	
Tomato, 3 medium slices	10	0	0	(1 vegetable)
Mayonnaise, low calorie, 2 tsp	30	3.3	99	(2/3 fat)
• Apple, 1 medium	8	0	0	(1 fruit)
• Water, 1 cup	0	0	0	(free)
Lunch total	**366**	**9**	**22**	
Dinner				
• Salmon, 3 ounces edible	155	7	40	(3 lean protein)
• Vegetable oil, 1 1/2 tsp	60	7	100	(1 1/2 fat)
• Baked potato, 3/4 medium	100	0	0	(1 bread/starch)
• Margarine, 1 tsp	34	4	100	(1 fat)
• Green beans, seasoned, with margarine, 1/2 cup	52	2	4	(1 vegetable) (1/2 fat)
• Carrots, seasoned, with margarine, 1/2 cup	52	2	4	(1 vegetable) (1/2 fat)
• White dinner roll, 1 medium	80	3	33	(1 bread/starch)
• Ice milk, 1/2 cup	92	3	28	(1 bread/starch) (1/2 fat)
• Iced tea, unsweetened, 1 cup	0	0	0	(free)
• Water, 2 cups	0	0	0	(free)
Dinner total	**625**	**28**	**38**	
Snack				
• Popcorn, 2 1/2 cups	69	0	0	(1 bread/starch)
• Margarine, 1/2 tsp	58	6.5	100	(1 1/2 fat)
Total	**1,613**	**50**	**28**	

Calories	1,613	Saturated fat, % kcals	8	
Total carbohydrate, % kcals	55	Cholesterol, mg	142	
Total fat, % kcals	29	Protein, % kcals	19	
*Sodium, mg	1,341			

Note: Calories have been rounded. Kcal = kilo calorie.
1,600: 100% RDA met for all nutrients except vitamin E 99%, iron 73%, and zinc 91%.
No salt added in recipe preparation or as seasoning. Consume at least 32 ounces of water.

SOURCE: "Appendix D. Traditional American Cuisine—1,600 Calories," in *The Practical Guide: Identification, Evaluation, and Treatment of Overweight and Obesity in Adults*, National Institutes of Health, National Heart, Lung, and Blood Institute, North American Association for the Study of Obesity, October 2000, http://www.nhlbi.nih.gov/guidelines/obesity/prctgd_b.pdf (accessed October 21, 2011).

were high in simple carbohydrates and indirectly promoted the observed increase in overweight and diabetes in the United States.

Low-Fat Diets

Low-fat diets reduce caloric intake by reducing fat consumption. Fat has 9 calories per gram, whereas protein and carbohydrates have 4 calories per gram. These diets rely on the high-fiber content of complex carbohydrates to satisfy dieters. High-fiber foods also slow the absorption of carbohydrates, so they do not provoke a rapid rise in blood sugar and insulin.

Table 5.13 shows some of the food substitutions that may be made to reduce the dietary fat content. Besides making substitutions, many fat-free or low-fat food products are available—from fat-free frozen desserts to reduced-fat peanut butter. However, dieters are often cautioned that fat-free or reduced-fat foods are not calorie-free and that their consumption will not result in weight loss when more of the reduced-fat foods are consumed than would be eaten of the full-fat versions. For example, eating twice as many baked tortilla chips would actually result in higher caloric intake than a single serving of regular tortilla chips. (See Table 5.14.)

Low-Fat versus Low-Carbohydrate Diets

In the absence of rigorous scientific research and studies demonstrating the long-term safety and effectiveness

TABLE 5.8

Sample reduced calorie menus, southern cuisine

	1,600 calories	1,200 calories
Breakfast		
• Oatmeal, prepared with 1% milk, low fat	1/2 cup	1/2 cup
• Milk, 1%, low fat	1/2 cup	1/2 cup
• English muffin	1 medium	—
• Cream cheese, light, 18% fat	1 T	—
• Orange juice	3/4 cup	1/2 cup
• Coffee	1 cup	1 cup
• Milk, 1%, low fat	1 oz	1 oz
Lunch		
• Baked chicken, without skin	2 oz	2 oz
• Vegetable oil	1 tsp	1/2 tsp
• Salad:		
Lettuce	1/2 cup	1/2 cup
Tomato	1/2 cup	1/2 cup
Cucumber	1/2 cup	1/2 cup
• Oil and vinegar dressing	2 tsp	1 tsp
• White rice	1/2 cup	1/4 cup
• Margarine, diet	1/2 tsp	1/2 tsp
• Baking powder biscuit, prepared with vegetable oil	1 small	1/2 small
• Margarine	1 tsp	1 tsp
• Water	1 cup	1 cup
Dinner		
• Lean roast beef	3 oz	2 oz
• Onion	1/4 cup	1/4 cup
• Beef gravy, water-based	1 T	1 T
• Turnip greens	1/2 cup	1/2 cup
• Margarine, diet	1/2 tsp	1/2 tsp
• Sweet potato, baked	1 small	1 small
• Margarine, diet	1/2 tsp	1/4 tsp
• Ground cinnamon	1 tsp	1 tsp
• Brown sugar	1 tsp	1 tsp
• Corn bread prepared with margarine, diet	1/2 medium slice	1/2 medium slice
• Honeydew melon	1/4 medium	1/8 medium
• Iced tea, sweetened with sugar	1 cup	1 cup
Snack		
• Saltine crackers, unsalted tops	4 crackers	4 crackers
• Mozzarella cheese, part skim, low sodium	1 oz	1 oz

Calories	1,653	Calories	1,225
Total carbohydrate, % kcals	53	Total carbohydrate, % kcals	50
Total fat, % kcals	28	Total fat, % kcals	31
*Sodium, mg	1,231	*Sodium, mg	867
Saturated fat, % kcals	8	Saturated fat, % kcals	9
Cholesterol, mg	172	Cholesterol, mg	142
Protein, % kcals	20	Protein, % kcals	21

1,600: 100% RDA met for all nutrients except vitamin E 97%, magnesium 98%, iron 78%, and zinc 90%.
1,200: 100% RDA met for all nutrients except vitamin E 82%, vitamin B₁ & B₂ 95%, vitamin B₃ 99%, vitamin B₆ 88%, magnesium 83%, iron 56%, and zinc 70%.
*No salt added in recipe preparation or as seasoning. Consume at least 32 ounces of water.
Kcal = kilo calorie.

SOURCE: "Appendix D. Southern Cuisine—Reduced Calorie," in *The Practical Guide: Identification, Evaluation, and Treatment of Overweight and Obesity in Adults*, National Institutes of Health, National Heart, Lung, and Blood Institute, North American Association for the Study of Obesity, October 2000, http://www.nhlbi.nih.gov/guidelines/obesity/prctgd_b.pdf (accessed October 21, 2011)

TABLE 5.9

Sample reduced calorie menus, Asian-American cuisine

	1,600 calories	1,200 calories
Breakfast		
• Banana	1 small	1 small
• Whole wheat bread	2 slices	1 slice
• Margarine	1 tsp	1 tsp
• Orange juice	3/4 tsp	3/4 tsp
• Milk 1%, low fat	3/4 cup	3/4 cup
Lunch		
• Beef noodle soup, canned, low sodium	1/2 cup	1/2 cup
• Chinese noodle and beef salad:		
Roast beef	3 oz	2 oz
Peanut oil	1 1/2 tsp	1 tsp
Soya sauce, low sodium	tsp	1 tsp
Carrots	1/2 cup	1/2 cup
Zucchini	1/2 cup	1/2 cup
Onion	1/4 cup	1/4 cup
Chinese noodles, soft type	1/4 cup	1/4 cup
• Apple	1 medium	1 medium
• Tea, unsweetened	1 cup	1 cup
Dinner		
• Pork stir-fry with vegetables:		
Pork cutlet	2 oz	2 oz
Peanut oil	1 tsp	1 tsp
Soya sauce, low sodium	1 tsp	1 tsp
Broccoli	1/2 cup	1/2 cup
Carrots	1 cup	1 cup
Mushrooms	1/4 cup	1/2 cup
• Steamed white rice	1 cup	1/2 cup
• Tea, unsweetened	1 cup	1 cup
Snack		
• Almond, cookies	2 cookies	—
• Milk 1%, low fat	1/2 cup	1/2 cup

Calories	1,609	Calories	1,220
Total carbohydrate, % kcals	56	Total carbohydrate, % kcals	55
Total fat, % kcals	27	Total fat, % kcals	27
*Sodium, mg	1,296	*Sodium, mg	1,043
Saturated fat, % kcals	8	Saturated fat, % kcals	8
Cholesterol, mg	148	Cholesterol, mg	117
Protein, % kcals	20	Protein, % kcals	21

1,600: 100% RDA net for all nutrients except zinc 95%, iron 87%, and calcium 93%
1,200: 100% RDA net for all nutrients except vitamin E 75%, calcium 84%, magnesium 98%, iron 66%, and zinc 77%.
*No salt added in recipe preparation or as seasoning. Consume at least 32 ounces of water.
Kcal = kilo calorie.

SOURCE: "Appendix D. Asian American Cuisine—Reduced Calorie," in *The Practical Guide: Identification, Evaluation, and Treatment of Overweight and Obesity in Adults*, National Institutes of Health, National Heart, Lung, and Blood Institute, North American Association for the Study of Obesity, October 2000, http://www.nhlbi.nih.gov/guidelines/obesity/prctgd_b.pdf (accessed October 21, 2011)

of low-carbohydrate and low-fat diets, many investigators and health professionals hesitate to proclaim one diet's superiority over all others. Nevertheless, there is consensus that even though some diets may produce greater initial weight loss, most perform similarly over time, and that the best predictor of successful weight loss is adherence to a diet.

In "Micronutrient Quality of Weight-Loss Diets That Focus on Macronutrients: Results from the A TO Z Study" (*American Journal of Nutrition*, vol. 92, no. 2, August 1, 2010), Christopher D. Gardner et al. of the Stanford University Medical School compare the micronutrient (vitamins and minerals) intake of 311 overweight or obese women who were randomly assigned to one of four popular diets: Atkins, Zone, Ornish, and LEARN

TABLE 5.10

Sample reduced calorie menus, Mexican-American cuisine

	1,600 calories	1,200 calories
Breakfast		
• Cantaloupe	1 cup	1/2 cup
• Farina, prepared with 1% low fat milk	1/2 cup	1/2 cup
• White bread	1 slice	1 slice
• Margarine	1 tsp	1 tsp
• Jelly	1 tsp	1 tsp
• Orange juice	1 1/2 cup	3/4 cup
• Milk, 1%, low fat	1/2 cup	1/2 cup
Lunch		
• Beef enchilada:		
Tortilla, corn	2 tortillas	2 tortillas
Lean roast beef	2 1/2 oz	2 oz
Vegetable oil	2/3 tsp	2/3 tsp
Onion	1 T	1 T
Tomato	4 T	4 T
Lettuce	1/2 cup	1/2 cup
Chili peppers	2 tsp	2 tsp
Refried beans, prepared with vegetable oil	1/4 cup	1/4 cup
• Carrots	5 sticks	5 sticks
• Celery	6 sticks	6 sticks
• Milk, 1%, low fat	1/2 cup	—
• Water	—	1 cup
Dinner		
• Chicken taco:		
Tortilla, corn	1 tortilla	1 tortilla
Chicken breast, without skin	2 oz	1 oz
Vegetable oil	2/3 tsp	2/3 tsp
Cheddar cheese, low fat and low sodium	1 oz	1/2 oz
Guacamole	2 T	2 T
Salsa	1 T	1 T
• Corn, seasoned with	1/2 cup	1/2 cup
margarine	1/2 tsp	—
• Spanish rice without meat	1/2 cup	1/2 cup
• Banana	1 large	1/2 large
• Coffee	1 cup	1/2 cup
• Milk, 1%	1 oz	1 oz

Calories	1,638	Calories		1,239
Total carbohydrate, % kcals	56	Total carbohydrate, % kcals		58
Total fat, % kcals	27	Total fat, % kcals		26
*Sodium, mg	1,616	*Sodium, mg		1,364
Saturated fat, % kcals	9	Protein, % kcals		8
Cholesterol, mg	153	Cholesterol, mg		91
Protein, % kcals	20	Protein, % kcals		19

1,600: 100% RDA met for all nutrients except vitamin in E 97% and zinc 84%.
1,200: 100% RDNA met for all nutrients except vitamin E 71%, vitamin B₁ & B₃ 91%, vitamin B₂ & iron 90%, and calcium 92%.
*No salt in recipe preparation or as seasoning. Consume at least 32 ounces of water.
Kcal = kilo calorie.

SOURCE: "Appendix D. Mexican American Cuisine—Reduced Calorie," in *The Practical Guide: Identification, Evaluation, and Treatment of Overweight and Obesity in Adults*, National Institutes of Health, National Heart, Lung, and Blood Institute, North American Association for the Study of Obesity, October 2000, http://www.nhlbi.nih.gov/guidelines/obesity/prctgd_b.pdf (accessed October 21, 2011)

TABLE 5.11

Sample reduced calorie menus, lacto-ovo vegetarian cuisine

	1,600 calories	1,200 calories
Breakfast		
• Orange	1 medium	1 medium
• Pancakes, made with 1% lowfat milk and egg whites	3 4" circles	2 4" circles
• Pancake syrup	2 T	1 T
• Margarine, diet	1 1/2 tsp	1 1/2 tsp
• Milk, 1%, lowfat	1 cup	1/2 cup
• Coffee	1 cup	1 cup
• Milk, 1%, lowfat	1 oz	1 oz
Lunch		
• Vegetable soup, canned, low sodium	1 cup	1/2 cup
• Bagel	1 medium	1/2 medium
• Processed American cheese, lowfat	3/4 oz	—
• Spinach salad:		
Spinach	1 cup	1 cup
Mushrooms	1/2 cup	1/2 cup
• Salad dressing, regular calorie	2 tsp	2 tsp
• Apple	1 medium	1 medium
• Iced tea, unsweetened	1 cup	1 cup
Dinner		
• Omelette:		
Egg whites	4 large eggs	4 large eggs
Green pepper	2 T	2T
Onion	2 T	2T
Mozzarella cheese, made from part skim milk, low sodium	1 oz	1/2 oz
Vegetable oil	1 T	1/2 T
• Brown rice, seasoned with	1/2 cup	1/2 cup
margarine, diet	1/2 tsp	1/2 tsp
• Carrots, seasoned with	1/2 cup	1/2 cup
Margarine, diet	1/2 tsp	1/2 tsp
• Whole wheat bread	1 slice	1 slice
• Margarine, diet	1 tsp	1 tsp
• Fig bar cookie	1 bar	1 bar
• Tea	1 cup	1 cup
• Honey	1 tsp	1 tsp
• Milk, 1%, lowfat	3/4 cup	3/4 cup

Calories	1,650	Calories		1,205
Total carbohydrate, % kcals	56	Total carbohydrate, % kcals		60
Total fat, % kcals	27	Total fat, % kcals		25
*Sodium, mg	1,829	*Sodium, mg		1,335
Saturated fat, % kcals	8	Saturated fat, % kcals		7
Cholesterol, mg	82	Cholesterol, mg		44
Protein, % kcals	19	Protein, % kcals		18

1,600: 100% RDA met for all nutrients except vitamin E 92%, vitamin B₃ 97%, vitamin B₆ 67%, iron 73%, and zinc 68%.
1,200: 100% RDA met for all nutrients except vitamin E 75%, vitamin B₁ 92%, vitamin B₃ 69%, vitamin B₆ 59%, iron 54%, and zinc 46%.
*No salt added in recipe preparation or as seasoning. Consume at least 32 ounces of water.
Kcal = kilo calorie.

SOURCE: "Appendix D. Lacto-Ovo Vegetarian Cuisine—Reduced Calorie," in *The Practical Guide: Identification, Evaluation, and Treatment of Overweight and Obesity in Adults*, National Institutes of Health, National Heart, Lung, and Blood Institute, North American Association for the Study of Obesity, June 1998, http://www.nhlbi.nih.gov/guidelines/obesity/practgde.htm (accessed October 21, 2011)

(eat less and exercise more with the help of various behavior-modification strategies while following the USDA guidelines of less than 30% fat and 55% to 60% carbohydrate). The researchers find that many significant differences in vitamin and mineral intakes were observed—not only differences between the groups in intake of micronutrients but also differences in the risk of inadequate intakes. A significant number of Atkins, LEARN, and Ornish dieters shifted from consuming the

estimated average requirement (EAR) prior to dieting to intakes below the EAR after eight weeks of dieting, which suggested an increased risk of inadequacy for several micronutrients. By contrast, the Zone dieters had improved intakes of several vitamins at eight weeks compared with pre-diet levels. Gardner et al. conclude, "Of the specific weight-loss diets that are defined largely

TABLE 5.12

Food exchange list

Within each group, these foods can be exchanged for each other. You can use this list to give yourself more choices.

Vegetables contain 25 calories and 5 grams of carbohydrate. One serving equals:
- 1/2 cup   Cooked vegetables (carrots, broccoli, zucchini, cabbage, etc.)
- 1 cup   Raw vegetables or salad greens
- 1/2 cup   Vegetable juice

If you're hungry, eat more fresh or steamed vegetables.

Fat free and very low fat milk contains 90 calories and 12 grams of carbohydrate per serving. One serving equals:
- 8 oz   Milk, fat free or 1% fat
- 1/4 cup   Yogurt, plain nonfat or low fat
- 1 cup   Yogurt, artificially sweetened

Very lean protein choices have 35 calories and 1 gram of fat per serving. One serving equals:
- 1 oz   Turkey breast or chicken breast, skin removed
- 1 oz   Fish fillet (flounder, sole, scrod, cod, haddock, halibut)
- 1 oz   Canned tuna in water
- 1 oz   Shellfish (clams, lobster, scallop, shrimp)
- 3/4 cup   Cottage cheese, nonfat or lowfat
- 2 each   Egg whites
- 1/4 cup   Egg substitute
- 1 oz   Fat free cheese
- 1/2 cup   Beans—cooked (black beans, kidney, chickpeas, or lentils): count as 1 starch/bread and 1 very lean protein

Medium fat proteins have 75 calories and 5 grams of fat per serving. One serving equals:
- 1 oz   Beef (any prime cut), corned beef, ground beef**
- 1 oz   Pork chop
- 1 each   Whole egg (medium)**
- 1 oz   Mozzarella cheese
- 1/4 cup   Ricotta cheese
- 4 oz   Tofu (note that this is a heart-healthy choice)

**Choose these very infrequently.

Fats contain 45 calories and 5 grams of fat per serving. One serving equals:
- 1 tsp   Oil (vegetable, corn, canola, olive, etc.)
- 1 tsp   Butter
- 1 tsp   Stick margarine
- 1 tsp   Mayonnaise
- 1 T   Reduced fat margarine or mayonnaise
- 1 T   Salad dressing
- 1 T   Cream cheese
- 2 T   Lite cream cheese
- 1/8   Avocado
- 8 large   Black olives
- 10 large   Stuffed green olives
- 1 slice   Bacon

Fruits contain 15 grams of carbohydrates and 60 calories. One serving equals:
- 1 small   Apple, banana, orange, nectarine
- 1 medium   Fresh peach
- 1   Kiwi
- 1/2   Grapefruit
- 1/2   Mango
- 1 cup   Fresh berries (strawberries, raspberries, or blueberries)
- 1 cup   Fresh melon cubes
- 1/8   Honeydew melon
- 4 oz   Unsweetened juice
- 4 tsp   Jelly or jam

Lean protein choices have 55 calories and 2 to 3 grams of fat per serving. One serving equals:
- 1 oz   Chicken—dark meat, skin removed
- 1 oz   Turkey—dark meat, skin removed
- 1 oz   Salmon, swordfish, herring, catfish, trout
- 1 oz   Lean beef (flank steak, London broil, tenderloin, roast beef)*
- 1 oz   Veal, roast, or lean chop*
- 1 oz   Lamb, roast, or lean chop*
- 1 oz   Pork, tenderloin, or fresh ham*
- 1 oz   Lowfat luncheon meats (with 3 grams or less of fat per ounce)
- 1/4 cup   4.5% cottage cheese
- 2 medium   Sardines

*Limit to 1 to 2 times per week.

Starches contain 15 grams of carbohydrate and 80 calories per serving. One serving equals:
- 1 slice   Bread (white, pumpernickel, whole wheat, rye)
- 2 slice   Reduced calorie or "lite" bread
- 1/4 (1 oz)   Bagel (varies)
- 1/2   English muffin
- 1/2   Hamburger bun
- 3/4 cup   Cold cereal
- 1/3 cup   Rice, brown or white—cooked
- 1/3 cup   Barley or couscous—cooked
- 1/3 cup   Legumes (dried beans, peas, or lentils)—cooked
- 1/2 cup   Pasta—cooked
- 1/2 cup   Bulgur—cooked
- 1/2 cup   Corn, sweet potato, or green peas
- 3 oz   Baked sweet or white potato
- 3/4 oz   Pretzels
- 3 cups   Popcorn, hot-air popped or microwave (80-percent light)

SOURCE: "Appendix E. Food Exchange List," in *The Practical Guide: Identification, Evaluation, and Treatment of Overweight and Obesity in Adults*, National Institutes of Health, National Heart, Lung, and Blood Institute, North American Association for the Study of Obesity, October 2000, http://www.nhlbi.nih.gov/guidelines/obesity/prctgd_b.pdf (accessed October 21, 2011)

by their macronutrient content (eg, "low-fat," "low-carb"), micronutrient intakes tend to be overlooked. Given the established roles of vitamins and minerals in acute and chronic health conditions, micronutrient adequacy should be an important consideration when assessing the overall quality of weight-loss diets."

Even though there is no single winner in the diet wars, research has dispelled some of the fears about the safety and effectiveness of low-carbohydrate diets. Low-carbohydrate diets appear to be safe and effective in the short term, but long-term outcomes are still unclear. Some results suggest that higher protein and fat intakes lead to lower total caloric intake by producing earlier satiety, but these diets have not been shown to alter fundamental eating behaviors, nor have they demonstrated, as many of their proponents argue, the ability to modify caloric balance such that weight loss persists when more calories are consumed than expended.

TABLE 5.13

Low calorie, lower fat food alternatives

Instead of...		Replace with...
• Evaporated whole milk		• Evaporated fat free (skim) or reduced fat (2%) milk
• Whole milk		• Low fat (1%), reduced fat (2%), or fat free (skim) milk
• Ice cream		• Sorbet, sherbet, lowfat or fat free frozen yogurt, or ice milk (check label for calorie content)
• Whipping cream		• Imitation whipped cream (made with fat free [skim] milk) or lowfat vanilla yogurt
• Sour cream		• Plain lowfat yogurt
• Cream cheese	**Dairy**	• Neufchatel or "light" cream cheese or fat free cream cheese
• Cheese (cheddar, Swiss, jack)	**Products**	• Reduced calorie cheese, low calorie processed cheese, etc.
		• Fat free cheese
• American cheese		• Fat free American cheese or other types of fat free cheeses
• Regular (4%) cottage cheese		• Lowfat (1%) or reduced fat (2%) cottage cheese
• Whole milk mozzarella cheese		• Part skim low-moisture mozzarella cheese
• Whole milk ricotta cheese		• Part skim milk ricotta cheese
• Coffee cream (half and half) or nondairy creamer (liquid, power)		• Low fat (1%) or reduced fat (2%) milk or nonfat dry milk power
• Ramen noodles		• Rice or noodles (spaghetti, macaroni, etc.)
• Pasta with white sauce (alfredo)	**Cereals, grains**	• Pasta with red sauce (marinara)
• Pasta with cheese sauce	**and pasta**	• Pasta with vegetables (primavera)
• Granola		• Bran flakes, crispy rice, etc.
		• Cooked grits or oatmeal
		• Whole grains (e.g., couscous, barley, bulgur, etc.)
		• Reduced fat granola
• Cold cuts or lunch meats (bologna, salami, liverwurst, etc.)		• Lowfat cold cuts (95% to 97% fat free lunch meats, lowfat pressed meats)
• Hot dogs (regular)		• Lower fat hot dogs
• Bacon or sausage		• Canadian bacon or lean ham
• Regular ground beef		• Extra lean ground beef such as ground round or ground turkey (read labels)
• Chicken or turkey with skin, duck, or goose		• Chicken or turkey without skin (white meat)
• Oil-packed tuna		• Water-packed tuna (rinse to reduce sodium content)
• Beef (chuck, rib, brisket)	**Meat, fish,**	• Beef (round, loin) (trimmed of external fat) (choose select grades)
• Pork (spareribs, untrimmed loin)	**and poultry**	• Pork tenderloin or trimmed, lean smoked ham
• Frozen breaded fish or fried fish (homemade or commercial)		• Fish or shellfish, unbreaded (fresh, frozen, canned in water)
• Whole eggs		• Egg whites or egg substitutes
• Frozen TV dinners (containing more than 13 gram of fat per serving)		• Frozen TV dinners (containing less than 13 grams of fat per serving and lower in sodium)
• Chorizo sausage		• Turkey sausage, drained well (read label)
		• Vegetarian sausage (made with tofu)
• Croissants, brioches, etc.		• Hard French rolls or soft "brown 'n serve" rolls
• Donuts, sweet rolls, muffins, scones, or pastries		• English muffins, bagels, reduced fat or fat free muffins or scones
• Party crackers		• Lowfat crackers (choose lower in sodium)
• Saltine or soda crackers (choose lower in sodium)	**Baked goods**	
• Cake (pound, chocolate, yellow)		• Cake (angel food, white, gingerbread)
• Cookies		• Reduced fat or fat free cookies (graham crackers, ginger snaps, fig bars) (compare calorie level)
• Nuts	**Snacks and**	• Popcorn (air-popped or light microwave), fruits, vegetables
• Ice cream, e.g., cones or bars	**sweets**	• Frozen yogurt, frozen fruit, or chocolate pudding bars
• Custards or puddings (made with whole milk)		• Puddings (made with skim milk)
• Regular margarine or butter		• Light-spread margarines, diet margarine, or whipped butter, tub or squeeze bottle
• Regular mayonnaise		• Light or diet mayonnaise or mustard
• Regular salad dressings	**Fats, oils, and**	• Reduced calorie or fat free salad dressings, lemon juice, or plain, herb-flavored, or
	salad dressings	wine vinegar
• Butter or margarine on toast or bread		• Jelly, jam, or honey on bread or toast
• Oils, shortening, or lard		• Nonstick cooking spray for stir-frying or sautéing
		• As a substitute for oil or butter, use applesauce or prune puree in baked goods
• Canned cream soups		• Canned broth-based soups
• Canned beans and franks	**Miscellaneous**	• Canned baked beans in tomato sauce
• Gravy (home made with fat and/or milk)		• Gravy mixes made with water or homemade with the fat skimmed off and fat free milk included
• Fudge sauce		• Chocolate syrup
• Avocado on sandwiches		• Cucumber slices or lettuce leaves
• Guacamole dip or refried beans with lard		• Salsa

SOURCE: "Appendix C. Instead of...Replace with...," in *The Practical Guide: Identification, Evaluation, and Treatment of Overweight and Obesity in Adults*, National Institutes of Health, National Heart, Lung, and Blood Institute, North American Association for the Study of Obesity, October 2000, http://www.nhlbi.nih.gov/guidelines/obesity/prctgd_b.pdf (accessed October 21, 2011)

TABLE 5.14

Calories in fat free or reduced fat and regular food

Fat free or reduced fat	Calories	Regular	Calories
Reduced fat peanut butter, 2 T	187	Regular peanut butter, 2 T	191
Cookies		Cookies	
Reduced fat chocolate chip cookies, 3 cookies (30 g)	118	Regular chocolate chip cookies, 3 cookies (30 g)	142
Fat free fig cookies, 2 cookies (30 g)	102	Regular fig cookies, 2 cookies (30 g)	111
Ice cream		Ice cream	
Nonfat vanilla frozen yogurt (1% fat), 1/2 cup	100	Regular whole milk vanilla frozen yogurt (3–4% fat), 1/2 cup	104
Light vanilla ice cream (7% fat), 1/2 cup	111	Regular vanilla ice cream (11% fat), 1/2 cup	133
Fat free caramel topping, 2 T	103	Caramel topping, homemade with butter, 2 T	103
Low fat granola cereal, approx. 1/2 cup (55 g)	213	Regular granola cereal, approx 1/2 cup (55 g)	257
Low fat blueberry muffin, 1 small (2 1/2 inch)	131	Regular blueberry muffin, 1 small (2 1/2 inch)	138
Baked tortilla chips, 1 oz.	113	Regular tortilla chips, 1 oz.	143
Low fat cereal bar, 1 bar (1.3 oz.)	130	Regular cereal bar, 1 bar (1.3 oz.)	140

SOURCE: "Fat Free or Reduced Fat [versus] Regular," in *The Practical Guide: Identification, Evaluation, and Treatment of Overweight and Obesity in Adults*, National Institutes of Health, National Heart, Lung, and Blood Institute, North American Association for the Study of Obesity, October 2000, http://www.nhlbi.nih.gov/guidelines/obesity/prctgd_b.pdf (accessed October 21, 2011)

CHAPTER 6
PHYSICAL ACTIVITY, DRUGS, SURGERY, AND OTHER TREATMENTS FOR OVERWEIGHT AND OBESITY

Lack of activity destroys the good condition of every human being, while movement and methodical physical exercise save it and preserve it.

—Plato

One credible hypothesis about the source of the epidemic of overweight and obesity in the United States is the progressive decrease in physical activity expended in daily life—for work, transportation, and household chores. Some researchers contend that the average caloric intake of Americans has not substantially increased; instead, by reducing daily physical activity, the caloric imbalance between calories consumed and expended has shifted to favor weight gain. Even though no data conclusively prove this hypothesis, there is some evidence to support it.

Among the studies that support the premise that Americans' sedentary lifestyle has precipitated the obesity epidemic is a landmark study that examined the diets of an Amish community in Ontario, Canada. In "Physical Activity in an Old Order Amish Community" (*Medicine and Science in Sports and Exercise*, vol. 36, no. 1, January 2004), David R. Bassett, Patrick L. Schneider, and Gertrude E. Huntington describe the "Amish paradox"— that despite a diet that is high in fat, calories, and refined sugar, the Amish community had a scant 4% obesity rate, compared with 31% in the general U.S. population. The researchers chose this particular Amish population because it has rejected technological advances such as automobiles and electricity, and its physically demanding lifestyle is comparable to the way Americans lived 150 years ago. (Other Amish communities that have assumed occupations less physically active than farming have obesity rates that are similar to those found in the general U.S. population.) Bassett, Schneider, and Huntington analyzed the daily routines of 98 Amish people and found that the men averaged 18,425 steps per day and the women 14,196 steps per day, compared with the recom-

mended 10,000 steps per day that most Americans struggle to achieve. The Amish men performed about 10 hours per week of vigorous exercise and the women spent 3.4 hours engaged in heavy lifting, shoveling, digging, shoeing horses, or tossing straw bales. The men devoted an additional 42.8 hours per week and the women an average of 39.2 hours to moderate physical activities such as gardening, performing farm-related chores, or doing laundry.

PHYSICAL ACTIVITY

In sharp contrast to the Amish farmers, many Americans are not physically active. The Centers for Disease Control and Prevention (CDC) defines in "How Much Physical Activity Do Adults Need?" (December 1, 2011, http://www.cdc.gov/physicalactivity/everyone/guidelines/adults.html) the minimum recommended physical activity level for adults as: (1) moderate-intensity physical activity for 150 minutes every week and muscle-strengthening activities on at least two days per week or (2) vigorous-intensity physical activity for 75 minutes or more every week and muscle-strengthening activities on at least two days per week. Figure 6.1 shows that the percentage of men and women who met the federal guidelines for aerobic and muscle-strengthening exercise increased between 1999 and 2009; however, less than 30% of Americans obtained the physical activity prescribed by the guidelines. In 2009 just 12% of men and 9% of women aged 65 years and older met the guidelines for leisure-time physical activity, compared with about 28% of men and 19% of women aged 18 to 44 years. Fewer women met the guidelines than men of the same age across all age groups.

According to the National Center for Health Statistics, in *Health, United States, 2010* (2011, http://www.cdc.gov/nchs/data/hus/hus10.pdf), the overall percentage of adults considered to be inactive (meeting

FIGURE 6.1

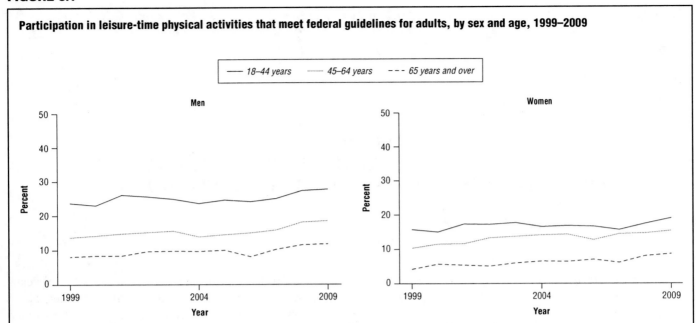

Participation in leisure-time physical activities that meet federal guidelines for adults, by sex and age, 1999–2009

SOURCE: "Figure 12. Participation in Leisure-Time Aerobic and Muscle-Strengthening Activities That Meet the 2008 Federal Physical Activity Guidelines for Adults 18 Years of Age and over, by Sex and Age: United States, 1999–2009," in *Health, United States, 2010: With Special Feature on Death and Dying,* Centers for Disease Control and Prevention, National Center for Health Statistics, 2011, http://www.cdc.gov/nchs/data/hus/hus10.pdf#listtables (accessed September 30, 2011)

neither the aerobic nor the muscle-strengthening activity guidelines) decreased from 56.6% in 1998 to 49.3% in 2009; however, inactivity was higher among specific groups. (See Table 6.1.) For example, the percentage of inactive adults was higher among non-Hispanic African-Americans (56.5%) and Hispanics (59%) than among non-Hispanic whites (45.6%) and Native Americans or Alaskan Natives (52.4%). Inactivity declined with increasing education, from 69.1% of people with no high school diploma to 42.1% of those with some college or more. Similarly, inactivity declined with increasing income: 62.2% of people 100% below the poverty level were inactive, compared with 38.3% of people 400% or more above the poverty level.

Figure 6.2 reveals that among adults aged 25 to 64 years who engaged in regular leisure-time physical activity in early 2011, comparable percentages of men and women reported regular physical activity. Figure 6.3 shows that in early 2011 non-Hispanic white adults (50.2%) were more likely than non-Hispanic African-American adults (39.2%) and Hispanic adults (35%) to participate in sufficient leisure-time physical activity to meet the federal guidelines.

Physical Activity and Weight Loss

Increasing physical activity and exercise is an important element of regimens that are intended to produce weight loss, even though the addition of exercise to a diet program generally does not produce substantially

greater weight loss—most of the weight that is lost is attributable to decreased caloric intake. By favorably affecting blood lipids, increased and sustained physical activity does offer many direct and indirect health benefits, including reducing risks for cardiovascular heart disease and type 2 diabetes beyond the risk reduction possible through diet alone. Physical activity lowers low-density lipoprotein (LDL) cholesterol and triglycerides, increases high-density lipoprotein (HDL) cholesterol, reduces abdominal fat as measured by waist circumference, and may protect against a decrease in muscle mass during weight loss.

Like those who have been inactive or sedentary, overweight people are advised to initiate physical activity slowly and gradually. Walking and swimming at a slow pace are ideal activities because they are enjoyable, easy to schedule, and less likely to produce injuries than many competitive sports. Table 6.2 is an example of a walking program that progressively increases physical activity. Furthermore, because the amounts of activity and the resulting health benefits are functions of the duration, intensity, and frequency of the activity, the same amounts of activity may be obtained in longer sessions of moderately intense activity such as brisk walking than in shorter sessions of more strenuous activity such as running. Table 6.3 shows how a moderate amount of activity—physical activity that uses about 150 calories of energy per day for a total of about 1,000 calories per week—can be obtained in a variety of ways. The table also indicates

TABLE 6.1

Participation in leisure-time physical activities that meet federal guidelines for adults, by selected characteristics, selected years 1998–2009

[Data are based on household interviews of a sample of the civilian noninstitutionalized population]

Characteristic	2008 physical activity guidelines for adults[a]							
	Aerobic activity and muscle-strengthening				Inactive			
	1998	2000	2008	2009	1998	2000	2008	2009
	Percent of adults that meet both the aerobic activity and muscle-strengthening guidelines				Percent of adults that meet neither the aerobic activity nor the muscle-strengthening guidelines			
18 years and over, age-adjusted[b, c]	14.3	15.0	18.4	19.1	56.6	54.7	52.7	49.3
18 years and over, crude[c]	14.5	15.1	18.1	18.8	56.3	54.6	52.9	49.5
Age								
18–44 years	18.9	18.9	22.3	23.3	50.7	49.1	47.6	43.6
18–24 years	23.8	23.8	26.1	25.2	46.5	44.5	44.3	40.0
25–44 years	17.4	17.3	21.0	22.6	51.9	50.6	48.7	44.9
45–64 years	11.4	12.8	16.3	16.8	58.8	57.6	54.7	51.8
45–54 years	13.2	14.5	17.9	18.0	56.9	55.4	53.1	50.5
55–64 years	8.6	10.1	14.2	15.4	61.8	61.0	56.9	53.5
65 years and over	5.5	6.8	9.5	10.0	71.0	67.0	65.1	62.2
65–74 years	7.0	8.4	11.3	12.8	65.6	60.3	60.8	54.6
75 years and over	3.5	4.9	7.5	6.6	77.8	75.0	69.9	71.3
Sex[b]								
Male	17.5	17.9	21.9	22.2	50.8	49.6	48.4	45.0
Female	11.4	12.3	15.0	16.2	61.9	59.4	56.6	53.2
Sex and age								
Male:								
18–44 years	23.0	23.0	27.3	27.7	44.3	43.0	43.1	38.9
45–54 years	16.1	16.0	20.0	18.9	52.9	52.7	50.0	48.1
55–64 years	9.4	11.3	15.5	18.0	58.2	58.7	54.1	50.0
65–74 years	9.5	9.4	11.6	13.8	58.9	55.3	56.4	50.1
75 years and over	4.9	7.1	11.4	9.1	69.5	66.7	62.3	65.4
Female:								
18–44 years	14.9	15.0	17.4	19.0	56.9	55.0	52.0	48.2
45–54 years	10.5	13.1	15.8	17.1	60.8	57.9	56.2	52.8
55–64 years	7.8	9.0	13.1	13.1	65.0	63.1	59.4	56.6
65–74 years	5.1	7.7	11.0	12.0	70.9	64.3	64.5	58.5
75 years and over	2.6	3.6	4.9	4.9	83.0	80.0	74.9	75.2
Race[b, d]								
White only	14.8	15.7	19.1	19.8	55.2	53.1	51.2	47.9
Black or African American only	11.7	12.2	15.2	17.5	65.7	64.6	61.5	56.8
American Indian or Alaska Native only	16.0	10.6	9.7	14.8	57.6	67.1	66.2	52.4
Asian only	13.5	14.1	14.6	13.9	59.1	55.0	52.5	54.7
Native Hawaiian or other Pacific Islander only	—				—		54.5	47.7
2 or more races	—	19.0	20.7	16.6	—	52.8	52.2	44.8
Hispanic origin and race[b, d]								
Hispanic or Latino	9.4	9.2	11.3	12.5	67.7	66.5	62.7	59.0
Mexican	8.7	8.1	11.0	11.8	69.5	67.0	61.6	58.3
Not Hispanic or Latino	14.9	15.8	19.6	20.3	55.3	53.2	50.8	47.6
White only	15.5	16.5	20.8	21.3	53.6	51.4	48.7	45.6
Black or African American only	11.7	12.2	14.9	17.8	65.8	64.6	61.6	56.5
Education[e, f]								
No high school diploma or GED	4.6	4.3	5.3	5.9	76.3	74.0	73.8	69.1
High school diploma or GED	8.6	9.5	11.0	10.4	64.6	61.7	62.5	59.6
Some college or more	18.2	18.9	22.9	24.5	48.0	47.1	44.8	42.1
Percent of poverty level[b, g]								
Below 100%	8.0	9.3	11.2	11.9	71.3	68.0	66.7	62.2
100%–199%	9.0	9.0	10.5	10.9	67.1	65.5	64.8	59.3
200%–399%	12.6	13.2	15.2	16.8	58.0	56.8	55.6	52.1
400% or more	20.2	20.5	26.5	27.1	46.2	45.0	40.7	38.3
Hispanic origin and race and percent of poverty level[b, d, g]								
Hispanic or Latino:								
Below 100%	4.6	4.4	8.9	6.5	78.0	75.2	71.0	65.4
100%–199%	7.0	5.0	6.1	7.8	71.2	72.2	70.9	67.9
200%–399%	11.1	10.2	10.8	15.2	63.8	63.1	59.4	55.1
400% or more	17.4	19.6	21.3	22.7	55.6	52.8	48.9	44.1

Physical Activity, Drugs, Surgery, and Other Treatments for Overweight and Obesity

TABLE 6.1

Participation in leisure-time physical activities that meet federal guidelines for adults, by selected characteristics, selected years 1998–2009 [CONTINUED]

[Data are based on household interviews of a sample of the civilian noninstitutionalized population]

| | 2008 physical activity guidelines for adults[a] | | | | | | | |
| | Aerobic activity and muscle-strengthening | | | | Inactive | | | |
Characteristic	1998	2000	2008	2009	1998	2000	2008	2009
Not Hispanic or Latino:								
White only:								
Below 100%	9.9	11.7	13.4	15.8	66.9	63.5	71.0	58.0
100%–199%	9.6	10.3	13.0	12.8	65.1	62.6	70.9	55.2
200%–399%	13.1	13.9	16.4	16.7	56.1	54.7	59.4	51.2
400% or more	20.2	21.0	27.6	28.2	45.2	43.7	48.9	36.5
Black or African American only:								
Below 100%	7.1	9.5	9.7	11.5	74.6	72.1	70.8	66.2
100%–199%	8.8	9.5	10.4	10.3	69.8	69.2	70.7	59.9
200%–399%	10.6	11.8	13.1	20.1	64.5	64.3	60.4	55.1
400% or more	21.2	17.6	25.6	27.8	54.2	54.9	46.5	45.3
Disability measure[b, h]								
Any basic actions difficulty or complex activity limitation	10.2	10.3	12.5	13.0	64.4	62.2	63.0	59.3
Any basic actions difficulty	9.8	10.3	12.4	13.1	64.8	62.1	63.3	59.4
Any complex activity limitation	7.7	7.2	8.2	9.2	71.9	71.2	72.2	67.4
No disability	16.0	17.0	21.3	22.1	52.5	50.6	46.9	43.4
Geographic region[b]								
Northeast	14.2	17.0	18.2	18.6	57.0	51.8	53.6	51.3
Midwest	15.0	16.4	20.1	19.9	54.9	53.4	50.1	48.9
South	11.8	12.1	16.7	18.3	61.4	59.7	56.4	51.9
West	18.5	16.7	19.2	20.0	49.5	50.1	48.8	43.8
Location of residence[b]								
Within MSA[i]	14.9	15.7	19.4	20.2	55.8	54.1	51.5	47.6
Outside MSA[i]	12.2	12.3	12.5	13.5	59.7	56.9	59.3	57.9

Data not shown have an RSE of greater than 30%.
—Data not available.

[a]Starting with *Health, United States, 2010*, measures of physical activity shown in this table changed to reflect the 2008 Federal Physical Activity Guidelines for Americans. This new table presents four measures of physical activity: the percentage of adults that fully met the 2008 federal guidelines for both aerobic activity and muscle strengthening; the percentage of adults that did not meet the aerobic activity guideline and did not meet the muscle-strengthening guideline (inactive); the percentage of adults who met the aerobic activity component; and the percentage of adults who met the muscle-strengthening component of the 2008 guidelines. The inactive category contains persons who were completely inactive in addition to those who had some activity but amounts were insufficient to meet the guidelines. The 2008 federal guidelines recommend that for substantial health benefits, adults perform at least 150 minutes (2 hours and 30 minutes) a week of moderate-intensity, or 75 minutes (1 hour and 15 minutes) a week of vigorous-intensity aerobic physical activity, or an equivalent combination of moderate-and vigorous-intensity aerobic activity. Aerobic activity should be performed in episodes of at least 10 minutes, and preferably, it should be spread throughout the week. The 2008 guidelines also recommend that adults perform muscle-strengthening activities that are moderate or high intensity and involve all major muscle groups on 2 or more days a week, because these activities provide additional health benefits.
[b]Estimates are age-adjusted to the year 2000 standard population using five age groups: 18–44 years, 45–54 years, 55–64 years, 65–74 years, and 75 years and over. Age-adjusted estimates in this table may differ from other age-adjusted estimates based on the same data and presented elsewhere if different age groups are used in the adjustment procedure.
[c]Includes all other races not shown separately, unknown education level, and unknown disability status.
[d]The race groups, white, black, American Indian or Alaska Native, Asian, Native Hawaiian or Other Pacific Islander, and 2 or more races, include persons of Hispanic and non-Hispanic origin. Persons of Hispanic origin may be of any race. Starting with 1999 data, race-specific estimates are tabulated according to the 1997 Revisions to the Standards for the Classification of Federal Data on Race and Ethnicity and are not strictly comparable with estimates for earlier years. The five single-race categories plus multiple-race categories shown in the table conform to the 1997 Standards. Starting with 1999 data, race-specific estimates are for persons who reported only one racial group; the category 2 or more races includes persons who reported more than one racial group. Prior to 1999, data were tabulated according to the 1977 Standards with four racial groups and the Asian only category included Native Hawaiian or Other Pacific Islander. Estimates for single-race categories prior to 1999 included persons who reported one race or, if they reported more than one race, identified one race as best representing their race. Starting with 2003 data, race responses of other race and unspecified multiple race were treated as missing, and then race was imputed if these were the only race responses. Almost all persons with a race response of other race were of Hispanic origin.
[e]Estimates are for persons 25 years of age and over and are age-adjusted to the year 2000 standard population using five age groups: 25–44 years, 45–54 years, 55–64 years, 65–74 years, and 75 years and over.
[f]GED is General Educational Development high school equivalency diploma.
[g]Percent of poverty level is based on family income and family size and composition using U.S. Census Bureau poverty thresholds. Missing family income data were imputed for 1997 and beyond.
[h]Any basic actions difficulty or complex activity limitation is defined as having one or more of the following limitations or difficulties: movement difficulty, emotional difficulty, sensory (seeing or hearing) difficulty, cognitive difficulty, self-care (ADL or IADL) limitation, social limitation, or work limitation. Starting with 2007 data, the hearing question, a component of the basic actions difficulty measure, was revised. Consequently, data prior to 2007 are not comparable with data for 2007 and beyond.
[i]MSA is metropolitan statistical area. Starting with 2006 data, MSA status is determined using 2000 census data and the 2000 standards for defining MSAs.
Note: Data for additional years are available.

SOURCE: Adapted from "Table 70. Participation in Leisure-Time Aerobic and Muscle-Strengthening Activities That Meet the 2008 Federal Physical Activity Guidelines for Adults 18 Years of Age and over, by Selected Characteristics: United States, 1998–2009," in *Health, United States, 2010: With Special Feature on Death and Dying*, Centers for Disease Control and Prevention, National Center for Health Statistics, 2011, http://www.cdc.gov/nchs/data/hus/hus10.pdf#listtables (accessed September 30, 2011)

FIGURE 6.2

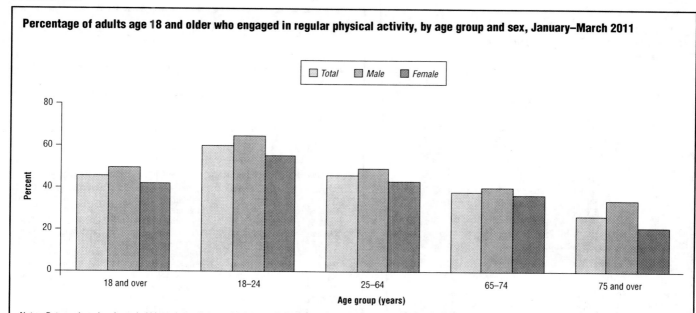

Percentage of adults age 18 and older who engaged in regular physical activity, by age group and sex, January–March 2011

Notes: Data are based on household interviews of a sample of the civilian noninstitutionalized population. Estimates in this figure are limited to leisure-time physical activity only. This measure reflects an estimate of leisure-time aerobic activity motivated by the 2008 federal *Physical Activity Guidelines for Americans*, which are being used for *Healthy People 2020 Objectives* (9). The 2008 guidelines refer to any kind of aerobic activity, not just to leisure-time aerobic activity, so the leisure-time aerobic activity estimates in this figure may be underestimates of the percentage of adults who met the 2008 guidelines for aerobic activity. This figure presents the percentage of adults who met the 2008 federal guidelines for aerobic activity. The 2008 federal guidelines recommend that for substantial health benefits, adults perform at least 150 minutes a week of moderate-intensity aerobic physical activity, or 75 minutes a week of vigorous-intensity aerobic physical activity, or an equivalent combination of moderate- and vigorous-intensity aerobic activity. The 2008 guidelines say that aerobic activity should be performed in episodes of at least 10 minutes, and preferably it should be spread throughout the week. The analyses excluded 1.9% of persons with unknown physical activity participation.

SOURCE: P. M. Barnes et al., "Figure 7.2. Percentage of Adults Aged 18 Years and Over Who Met the 2008 Federal Physical Activity Guidelines for Aerobic Activity through Leisure-Time Activity, by Age Group and Sex: United States 1997–March 2011," in *Early Release of Selected Estimates Based on Data from the January–March 2011 National Health Interview Survey*, Centers for Disease Control and Prevention, National Center for Health Statistics, September 2011, http://www.cdc.gov/nchs/data/nhis/earlyrelease/201109_07.pdf (accessed September 30, 2011)

how performing common household chores, and even self-care activities such as using a wheelchair, may be used to fulfill requirements for moderate amounts of physical activity. Changing routines to include walking up stairs rather than taking an elevator or parking farther than usual from work or school are ways to increase physical activity incrementally. Even reducing sedentary time, such as hours spent in front of the television or computer, can serve to increase energy expenditure.

Table 6.3 also shows the relationship between the intensity and duration of physical activities by comparing the amount of time an adult must spend performing each activity to expend 150 calories. It is interesting to note that just five additional minutes of walking at a moderate pace expends the same number of calories as walking at a brisk pace.

In "Effect of Exercise Intensity on Abdominal Fat Loss during Calorie Restriction in Overweight and Obese Postmenopausal Women: A Randomized, Controlled Trial" (*American Journal of Clinical Nutrition*, vol. 89, no. 4, April 2009), Barbara J. Nicklas et al. examine the weight-loss benefits of even moderate exercise. The researchers assigned 112 women to one of three regimes: calorie restriction (CR) only, CR plus moderate-intensity aerobic exercise, or CR plus vigorous-intensity exercise. Nicklas et al. find that the average weight loss was not significantly different across the three groups. However, women in the CR only group lost more lean muscle mass than did the exercisers, which suggests that exercise more effectively produces fat loss and preserves lean muscle mass.

Donal J. O'Gorman and Anna Krook observe in "Exercise and the Treatment of Diabetes and Obesity" (*Medical Clinics of North America*, vol. 95, no. 5, September 2011) that there is a significant dose-response to the effect of exercise and that recommendations such as the minimum amount of physical activity needed to maintain or improve cardiovascular health are not sufficient to prevent weight gain or promote weight loss. The researchers suggest that exercise recommendations for people seeking to lose weight may have to be revised upward to achieve these objectives. O'Gorman and Krook also reiterate that "exercise by itself exerts clinically beneficial effects in both lean and obese subjects, even in the absence of effects on weight—it exerts an effect on metabolism and changes in gene expression (regulation of the process by which the heritable effects of a gene are displayed)."

FIGURE 6.3

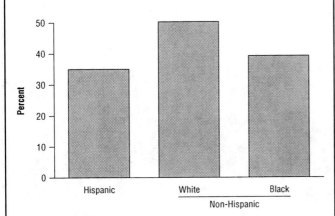

Percentage of adults aged 18 and older who engaged in regular physical activity, by race/ethnicity, January–March 2011

Notes: Data are based on household interviews of a sample of the civilian noninstitutionalized population. Estimates in this figure are limited to leisure-time physical activity only. This measure reflects an estimate of leisure-time aerobic activity motivated by the 2008 federal *Physical Activity Guidelines for Americans*, which are being used for *Healthy People 2020 Objectives* (9). The 2008 guidelines refer to any kind of aerobic activity, not just to leisure-time aerobic activity, so the leisure-time aerobic activity estimates in this figure may be underestimates of the percentage of adults who met the 2008 guidelines for aerobic activity. This figure presents the percentage of adults who met the 2008 federal guidelines for aerobic activity. The 2008 federal guidelines recommend that for substantial health benefits, adults perform at least 150 minutes a week of moderate-intensity aerobic physical activity, or 75 minutes a week of vigorous-intensity aerobic physical activity, or an equivalent combination of moderate- and vigorous-intensity aerobic activity. The 2008 guidelines say that aerobic activity should be performed in episodes of at least 10 minutes, and preferably it should be spread throughout the week. The analyses excluded 1.9% of persons with unknown physical activity participation. Estimates are age-sex-adjusted using the projected 2000 U.S. population as the standard population and using five age groups: 18–24, 25–34, 35–44, 45–64, and 65 and over.

SOURCE: P. M. Barnes et al., "Figure 7.3. Age-Sex-Adjusted Percentage of Adults Aged 18 Years and Over Who Met the 2008 Federal Physical Activity Guidelines for Aerobic Activity through Leisure-Time Activity, by Race/Ethnicity: United States 1997–March 2011," in *Early Release of Selected Estimates Based on Data from the January–March 2011 National Health Interview Survey*, Centers for Disease Control and Prevention, National Center for Health Statistics, September 2011, http://www.cdc.gov/nchs/data/nhis/earlyrelease/201109_07.pdf (accessed September 30, 2011)

TABLE 6.2

A sample walking program

	Warm up	Exercising	Cool down	Total time
Week 1				
Session A	Walk 5 min.	Then walk briskly 5 min.	Then walk more slowly 5 min.	15 min.
Session B	Repeat above pattern			
Session C	Repeat above pattern			

Continue with at least three exercise sessions during each week of the program.

Week 2	Walk 5 min.	Walk briskly 7 min.	Walk 5 min.	17 min.
Week 3	Walk 5 min.	Walk briskly 9 min.	Walk 5 min.	19 min.
Week 4	Walk 5 min.	Walk briskly 11 min.	Walk 5 min.	21 min.
Week 5	Walk 5 min.	Walk briskly 13 min.	Walk 5 min.	23 min.
Week 6	Walk 5 min.	Walk briskly 15 min.	Walk 5 min.	25 min.
Week 7	Walk 5 min.	Walk briskly 18 min.	Walk 5 min.	28 min.
Week 8	Walk 5 min.	Walk briskly 20 min.	Walk 5 min.	30 min.
Week 9	Walk 5 min.	Walk briskly 23 min.	Walk 5 min.	33 min.
Week 10	Walk 5 min.	Walk briskly 26 min.	Walk 5 min.	36 min.
Week 11	Walk 5 min.	Walk briskly 28 min.	Walk 5 min.	38 min.
Week 12	Walk 5 min.	Walk briskly 30 min.	Walk 5 min.	40 min.

Week 13 on: Gradually increase your brisk walking time to 30 to 60 minutes, three or four times a week. Remember that your goal is to get the benefits you are seeking and enjoy your activity.

SOURCE: "A Sample Walking Program," in *The Practical Guide: Identification, Evaluation, and Treatment of Overweight and Obesity in Adults*, National Institutes of Health, National Heart, Lung, and Blood Institute, North American Association for the Study of Obesity, October 2000, http://www.nhlbi.nih.gov/guidelines/obesity/prctgd_b.pdf (accessed November 1, 2011)

changes made by subjects who lost as much as 30 pounds (13.6 kg), those who lost just a few pounds, and those who gained weight. King et al. suggest their results demonstrate that there is considerable variability in the body's compensatory responses to exercise. In other words, moderate exercise may cause some people to lose weight, whereas others find their weight is unchanged or even increases.

O'Gorman and Krook assert that there has been relatively little rigorous research to evaluate the effect of exercise on weight loss. Many studies call for about 150 minutes of exercise per week, or 30 minutes of physical activity on all or most days of the week. O'Gorman and Krook observe that this amount of exercise is only equivalent to a 150- to 200-calorie energy expenditure per day or about 700 to 1,000 calories per week. As such, it is not surprising that this level of exercise does not compare favorably in terms of weight loss with diets that result in a 500-calorie-per-day reduction, or about 3,500 calories per week. O'Gorman and Krook report that there have been just two studies that matched the energy expenditure of exercise with that of a calorie-restricted diet. When exercise and diet both resulted in a deficit of 500 or 700 calories per day, both regimens produced comparable weight loss. O'Gorman and Krook conclude that "exercise is an effective weight-loss strategy but the

RESEARCHERS RECONSIDER THE ROLE OF EXERCISE IN WEIGHT LOSS AND MAINTENANCE. Regular exercise and high levels of physical activity help maintain weight loss over time. However, does strenuous exercise really cause weight loss?

In an effort to answer this question, Neil A. King et al. asked 35 overweight people to exercise vigorously enough to burn 500 calories per day for 12 weeks and reported their findings in "Individual Variability Following 12 Weeks of Supervised Exercise: Identification and Characterization of Compensation for Exercise-Induced Weight Loss" (*International Journal of Obesity*, vol. 32, no. 1, January 2008). Even though many of the subjects lost weight during the study, five gained weight—and there was not much variability between the dietary

TABLE 6.3

Examples of moderate amounts of physical activity

Common chores	Sporting activities	
Washing and waxing a car for 45–60 minutes	Playing volleyball for 45–60 minutes	Less vigorous more time*
Washing windows or floors for 45–60 minutes	Playing touch football for 45 minutes	
Gardening for 30–45 minutes	Walking 1 3/4 miles in 35 minutes (20 min/mile)	
Wheeling self in wheelchair for 30–40 minutes	Basketball (shooting baskets) for 30 minutes	
Pushing a stroller 1 1/2 miles in 30 minutes	Bicycling 5 miles in 30 minutes	
Raking leaves for 30 minutes	Dancing fast (social) for 30 minutes	
Walking 2 miles in 30 minutes (15 min/mile)	Water aerobics for 30 minutes	
Shoveling snow for 15 minutes	Swimming laps for 20 minutes	
Stairwalking for 15 minutes	Basketball (playing a game) for 15–20 minutes	
	Jumping rope for 15 minutes	
	Running 1 1/2 miles in 15 minutes	More vigorous, less time

Note: A moderate amount of physical activity is roughly equivalent to physical activity that uses approximately 150 calories of energy per day, or 1,000 calories per week.
*Some activities can be performed at various intensities; the suggested durations correspond to expected intensity of effort.

SOURCE: "Appendix H. Examples of Moderate Amounts of Physical Activity," in *The Practical Guide: Identification, Evaluation, and Treatment of Overweight and Obesity in Adults*, National Institutes of Health, National Heart, Lung, and Blood Institute, North American Association for the Study of Obesity, October 2000, http://www.nhlbi.nih.gov/guidelines/obesity/prctgd_b.pdf (accessed November 1, 2011)

TABLE 6.4

A guide to selecting weight loss treatment by body mass index (BMI)

Treatment	BMI category				
	25–26.9	27–29.9	30–34.9	35–39.9	≥40
Diet, physical activity, and behavior therapy	With comorbidities	With comorbidities	+	+	+
Pharmacotherapy		With comorbidities	+	+	+
Surgery				With comorbidities	

• Prevention of weight gain with lifestyle therapy is indicated in any patient with a BMI ≥25 kg/m², even without comorbidities, while weight loss is not necessarily recommended for those with a BMI of 25–29.9 kg/m² or a high waist circumference, unless they have two or more comorbidities.
• Combined therapy with a low-calorie diet (LCD), increased physical activity, and behavior therapy provide the most successful intervention for weight loss and weight maintenance.
• Consider pharmacotherapy only if a patient has not lost 1 pound per week after 6 months of combined lifestyle therapy.

The + represents the use of indicated treatment regardless of comorbidities.

SOURCE: "Table 3. A Guide to Selecting Treatment," in *The Practical Guide: Identification, Evaluation, and Treatment of Overweight and Obesity in Adults*, National Institutes of Health, National Heart, Lung, and Blood Institute, North American Association for the Study of Obesity, October 2000, http://www.nhlbi.nih.gov/guidelines/obesity/prctgd_b.pdf (accessed November 2, 2011)

accumulated energy expenditure required for weight reduction may be greater than the general recommendations."

EXERCISE MAY COUNTER GENES THAT INCREASE THE RISK OF OBESITY. A gene variant known as FTO (fat mass and obesity associated) is known to increase the risk of obesity by 20% to 30%. In "Physical Activity Attenuates the Influence of FTO Variants on Obesity Risk: A Meta-analysis of 218,166 Adults and 19,268 Children" (*PLoS Medicine*, vol. 8, no. 11, November 2011), Tuomas O. Kilpeläinen et al. analyze the results of 45 research studies of adults and nine studies conducted with children and adolescents to determine whether physical activity modifies or reduces the risk that is associated with the FTO gene. The researchers find that moderate physical activity—about an hour per day, five days per week—moderated the influence of the gene. Among physically active adults with the FTO gene variant, the risk of obesity was reduced by about 30%. Kilpeläinen et al. conclude that physical activity "is a

particularly effective way of controlling body weight in individuals with a genetic predisposition towards obesity and thus contrast with the determinist view held by many that genetic influences are unmodifiable."

MEDICATION

Pharmacotherapy for weight loss involves the use of prescription drugs as one of several strategies including diet, physical activity, behavioral therapy, counseling, and participation in group-support programs that in combination can work to achieve weight loss. Adding weight-loss medications to a comprehensive treatment program consisting of diet, physical activity, and counseling can increase weight loss by 5 to 20 pounds (2.3 to 9.1 kg) during the first six months of treatment. The decision to add prescription drugs to a treatment program takes into account the individual's body mass index (BMI; body weight in kilograms divided by height in meters squared), other medical problems, and coexisting risk factors. Table 6.4 shows the

TABLE 6.5

Prescription drugs that may be used for weight loss

Generic name	Food and Drug Administration approval for weight loss	Drug type	Common side effects
Phentermine	Yes; short term (up to 12 weeks) for adults	Appetite suppressant	Increased blood pressure and heart rate, sleeplessness, nervousness
Diethylpropion	Yes; short term (up to 12 weeks) for adults	Appetite suppressant	Dizziness, headache, sleeplessness, nervousness
Phendimetrazine	Yes; short term (up to 12 weeks) for adults	Appetite suppressant	Sleeplessness, nervousness
Orlistat	Yes; long term (up to 1 year) for adults and children age 12 and older	Lipase inhibitor	Gastrointestinal issues (cramping, diarrhea, oily spotting), rare cases of severe liver injury reported
Bupropion	No	Depression treatment	Dry mouth, insomnia
Topiramate	No	Seizure treatment	Numbness of skin, change in taste
Zonisamide	No	Seizure treatment	Drowsiness, dry mouth, dizziness, headache, nausea
Metformin	No	Diabetes treatment	Weakness, dizziness, metallic taste, nausea

SOURCE: "Medications That Promote Weight Loss," in *Prescription Medications for the Treatment of Obesity*, NIDDK Weight-Control Information Network, National Institutes of Health, December 2010, http://win.niddk.nih.gov/publications/prescription.htm#meds (accessed November 3, 2011)

therapies that are appropriate for people with differing BMIs and takes into account the presence of comorbidities (the coexistence of two or more diseases) such as diabetes, severe obstructive sleep apnea, or heart disease.

Most drugs used for weight loss are anorexiants (appetite suppressants), which act on neurotransmitters (chemical substances that convey impulses from one nerve cell to another) in the brain. Anorexiant drugs vary depending on which neurotransmitters they affect: some affect catecholamines such as dopamine and norepinephrine; others affect serotonin; and a third class of drugs acts on more than one neurotransmitter. The drugs, which include phentermine, diethylpropion, and phendimetrazine, act by increasing the secretion of dopamine, norepinephrine, or serotonin, by inhibiting reuptake of neurotransmitters, or by inducing a combination of both mechanisms. Table 6.5 offers an overview of the drugs that may be prescribed for weight loss.

Another class of weight-loss drugs blocks the absorption of fat. Orlistat, which was approved by the U.S. Food and Drug Administration (FDA) in 1999, decreases fat absorption in the digestive tract by about one-third. Because it also inhibits absorption of water and vitamins, some users suffer from cramping and diarrhea.

The determination of which type of drug to prescribe is based on individual patient characteristics: anorexiant drugs work best for people who are preoccupied with food and feel constantly hungry, orlistat may be effective for those who are unwilling to reduce fat from their diet, and phentermine may help reduce food cravings. Even though drug therapy has not demonstrated remarkable effectiveness, only modestly enhancing weight loss over diet alone, consumer demand for weight-loss drugs is high. In February 2007 the FDA approved the over-the-counter (nonprescription) sale of orlistat.

Several weight-loss drugs that appeared effective and were popular among consumers have been withdrawn from the U.S. market due to the number and severity of adverse side effects associated with their use. During the 1990s a combination of two drugs—phentermine and fenfluramine, commonly known as "phen-fen"—was prescribed for long-term use (more than three months). However, rare but unacceptable side effects, including serious damage to the heart valves, prompted the withdrawal of fenfluramine and a similar drug, dexfenfluramine, in September 1997. Phentermine is still approved for short-term use.

Rimonabant acts on the endocannabinoid system to block the so-called munchie receptor, which is believed to stimulate appetite among people who smoke marijuana. Because it blocks cravings, rimonabant was used to aid in weight loss. The drug was originally approved for use in Europe, but the FDA refused to grant marketing approval for it in the United States, largely due to reports of adverse side effects with its use, which were addressed in *Rimonabant Briefing Document* (June 13, 2007, http://www.fda.gov/ohrms/dockets/AC/07/briefing/2007-4306b1-fda-backgrounder.pdf). In November 2008 marketing of rimonabant was suspended in the United Kingdom due to safety concerns, and in January 2009 the European Medicines Agency withdrew its approval of the drug. Data revealed that people taking rimonabant had twice the risk of psychiatric disorders, compared with those taking a placebo.

Research Focuses on New Weight-Loss Drugs

By January 2012 only one weight-loss drug, orlistat, was FDA-approved for long-term use (up to one year), and evidence indicates that many users experience so-called rebound weight gain when this drug is discontinued. Regardless, many new drugs were in various stages of development during 2011.

Andrew Pollack reports in "F.D.A. Declines to Approve Diet Drug" (*New York Times*, February 1, 2011) that the last weight-loss drug approved by the

FDA was Xenical in 1999 and during the first months of 2011 the FDA had not approved any of the three most recent antiobesity drugs submitted for review. One of the new drugs, Contrave, is a new formulation that combines two drugs: the antidepressant buproprian and naltrexone (a drug used to help people stop drinking alcohol and using street drugs). Contrave helped study subjects lose weight, but it also increased their pulse and heart rates, which means that it might increase the risk for heart attack or stroke. In light of this finding, the FDA called on Contrave's maker, Orexigen Therapeutics, to conduct a long-term study to ensure that the drug does not pose undue cardiovascular risk, and Orexigen Therapeutics agreed to conduct the study. The FDA's concerns about Contrave are similar to the cardiovascular concerns that prompted it to withdraw Meridia from the market in October 2010. These experiences underscore the fact that the most significant challenge in developing effective weight-loss drugs is ensuring their safety, especially because people may have to use them over the course of several years to produce the desired weight loss.

According to Priya Sumithran et al., in "Long-Term Persistence of Hormonal Adaptations to Weight Loss" (*New England Journal of Medicine*, vol. 365, no. 17, October 27, 2011), effective drug therapy may have to be long term and focus on the endocrine system, possibly by using hormone manipulation. The researchers assert that hormones play a key role in regulating body weight, particularly in terms of regaining lost weight. Sumithran et al. find that obese people who have lost weight experience a shift in their levels of appetite-regulating hormones, which increases their hunger and provides a physiological trigger to consume more food.

WEIGHT-LOSS DRUG IS AVAILABLE WITHOUT A PRESCRIPTION. In February 2007 orlistat was approved for nonprescription sales, and in 2008 consumers began buying 60-milligram capsules sold under the brand names Alli and Xenical. The introduction of orlistat as an over-the-counter product made it the only FDA-approved product for weight loss since phenylpropanolamine was withdrawn by the FDA. Phenylpropanolamine is an amphetamine-like drug that constricts blood vessels and is used in some nasal decongestants. Because it has an appetite suppressant effect, it was used in diet pills that were sold without a prescription until 2005, when the FDA removed it from over-the-counter sales because it increased the risk of stroke. According to the FDA, in "Early Communication about an Ongoing Safety Review Orlistat (Marketed as Alli and Xenical)" (August 24, 2009, http://www.fda.gov/Drugs/DrugSafety/), in 2009 it analyzed 32 reports of serious liver injuries in users of orlistat and an undisclosed number of suspected cases of liver injury possibly related to the drug. The FDA advised orlistat users to consult their health care professional if they have symptoms such as weakness, fatigue, fever, brown urine, or yellowing of the skin or whites of the eyes, which may indicate the presence of liver problems. The FDA did not advise health care professionals to change their prescribing practices with orlistat.

Faheem Asem Ahmad and Sajid Mahmud indicate in "Acute Pancreatitis Following Orlistat Therapy: Report of Two Cases" (*Journal of the Pancreas*, vol. 11, no. 1, January 8, 2010) that in 2009 there were two published reports linking use of orlistat to cases of acute pancreatitis (sudden inflammation of the pancreas, which can produce severe abdominal pain and can have serious consequences including death). For this reason, Ahmad and Mahmud suggest that people taking orlistat should seek immediate medical care if they develop severe acute abdominal pain following use of the drug.

SURGERY

Weight-loss surgery is considered a treatment option only for people for whom all other treatment methods have failed and who suffer from clinically severe obesity—BMI of 40 or greater or BMI of 35 or greater in the presence of comorbidities. (Clinically severe obesity was formerly known as morbid obesity, indicating its potential to cause disease.) Two types of surgical procedures have been demonstrated to be effective in producing weight loss maintained for five years: restrictive techniques, which restrict gastric volume, and malabsorptive procedures, which not only limit food intake but also alter digestion. An example of the first type is banded gastroplasty, in which an inflatable band that can be adjusted to different diameters is placed around the stomach. (See Figure 6.4.) The Roux-en-Y gastric bypass is an example of the second type. On average, patients

FIGURE 6.4

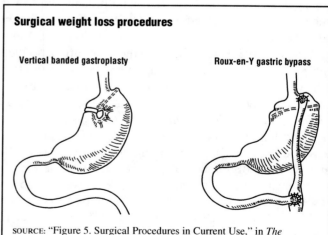

Surgical weight loss procedures

Vertical banded gastroplasty   Roux-en-Y gastric bypass

SOURCE: "Figure 5. Surgical Procedures in Current Use," in *The Practical Guide: Identification, Evaluation, and Treatment of Overweight and Obesity in Adults*, National Institutes of Health, National Heart, Lung, and Blood Institute, North American Association for the Study of Obesity, October 2000, http://www.nhlbi.nih.gov/guidelines/obesity/prctgd_b.pdf (accessed November 3, 2011) maintain a weight loss of 25% to 40% of their preoperative body weight after these procedures.

The surgery not only improves patients' quality of life by causing weight loss and the resolution of many weight-related conditions such as sleep apnea, joint pain, and diabetes but also reduces their risk of death. Lars Sjöström et al. find in "Effects of Bariatric Surgery on Mortality in Swedish Obese Subjects" (*New England Journal of Medicine*, vol. 357, no. 8, August 23, 2007), a study following 2,010 bariatric surgery patients and a control group consisting of 2,037 obese subjects who did not have surgery, that bariatric surgery was associated with a reduction in overall mortality (death).

Because the surgical procedures are not without risk, physicians generally recommend surgery only when the risks of obesity far outweigh the risks associated with the surgery. The National Heart, Lung, and Blood Institute (NHLBI) explains that surgical complications vary, depending on the weight and overall health of the surgical patient. According to Daniel Leslie, Todd A. Kellogg, and Sayeed Ikramuddin, in "Bariatric Surgery Primer for the Internist: Keys to the Surgical Consultation" (*Medical Clinics of North America*, vol. 91, no. 3, May 2007), young people without comorbidities and a BMI equal to or less than 50 have the lowest reported mortality rates—less than 1%. Not unexpectedly, those with a BMI equal to or greater than 60 with comorbidities such as diabetes or high blood pressure have higher mortality rates.

People who undergo weight-loss surgeries require lifelong medical monitoring. After surgery, they are no longer able to eat in the way to which they were accustomed. Those who have undergone gastric bypass experience "dumping syndrome" with symptoms such as sweating, palpitations, lightheadedness, and nausea when they ingest significant amounts of calorie-dense food. Over time, most become conditioned not to eat such foods. Patients who have had gastric restriction surgery are unable to eat more than a limited amount of food during a single sitting without vomiting, so they must eat several small meals per day to maintain adequate nutrition. Those who do not adhere to a prescribed regimen of vitamins and minerals may develop vitamin and iron deficiencies. There are also postoperative and long-term complications following surgery such as wound infections, hernias at the incision site, and gallstones. Generally, however, patients fare extremely well, experiencing dramatic improvement and even complete resolution of diabetes, hypertension (high blood pressure), and infertility, as well as improved mobility, self-esteem, and overall quality of life.

Robin Schroeder, Jordan M. Garrison Jr., and Mark S. Johnson explain in "Treatment of Adult Obesity with Bariatric Surgery" (*American Family Physician*, vol. 84, no. 7, October 1, 2011) that even though there have been no long-term randomized controlled trials (studies that randomly assign some people to have the surgery and others to forgo it), currently available research shows that bariatric surgery significantly improves and frequently eliminates many obesity-related conditions (e.g., diabetes, hypertension, hyperlipidemia [elevated blood lipids]) and has a beneficial effect on mortality. More than 90% of bariatric surgeries are performed laparoscopically (using a thin tube that is inserted in a small incision to insert instruments and perform the procedure), which results in fewer wound complications, shorter hospital stays, and more rapid recovery than open surgery.

Number of Weight-Loss Surgeries Soars

Schroeder, Garrison, and Johnson report that the number of bariatric surgical procedures performed in the United States rose from 13,365 in 1998 to more than 200,000 in 2008. According to the American Society for Metabolic and Bariatric Surgery (ASMBS), in the fact sheet "Metabolic and Bariatric Surgery" (May 2011, http://s3.amazonaws.com/publicASMBS/MediaPressKit/MetabolicBariatricSurgeryOverviewJuly2011.pdf), approximately 220,000 people had bariatric surgery in 2009. In the fact sheet "Access to Care: Morbid Obesity and Metabolic and Bariatric Surgery" (May 2011, http://s3.amazonaws.com/publicASMBS/MediaPressKit/ASMBS%20fact%20sheet%20-%20Access%20to%20Care%20-%202011.pdf), the ASMBS states that just 1% of the population of people with obesity who are candidates for bariatric surgery receive surgical treatment. The ASMBS also observes that in February 2011 the FDA lowered the BMI requirements for gastric banding to include people with a BMI of between 30 and 40 and at least one obesity-related condition, which dramatically increases the number of people who are eligible for such procedures. With the number of candidates for bariatric surgery increasing, the number of procedures is expected to continue to grow, even in view of the risks that are related to surgery.

BENEFITS OFTEN OUTWEIGH RISKS. David R. Flum et al. find in "Perioperative Safety in the Longitudinal Assessment of Bariatric Surgery" (*New England Journal of Medicine*, vol. 361, no. 5, July 30, 2009), a study of 4,776 bariatric surgery patients, that in the short term (30 days after the surgical procedures were performed) "the overall risk of death and other adverse outcomes after bariatric surgery was low and varied considerably according to patient characteristics," such as higher BMI, coexisting medical conditions, and the type of bariatric surgery performed. Flum et al. conclude that "bariatric surgery appears to be the only intervention that consistently results in substantial, sustained weight loss. The safety of such surgery is an important consideration, and our study shows that the incidence of death and adverse events within 30 days after bariatric surgery is low but is varied among different risk groups."

According to Malcolm K. Robinson, in the editorial "Surgical Treatment of Obesity—Weighing the Facts" (*New England Journal of Medicine*, vol. 361, no. 5, July 30, 2009), newer bariatric surgery techniques carry fewer risks than the older ones did and laparoscopic surgeries, which are performed through smaller incisions than traditional open surgeries and entail shorter hospital stays, have been proven effective. Robinson also observes that bariatric surgery "reduces medication use, outpatient visits, and hospitalizations over time. This ultimately may make surgery less costly than the current, less effective nonsurgical treatments of obesity."

BARIATRIC SURGERY CAN BENEFIT THE WHOLE FAMILY. In "Halo Effect for Bariatric Surgery" (*Archives of Surgery*, vol. 146, no. 10, October 2011), Gavitt A. Woodard et al. of the Stanford University School of Medicine look at changes in weight and health behaviors of 35 patients who underwent bariatric surgery and their families for one year. The researchers find that one year after surgery the families (spouses, children, and other relatives of the surgical patients) lost significant amounts of weight, increased their activity levels, and adopted other healthy behaviors. They drank less alcohol, watched less television, and reported fewer instances of emotional eating. Woodard et al. conclude that "this study demonstrates that performing a gastric bypass operation on 1 patient has a halo of positive effect on the weight, eating habits, activity levels, and health behaviors of the entire family."

COUNSELING AND BEHAVIORAL THERAPY

Weight-loss counseling and behavioral therapy aim to assist people to develop the skills needed to identify and modify eating and activity behaviors and to change thinking patterns that undermine weight-control efforts. Behavioral strategies include self-monitoring of weight, food intake, and physical activity; identifying and controlling stimuli that provoke overeating; identifying and solving problems; and using family and social support systems to reinforce weight-control efforts. Counseling and behavioral therapy are often perceived as necessary components of comprehensive weight-loss treatment, but are also viewed as labor intensive because educating and supporting people seeking to lose weight is time consuming. The effort also requires the active participation of everyone who may be involved in treatment: the affected individuals, their families, physicians, nurses, nutritionists, dieticians, exercise instructors, and mental health professionals. In view of the considerable resources that must be allocated to deliver counseling and behavioral therapy, it is important to know if these approaches promote weight loss effectively.

Erin S. LeBlanc et al. considered the evidence supporting the efficacy of counseling and behavioral therapy as well as other treatment methods and reported their findings in "Effectiveness of Primary Care–Relevant Treatments for Obesity in Adults: A Systematic Evidence Review for the U.S. Preventive Services Task Force" (*Annals of Internal Medicine*, vol. 155, no. 7, October 4, 2011). The researchers report that counseling to promote change in diet, exercise, or both, and behavioral therapy to help patients acquire the skills, motivations, and support to change diet and exercise patterns enabled obese patients to achieve modest but clinically significant and sustained (one to two years) weight loss. Furthermore, LeBlanc et al. observe that because control groups also frequently received some form of counseling, education, or support, they might have underestimated the effectiveness of counseling.

Not unexpectedly, more intensive programs, with higher numbers of treatment sessions and/or more frequent contact, were generally more successful and produced greater weight loss, as were those that incorporated behavioral therapy. Behavioral therapy–based treatments resulted in 6.6 pounds (3 kg) greater weight loss, compared with control groups, after 12 to 18 months. LeBlanc et al. also indicate that weight-loss treatment reduced diabetes incidence among people with prediabetes.

Pharmacotherapy also improved weight loss. People who received drug treatment (orlistat) along with behavioral intervention had greater weight loss, compared with those who were given a placebo. LeBlanc et al. conclude that behavioral weight-loss interventions, with or without pharmacotherapy, produce clinically meaningful weight loss.

Comparing Weight-Loss Using a Clinic-Based Program and a Commercial Program

According to Steven Fox, in "Advantages Seen with Clinic-Based Weight-Loss Programs" (*Medscape Medical News*, October 19, 2011), Adam Tsai et al. conducted a pilot study in Denver, Colorado, and presented their findings at the Obesity Society 29th Annual Scientific Meeting in Orlando, Florida, in 2011. The researchers indicated that some clinic-based weight-loss programs may produce better outcomes than commercial weight-loss programs.

Tsai et al. compared the efficacy of two programs: Weight Watchers and a clinic-based individualized treatment approach. Study subjects were randomly assigned to attend Weight Watchers for 17 weeks or to receive 12 individual counseling sessions lasting from 20 to 30 minutes with a nurse nutritionist. Subjects assigned to the clinic program were offered the option of using meal replacements or using the weight-loss medication phentermine. Four months after completing the programs, the subjects were evaluated for weight loss, blood pressure, waist circumference, and health-related quality of life.

Tsai et al. find that the subjects in the clinic-based group lost significantly more weight than those in the commercial weight-loss program. However, no significant differences in blood pressure, waist circumference, or health-related quality of life were found between the two groups of subjects.

Comparing Weight-Loss Counseling from a Primary Care Physician and a Commercial Program

Interestingly, the results of a study comparing people receiving weight-loss guidance from a primary care physician and those participating in Weight Watchers indicate that the commercial program yields better results. Susan A. Jebb et al. find in "Primary Care Referral to a Commercial Provider for Weight Loss Treatment versus Standard Care: A Randomised Controlled Trial" (*Lancet*, vol. 378, no. 9801, October 22, 2011) that after 12 months subjects attending Weight Watchers lost twice as much weight as those who received physician guidance (15 pounds [6.8 kg] versus 7 pounds [3.2 kg]). Participants in the Weight Watchers group also had greater reductions in waist circumference and fat mass. Jebb et al. conclude that "referral by a primary health-care professional to a commercial weight loss programme that provides regular weighing, advice about diet and physical activity, motivation, and group support can offer a clinically useful early intervention for weight management in overweight and obese people that can be delivered at large scale."

Weight-Loss Counseling Online

An expanding array of diet, counseling, and support group programs are available on the Internet; however, little research has compared them or determined their efficacy. In the landmark study "A Randomized Trial Comparing Human E-Mail Counseling, Computer-Automated Tailored Counseling, and No Counseling in an Internet Weight Loss Program" (*Archives of Internal Medicine*, vol. 166, no. 15, August 2006), Deborah F. Tate, Elizabeth H. Jackvony, and Rena R. Wing sought to determine whether computer-generated feedback, delivered via the Internet, would prove to be a viable alternative to human counseling via e-mail. They compared the effects of custom-tailored computer-automated interactions with an Internet program that provided weight-loss counseling from a human via e-mail.

Participants were randomly selected to be in one of three treatment groups: human e-mail counseling, computer-automated feedback, or no counseling. All the subjects received one weight-loss group session, coupons for meal replacements, and access to an interactive website, but the human e-mail counseling and computer-automated feedback groups also had access to an e-diary and a message board. The human e-mail counseling group received weekly e-mail feedback from a counselor,

the computer-automated feedback group received automated, custom-tailored messages, and the control group did not receive any counseling. Recommendations included calorie-restricted diets of between 1,200 and 1,500 calories per day, daily exercise equivalent to walking for 30 minutes, and instructions about how to use meal replacement products. All the participants were encouraged to self-monitor their diet and exercise using diaries and calorie books. Both groups accessed the same website, which featured weekly reporting and graphs of weight, weekly e-mail prompts to report weight, weekly weight-loss tips via e-mail, recipes, and a weight-loss e-buddy network system that enabled users to interact with other dieters with similar characteristics via e-mail.

The primary outcome measure used to compare the groups was change in body weight from baseline and at three and six months. Both the human and automated e-counseling groups had greater reductions in weight than the control group at each weigh-in. Tate, Jackvony, and Wing conclude that automated computer feedback was as effective as human e-mail counseling.

In "Minimal In-Person Support as an Adjunct to Internet Obesity Treatment" (*Annals of Behavioral Medicine*, vol. 33, no. 1, February 2007), Nicci Micco et al. of the University of Vermont, Burlington, confirm the efficacy of online counseling for weight loss. The researchers compared the weight loss of people using Internet-only behavioral weight-loss treatment with people using the same program and having monthly in-person meetings. Over 120 subjects were randomly assigned to either an Internet-only or an Internet and in-person treatment plan. All the subjects participated in a 12-month behavioral weight-loss program that was conducted over the Internet. The online groups met weekly for the first six months and biweekly for the remaining six months. The Internet and in-person group had access to the same website as the Internet-only group but once a month subjects had an in-person meeting instead of an online chat. Micco et al. find that there were no significant differences in weight loss between the two groups and conclude that "dynamic, socially supportive, and interactive elements of the Web site may have obviated the need for further interpersonal behavioral counseling."

Patricia A. Hageman et al. describe in "Web-Based Interventions for Weight Loss and Weight Maintenance among Rural Midlife and Older Women: Protocol for a Randomized Controlled Trial" (*BMC Public Health*, vol. 11, June 30, 2011) a study comparing behavior-change interventions for weight loss and maintenance that use a website only, a website with peer support, and a website with professional e-mail counseling to facilitate initial weight-loss maintenance among the study participants. The study will include more than 300 rural women aged 45 to 69 years with BMIs of between 28 and 45 and will compare changes in body weight and achievement of healthy eating and activity targets at six, 18, and 30 months. Hageman et al. hypothesize that the women who receive either peer-led online support or professional weight-loss counseling will achieve better weight loss and weight maintenance outcomes than the group that only uses the interactive website. Nonetheless, should any of these interventions prove to be effective, they may offer a practical, cost-effective way to help residents of rural communities gain access to weight management programs.

Complementary and Alternative Therapies

Many complementary and alternative medicine practices such as yoga, Dahn (a holistic mind-body training method), and mindful eating (which teaches greater awareness of bodily sensations such as hunger and satiety [the feeling of fullness or satisfaction after eating] and helps people to identify "emotional eating") have been used to promote weight loss. However, acupuncture (the Chinese practice of inserting extremely thin, sterile needles into any of 360 specific points on the body) and hypnosis are the only alternative medical practices that have been studied as potential treatments for obesity. Several studies report that acupuncture does not appear to have any benefit greater than a placebo.

Hypnosis is an altered state of consciousness. It is a state of heightened awareness and suggestibility and enables focused concentration that may be used to alter perceptions of hunger and satiety and to modify behavior. Hypnosis is considered a mainstream treatment for addictions and overeating. Regardless, there are conflicting data about its effectiveness—some studies find that it adds little, if any, benefit beyond that of a placebo, whereas others conclude that hypnosis may have some initial benefit for people seeking weight loss, but that it has little sustained effect.

In "Pilot Study: Mindful Eating and Living (MEAL): Weight, Eating Behavior, and Psychological Outcomes Associated with a Mindfulness-Based Intervention for People with Obesity" (*Complementary Therapies in Medicine*, vol. 18, no. 6, December 2010), Jeanne Dalon et al. report the results of a pilot study of a six-week group program that provides mindfulness training—meditation, mindful eating, and group discussion, with emphasis on awareness of body sensations, emotions, and triggers to overeat—to people who are obese. The researchers find that subjects receiving this intervention showed statistically significant increases in measures of mindfulness and thoughtful restraint around eating, and statistically significant decreases in weight, impulsive and binge eating, depression, and perceived stress. Dalon et al. conclude that this pilot study suggests that an "eating focused mindfulness-based intervention can result in significant changes in weight, eating behavior, and psychological distress in obese individuals."

According to Asker E. Jeukendrup and Rebecca Randell of the University of Birmingham, in "Fat Burners: Nutrition Supplements That Increase Fat Metabolism" (*Obesity Reviews*, vol. 12, no. 10, October 2011), a number of nutritional supplements such as caffeine, carnitine, chromium, conjugated linoleic acid, forskolin, fucoxanthin, green tea, and kelp are promoted as "fat burners" and are being used to promote weight loss. Jeukendrup and Randell observe that some of these supplements have demonstrated some benefit but have not yet been rigorously tested. Caffeine and green tea have demonstrated fat metabolism–enhancing properties; however, evidence is lacking for the others. As a result, health care professionals cannot definitively recommend their use.

MIGHT WEIGHT LOSS BE HARMFUL?

Successful weight-loss treatments generally result in reduced blood pressure, reduced triglycerides, reduced total cholesterol and LDL cholesterol, and increased HDL cholesterol. Weight loss of as little as 5% to 10% of initial weight produces measurable health benefits and may prevent illnesses among people at risk. These findings suggest that treatment should not exclusively focus on the medical consequences of obesity, but that obesity itself should be treated. National Institutes of Health guidelines recommend weight loss for people with a BMI greater than 30 and for people with a BMI greater than 25 with two or more obesity-related risk factors. The guidelines also recommend that for people with a BMI of between 25 and 30 without other risk factors, the focus should be on prevention of further weight gain, rather than on weight loss.

In "Weight Cycling and Mortality among Middle-Aged or Older Women" (*Archives of Internal Medicine*, vol. 169, no. 9, May 11, 2009), Alison E. Field, Susan Malspeis, and Walter C. Willett of the Harvard School of Public Health report that the health risks of weight cycling (the repeated loss and regain of body weight) are not as serious as previously assumed. The researchers analyzed the relationship between mortality, intentional weight loss, and mild or severe weight cycling. Subjects who said they had intentionally lost at least 20.1 pounds (9.1 kg) at least three times were classified as severe weight cyclers, and those who had intentionally lost at least 9.9 pounds (4.5 kg) at least three times were classified as mild weight cyclers. Field, Malspeis, and Willett find that during the 12 years of follow-up there was no increase in mortality associated with either mild or severe weight cyclers.

Kevin Y. Taing, Chris I. Ardern, and Jennifer L. Kuk question whether weight cycling increases the risk of death. In "Effect of the Timing of Weight Cycling during Adulthood on Mortality Risk in Overweight and Obese Postmenopausal Women" (*Obesity*, July 14, 2011), the researchers analyze data of 47,473 overweight and obese women aged 50 to 79 years. The women were classified as stable (WgtV) or weight-gainer or -loser (WgtC) based on weight changes during early adulthood (18 to 35 years), middle age (35 to 50 years), and later (50 years to current age) adulthood. Those with weight changes of less than 5% during all three periods were classified as being stable weight. Weight-gainers were those with at least one period of weight gain (greater than 5%) without a period of weight loss (greater than or equal to 5%), and weight-losers were those with at least one period of weight loss without a period of weight gain. Those who experienced both a period of weight gain and loss were termed WgtC. Those classified as WgtC and WgtV throughout adulthood did not have higher mortality risk than weight-stable women when the age period of weight change was not considered. However, when the age periods were analyzed, increased mortality risk was observed for every 11 pounds (5 kg) of weight gain during early or middle age or for every 11 pounds of weight loss since middle age or late adulthood. Taing, Ardern, and Kuk suggest that simply looking at WgtC and WgtV by weight changes across adulthood may not accurately assess mortality risk—the age at which the weight changes occur may influence whether the weight change poses increased risk.

Is It Really Dangerous to Be Overweight?

The health risks and consequences of obesity are well understood, but the risk of mortality associated with overweight remains unclear. In "BMI and Mortality: Results from a National Longitudinal Study of Canadian Adults" (*Obesity*, vol. 18, no. 1, January 2010), Heather M. Opana et al. estimate the relationship between BMI and mortality in a representative sample of 11,326 adults. The researchers find that overweight (BMI 25 to 30) was associated with a significantly decreased risk of death, whereas underweight (BMI less than 18.5) was associated with a significantly increased risk of death, as was class II obesity (BMI greater than 35). Interestingly, class I obesity (BMI 30 to 35) was found to not have an increased risk of mortality. Opana et al. conclude that "when compared to the acceptable BMI category, overweight appears to be protective against mortality."

David Faeh et al. analyzed data from 9,853 Swiss men and women aged 25 to 74 years to determine the relationship between BMI and mortality and published their findings in "Obesity but Not Overweight Is Associated with Increased Mortality Risk" (*European Journal of Epidemiology*, vol. 26, no. 8, August 2011). The researchers indicate that obesity, but not overweight, was associated with an increased mortality risk, which was largely attributable to an increased risk of death from cardiovascular disease and cancer. Faeh et al. conclude that public health interventions should "focus on preventing normal- and overweight persons from becoming obese."

CHAPTER 7
THE ECONOMICS OF OVERWEIGHT AND OBESITY

The economic impact of obesity is considerable. In "Financial Implications of Obesity" (*Orthopedic Clinics of North America*, vol. 42, no. 1, January 2011), George V. Russell, Christine W. Pierce, and Loren Nunley assert that "obesity outranks both smoking and drinking in its deleterious effects on health and health costs." Smoking and drinking are associated with a 21% increase in health care costs, compared with the 36% increase attributable to obesity. In 2008 obesity was responsible for approximately $147 billion in direct health care costs, which are those incurred for diagnostic and treatment services and for preventive measures. Examples of direct health care costs are physician office visits, hospital and nursing home charges, prescription drug costs, and special hospital beds to accommodate obese patients. The indirect costs of overweight and obesity are measured in terms of decreased earnings: lost wages and lower productivity resulting from the inability to work because of illness or disability, as well as the value of future earnings lost by premature mortality (death). Estimates of indirect costs vary, but several studies suggest that the monetary loss resulting from lost productivity is several times larger than health care costs.

According to Y. Claire Wang et al., in "Health and Economic Burden of the Projected Obesity Trends in the USA and the UK" (*Lancet*, vol. 378, no. 9793, August 27, 2011), the economic losses attributable to health care costs and lost productivity are projected to increase. By 2020 three out of four Americans will be overweight or obese and by 2030 there will be an additional 65 million obese adults in the United States. Obesity-related health care costs are attributable not only to increased risk for type 2 diabetes, cardiovascular diseases, and several forms of cancer but also to costly and disabling conditions such as osteoarthritis, asthma, infertility, and sleep apnea. Along with health care costs and lost productivity, there are indirect costs as a result of decreased years of

disability-free life, increased mortality before retirement, early retirement, and disability benefits.

There are other economic consequences and personal costs of obesity: obese workers may earn less than their healthy-weight counterparts because of job discrimination. Many insurance companies, particularly in the life insurance sector, charge higher premiums with increasing degrees of overweight. When obesity compromises physical functioning and limits activities of daily living, affected individuals may require assistance from home health aides, durable medical equipment such as walkers or wheelchairs, or other costly adaptations to accommodate disability.

THE HIGH COST OF OVERWEIGHT AND OBESITY

Because overweight and obesity have been linked to an increased risk for many chronic conditions, it may be argued that some percentage of the costs attributed to arthritis, cancer, diabetes, heart disease, and stroke are also attributable to obesity. It is important to remember that estimates of the medical care costs, direct and indirect as well as total cost of overweight and obesity in the United States, vary depending on how the conditions are defined, whether overweight and obesity are considered together or separately, and which costs and obesity-related conditions are included in the estimates and projections.

According to Eric A. Finkelstein et al., in "Annual Medical Spending Attributable to Obesity: Payer- and Service-Specific Estimates" (*Health Affairs*, vol. 28, no. 5, September–October 2009), annual medical care expenditures attributable to overweight and obesity doubled between 1998 and 2006. During this period obesity (a body mass index [BMI; body weight in kilograms divided by height in meters squared] of greater than 30) increased by 39%, prompting an 89% increase in health care costs attributable to obesity. Finkelstein et al. estimate that the direct cost of overweight and obesity in 2006 was 9.1% of the total U.S. health care expenditures, up from 6.5% in 1998. Of this 9.1%, 3.7% was attributable to overweight and 5.3% to obesity. An obese person incurred about 42% more costs than a healthy-weight person, which translates into $1,429 more (per obese person) per year for medical care. The majority of these dollars are spent treating obesity-related diseases and disorders.

According to Finkelstein et al., the estimated increase associated with being overweight was 14.5% ($247) and ranged from 11.4% ($53) for out-of-pocket spending to 15.1% ($271) for Medicaid (a federal and state health care program for people below the poverty level). The average increase in annual medical spending associated with obesity was 37.4% ($732) and ranged from 26.1% ($125) for out-of-pocket spending to 36.8% ($1,486) for Medicare (a medical insurance program for older adults and people with disabilities) and 39.1% ($864) for Medicaid. Obesity was responsible for nearly $40 billion of increased medical spending through 2006, including $7 billion in Medicare prescription drug costs.

Finkelstein et al. observe that the lifetime costs of overweight and obesity borne by the government are likely to be greater than the lifetime costs imposed by smokers. Furthermore, the results of this study reveal that obese people who live to age 65 have much larger annual Medicare expenditures than their normal-weight peers. According to Catharine Paddock, in "Obesity Healthcare Costs US 147 Billion Dollars a Year, New Study" (Medical News Today, July 28, 2009), Eric A. Finkelstein asserts that because medical care spending attributable to overweight and obesity rivals spending attributable to smoking, "the medical costs attributable to obesity are almost entirely a result of costs generated from treating the diseases that obesity promotes," and suggests "that as long as obesity prevails to the extent that it does today, it will continue to be a significant burden on health care."

Wang et al. concur with Finkelstein et al. and offer projections for 2030 that are based on current trends of BMI in the U.S. population. The researchers forecast an excess of 8 million cases of diabetes, 6 million to 8 million cases of heart disease and stroke, and more than 1.5 million cases of cancer. This forecast translates into an increase in annual medical costs of treating obesity-related disorders from $28 billion per year in 2020 to $66 billion per year in 2030.

The Impact of Obesity Costs on a State Economy

The high costs of obesity have prompted states to fund obesity prevention and control efforts. For example, in "State- and Payer-Specific Estimates of Annual Medical Expenditures Attributable to Obesity" (Obesity, vol. 20, no. 1, January 2012), Justin G. Trogdon et al. report

that from 22% of the state-level costs of obesity in Virginia to 55% of the costs in Rhode Island are financed by Medicare and Medicaid. The researchers calculate that without obesity-related expenses, the states' annual medical expenditures would be reduced by 6.7% to 10.7%.

In "Paying for Obesity: A Changing Landscape" (Pediatrics, vol. 123, suppl. 5, June 1, 2009), Lisa A. Simpson and Julie Cooper report that the costs of obesity to states through their Medicaid budgets are considerable, "with estimates ranging from $23 million in Wyoming to $3.5 billion in New York in 2003." Most states use one of two strategies to pay for obesity-related medical care:

- Medicaid-focused interventions that include reimbursement and/or specific weight-management programs or incentives, which vary from state to state. In some states health professionals are "paid at least as well for obesity and its related comorbidities as for other conditions they treat," while in other states claims for obesity-related care, especially nutritional counseling, are rejected.

- Public employee benefit programs with obesity-prevention and weight-loss programs that help states reduce the cost impact of overweight and obese workers. Arkansas and Kentucky are among the states that have implemented weight-education programs for state employees.

Hospital Costs of Childhood and Adolescent Obesity

Because most research about obesity-related medical care costs focus on costs incurred as a result of treating adults, Leonardo Trasande et al. decided to look at the economic consequences of childhood obesity and reported their findings in "Effects of Childhood Obesity on Hospital Care and Costs, 1999–2005" (Health Affairs, vol. 28, no. 4, July–August 2009). Using data from a nationally representative sample of 3.1 million U.S. hospital discharges of children and adolescents aged two to 19 years between 1999 and 2005, the researchers note trends in obesity-associated hospitalizations, charges, and costs. They find that hospitalizations of children attributable to obesity nearly doubled between 1999 and 2005 and that the resulting costs rose from $125.9 million in 2001 to $237.6 million in 2005. Trasande et al. also report that Medicaid assumed a large share of the cost of hospitalizations for obesity-related conditions in children and adolescents, such as diabetes and hypertension (high blood pressure), and that private payers paid a greater portion of hospital costs related to the direct treatment of obesity, such as nutritional counseling, drug therapy, and weight-loss surgery.

In 2009 the National Association of Children's Hospitals and Related Institutions FOCUS on a Fitter Future Group sought to guide medical providers, patients, and payers to better serve obese children and adolescents. In

"Payment for Obesity Services: Examples and Recommendations for Stage 3 Comprehensive Multidisciplinary Intervention Programs for Children and Adolescents" (*Pediatrics*, vol. 128, suppl. 2, September 1, 2011), Wendy Slusser et al. explain that "health insurers and hospitals often have to evaluate coverage of obesity care services on a case-by-case basis, which creates a barrier between patients and providers." The researchers interviewed several hospital-based programs and find that most programs fell short of operating expenses. For example, the Duke Children's Health Lifestyles Program is funded by grants and clinic-visit payments and revenue is about 10% less than operating expenses each year. Approximately 40% of reimbursement is from Medicaid, 30% from private insurance such as BlueCross, BlueShield, and Aetna, 20% from managed care plans, and 10% from the Duke employee health plan.

Slusser et al. observe that recent research demonstrates that obesity interventions, especially those with intensive treatment regimens, are effective. The results of these studies support the premise that effective treatment approaches obesity as a chronic condition that requires ongoing care. The U.S. Preventive Services Task Force reviewed childhood and adolescent obesity interventions and found that medium- to high-intensity comprehensive behavioral interventions were most effective in the treatment of obesity. Slusser et al. indicate that "no statewide or national efforts are testing models of payment packages for children treated by a multidisciplinary team.... However, these efforts are desperately needed, given the near-doubling of hospital admissions and an associated increase in costs from $125.9 million in 1999 (adjusted for inflation) to $237.6 million in 2005 among US children aged 2 to 19 years with a diagnosis of obesity." They assert that intensive obesity interventions should be reimbursed, consistent with the White House Task Force on Childhood Obesity report *Solving the Problem of Childhood Obesity within a Generation: White House Task Force on Childhood Obesity Report to the President* (May 2010, http://www.letsmove.gov/white-house-task-force-childhood-obesity-report-president), which states that "federally funded and private insurance plans should cover services necessary to prevent, assess, and provide care to overweight and obese children."

Insurance Coverage for Obesity Treatment

Even though Medicare and Medicaid spend billions of dollars on obesity-related illnesses, neither entitlement program covers treatment for obesity itself. Medicaid does not cover obesity treatment, and under Medicare hospital and physician services for obesity are generally excluded. Historically, Medicare has covered treatment when obesity results from a disease such as hypothyroidism (a deficiency of the thyroid hormone, which is produced by the thyroid gland) or Cushing's disease (a condition in which excess cortisol, a hormone released in response to stress, is secreted by the pituitary gland) and when weight loss is medically necessary to treat a disease such as diabetes, hypertension, or heart disease. It also provides coverage for surgical treatment of obesity when it is medically appropriate and the surgery is to correct an illness that caused the obesity or was aggravated by the obesity.

Until 2004 Medicare justified excluding coverage for obesity treatment by asserting that obesity is not a disease. However, in October 2004 the Centers for Medicare and Medicaid Services (CMS), which administers Medicare, indicated in *CMS Manual System: Pub. 100-03 Medicare National Coverage Determinations* (http://www.cms.hhs.gov/transmittals/downloads/R23NCD.pdf) that it eliminated language ("obesity itself cannot be considered an illness") from its policy that had been used to deny coverage for weight-loss treatment. Even though the CMS did not technically name obesity a disease, this language allows consumers and health professionals to seek Medicare reimbursement for weight-loss programs and treatment. Industry observers speculate that private insurance companies will follow Medicare's lead and will extend coverage for weight-loss treatments.

The Medicare Prescription Drug, Improvement, and Modernization Act of 2003 excludes drugs that are used for weight loss. However, the CMS explains in "Medicare Program; Policy and Technical Changes to the Medicare Prescription Drug Benefit" (*Federal Register*, vol. 73, no. 73, April 15, 2008) that weight-loss drugs may be covered by Medicare when they are prescribed for a "medically accepted indication," such as clinically severe obesity. Regardless, in *Your Guide to Medicare Prescription Drug Coverage* (December 2011, http://www.medicare.gov/Publications/Pubs/pdf/11109.pdf), the CMS explains that even though some plans may choose to cover weight-loss drugs, Medicare drug plans are not required to cover them.

In view of the high prevalence of obesity among the populations covered by Medicaid (the poor and minorities) and the significant Medicaid expenditures for obesity-related illnesses, many health care industry observers believe it is shortsighted that some states specifically exclude coverage of antiobesity products in their Medicaid programs. For example, in "Coverage of Obesity Treatment: A State-by-State Analysis of Medicaid and State Insurance Laws" (*Public Health Reports*, vol. 125, no. 4, July–August 2010), Jennifer S. Lee et al. of George Washington University report that in 2010 just eight state Medicaid programs offered coverage of obesity treatment for adults and just 10 states reimbursed for obesity treatment for children. According to Christine C. Ferguson of the George Washington University, in "State Survey of Coverage of Obesity Interventions Finds Coverage of Treatment Options Limited for Overweight and Obese

Populations across the United States" (May 2011, http://www.stopobesityalliance.org/wp-content/assets/2011/05/Spring-2011-Obesity-and-the-States-Bulletin-FINAL.pdf), coverage varies widely. For example, California covers weight-loss drugs and the full spectrum of bariatric surgical procedures, while Arizona excludes weight-loss drugs and bariatric surgical procedures from coverage. Some health care analysts and advocacy groups, including the Obesity Society (formerly the American Obesity Association), contend that it is difficult to reconcile limited coverage of obesity in light of Medicaid coverage for inpatient and outpatient alcohol detoxification and rehabilitation, chemical dependency treatment and drug rehabilitation, and services for sexual impotence.

Some states require that private insurance companies pay for obesity treatment. For example, Alexis Macias indicates in "Covering Patients through Insurance Mandates" (*Bulletin of the American College of Surgeons*, vol. 96, no. 7, 2011) that six states (Arkansas, Georgia, Indiana, Maryland, New Hampshire, and Virginia) require insurers to pay for surgical treatment of obesity and 17 states have chosen not to cover bariatric surgery but do provide "financial incentives to participants for adhering to health promotion programs."

The Pharmacy Benefit Management Institute (PBMI), an independent organization that is not affiliated with any employee benefits program or pharmaceutical manufacturer, periodically surveys employers to determine the extent, cost, and coverage of their pharmacy benefits and publishes the survey data and trends in *Prescription Drug Benefit Cost and Plan Design Report*. The PBMI explains in *2011–2012 Prescription Drug Benefit Cost and Plan Design Report* (2011, http://www.benefitdesignreport.com/Portals/0/2011-2012_takeda_bdr.pdf) that in 2011 it queried 274 companies that provided coverage to 5.2 million beneficiaries. The institute finds that a majority (76%) of employers continued to exclude weight-loss drugs from their coverage in 2011. Just 28% of employers surveyed offered complete, unlimited coverage of weight-loss drugs.

The reluctance to cover antiobesity drugs is driven by concern about cost, in that many payers may determine that the rising prevalence of obesity and its comorbidities require higher prescription drug costs than drug treatment of obesity itself. For example, in "Health-Care Expenditures of Overweight and Obese Males and Females in the Medical Expenditures Panel Survey by Age Cohort" (*Obesity*, vol. 19 , no. 1, January 2011), Janice F. Bell et al. find that when compared with the health care expenditures of normal-weight people, the health care expenditures of overweight and obese people were higher, and the increased spending was primarily for more ambulatory care (outpatient visits to physicians and clinics) and prescription drugs.

OVERWEIGHT WORKERS MAY PAY MORE FOR HEALTH INSURANCE COVERAGE. Federal regulations reported in "Nondiscrimination and Wellness Programs in Health Coverage in the Group Market; Final Rules" (*Federal Register*, vol. 71, no. 239, December 13, 2006), which took effect on July 1, 2007, for some groups and on January 1, 2008, for others, permit companies to charge overweight employees more for their health insurance than their healthy-weight peers.

Jilian Mincer reports in "Insight: Firms to Charge Smokers, Obese More for Healthcare" (Reuters, October 30, 2011) that some companies have decided to charge workers who are obese higher insurance premiums beginning in 2013. Mincer observes that the percentage of companies imposing penalties for workers who are obese rose from 8% in 2009 to 19% in 2011 and that this percentage was expected to approach 40% in 2012. A survey conducted in June 2011 suggests that by 2016 nearly half of all employers will impose financial penalties on workers who fail to take action to lose weight. LuAnn Heinen, the vice president of the National Business Group on Health, explains that "nothing else has worked to control health trends." Critics of employers taking these actions worry that these penalties will disproportionately and unfairly burden low-income workers, who are more likely to be overweight or obese and less likely to have the necessary resources to improve their diets and gain access to exercise programs.

Some states favor charging obese public employees more for their health coverage. For example, the article "State to Hit Obese Workers with 'Fat Fee'" (Associated Press, August 26, 2008) indicates that in August 2008 Alabama's public employee health plan became the first to approve higher premiums for overweight. The fee went into effect in January 2010. In "Manchin Distances Himself from Overweight PEIA Proposal" (*Charleston [WV] Gazette*, October 28, 2009), Phil Kabler reports that in October 2009 the West Virginia Public Employees Insurance Agency voted to make the proposal to charge higher premiums to overweight employees. Other states, including North Carolina, have followed suit.

In "Fat Tax" (*New York Times*, August 12, 2009), David Leonhardt describes measures that go further than charging overweight and obese workers more for health insurance and health care services. Leonhardt explains that if it were up to Delos M. Cosgrove, the chief of the Cleveland Clinic in Cleveland, Ohio, "he would...stop hiring obese people." Cosgrove asserts that the U.S. antiobesity campaign lacks the urgency of previous public health initiatives such as smoking cessation. He states, "We should declare obesity a disease and say we're going to help you get over it." Cosgrove's approach— making value judgments and limiting people's choices— is unlikely to be enacted by U.S. companies, but Leonhardt observes that the impulse driving Cosgrove's approach indicates that "not even one of the nation's most prestigious hospitals can do much to reduce obesity."

FUNDING OBESITY RESEARCH

Since the 1970s considerable progress has been made in identifying the causes of obesity and developing treatments. Despite the enhanced understanding of the origins of obesity, increasing numbers of Americans continue to become overweight and obese. The Obesity Society, along with myriad medical professional organizations and advocacy groups, contends that public funding for obesity research is woefully inadequate in view of the size and scope of this public health problem. Besides insufficient National Institutes of Health (NIH) funding for obesity research, the Obesity Society cites inequities in research grants that are awarded by the NIH. Even though the NIH has awarded more grants to obesity research than in past years, obesity still receives a disproportionately small share of grant funding.

Table 7.1 shows NIH funding for a variety of diseases and research areas for fiscal years (FYs) 2007 to 2010 as well as estimates for FYs 2011 and 2012. Funding for obesity research has increased very slightly, from $824 million in FY 2010 to a projected $837 million in FY 2012.

WEIGHING THE PRICE THAT EMPLOYERS PAY

Obese employees incur substantially higher health care costs than normal-weight employees. Obesity significantly increases health expenditures and absenteeism. Kenneth E. Thorpe, Lydia Ogden, and Katya Galactionova of the National Business Group on Health, a consortium of large employers that researches and develops solutions to health-service delivery challenges, state in *Weighty Matters: How Obesity Drives Poor Health and Health Spending in the U.S.* (February 2009, http://www.businessgrouphealth.org/pdfs/NBGH%20Weighty Matters_Final.pdf) that even though the average per capita spending for health care rose by 40% between 1997 and 2005, for conditions associated with obesity, spending increased by 55%. More than one-quarter (27%) of the increase in inflation-adjusted health expenditures among working-age Americans is attributable to obesity. In 2005 normal-weight adults accounted for $170.6 million in health care spending, while spending for overweight adults was $168.6 million and obese adults accounted for $177.5 million.

In *Obesity and Its Relation to Mortality and Morbidity Costs* (December 2010, http://www.soa.org/files/pdf/research-2011-obesity-relation-mortality.pdf), Donald F. Behan and Samuel H. Cox estimate the costs of overweight and obesity related to the loss of productivity caused by excess mortality. Using average earnings of $35,700, and employee benefits of 19.4%, Behan and Cox calculate an average lifetime cost of $20,600 per overweight or obese worker, which when applied to the population of working-age Americans, results in an annual cost of $44 billion. Absenteeism attributable to overweight and obesity results in a cost of $43 billion per year and workers' compensation claims cost $10 billion per year.

Dan Witters and Sangeeta Agrawal of the Gallup Organization report in *Unhealthy U.S. Workers' Absenteeism Costs $153 Billion* (October 17, 2011, http://www.gallup.com/poll/150026/Unhealthy-Workers-Absenteeism-Costs-153-Billion.aspx) that overweight and obese workers with chronic health conditions miss 450 million more days of work than their normal-weight peers who do not have chronic health conditions. Witters and Agrawal estimate that the annual cost of lost productivity attributable to absenteeism among people who are overweight or obese and have one or two chronic conditions is more than $32 billion.

According to the Conference Board, in *Weights and Measures: What Employers Should Know about Obesity* (April 2008), U.S. companies pay $45 billion per year for medical care costs to treat obesity-related diseases, lower productivity, and absenteeism. The Conference Board states that obesity is associated with a 36% increase in spending on health care services, more than smoking or problem drinking. It also observes that 40% of U.S. companies have weight-reduction or weight-management programs, and an additional 24% planned to launch such programs during 2008.

Donald Liebenson reports in "The Crippling Costs of Obesity in the Workplace" (*Fiscal Times*, July 14, 2010) that one of the largest providers of health care in the Midwest attributed $6 million to obesity-related costs in 2009. Costs associated with obesity were six times higher than those related to smoking.

Obesity-Related Disability

Behan and Cox estimate that the total cost caused by the loss of productivity due to excess deaths and disability attributable to overweight and obesity, along with the cost of work-related injuries associated with overweight and obesity, is about $177 billion per year. Of this total, employment disability and absenteeism caused by physical disability related to overweight or obesity costs U.S. employers approximately $115 billion.

In "Smoking Kills, Obesity Disables: A Multistate Approach of the US Health and Retirement Survey" (*Obesity*, vol. 17, no. 4, April 2009), Mieke Reuser, Luc G. Bonneux, and Frans J. Willekens estimate life expectancy with and without disability at age 55 years for different BMIs. Compared with high normal weight

TABLE 7.1

Estimates of funding for various research, conditions, and disease categories, fiscal years 2007–12

Research/disease areas (Dollars in millions and rounded)	Fiscal year 2007 actual NIH historical method[i]	Fiscal year 2007 actual NIH revised method	Fiscal year 2008 actual	Fiscal year 2009 actual (Non-ARRA)	Fiscal year 2009 actual (ARRA)[k]	Fiscal year 2010 actual (Non-ARRA)	Fiscal year 2010 actual (ARRA)[k]	Fiscal year 2011 Estimated	Fiscal year 2012 Estimated
Acute respiratory distress syndrome	$48	$87	$82	$103	$17	$110	$22	$110	$112
Adolescent sexual activity	—	**	N/A	N/A	N/A	$80	$7	$80	$81
Agent Orange & dioxin	$18	$15	$13	$13	$2	$11	$1	$11	$11
Aging	$2,462	$1,879	$1,965	$3,015	$554	$2,517	$443	$2,517	$2,562
Alcoholism	$521	$443	$452	$441	$75	$454	$65	$454	$461
Allergic rhinitis (hay fever)	$5	$7	$6	$4	$1	$3	$1	$3	$3
ALS	$39	$40	$43	$43	$13	$47	$12	$47	$47
Alzheimer's disease	$645	$411	$412	$457	$77	$450	$79	$450	$458
American Indians/Alaska Natives	$141	$159	$142	$169	$19	$151	$16	$150	$154
Anorexia	$12	$8	$7	$8	$2	$9	$2	$9	$9
Anthrax	$105	$160	$134	$102	$13	$118	$12	$118	$121
Antimicrobial resistance	$269	$209	$228	$251	$52	$356	$66	$350	$358
Aphasia	$14	$20	$22	$22	$3	$21	$1	$21	$21
Arctic	$19	$25	$22	$28	$6	$34	$3	$34	$34
Arthritis	$339	$222	$232	$246	$65	$249	$59	$249	$253
Assistive technology	$184	$192	$215	$249	$43	$250	$48	$250	$254
Asthma	$294	$252	$246	$284	$51	$244	$33	$244	$248
Ataxia telangiectasia	$11	$14	$13	$13	$2	$12	$1	$12	$12
Atherosclerosis	$347	$468	$460	$495	$112	$544	$104	$544	$553
Attention Deficit Disorder (ADD)	$107	$61	$60	$71	$13	$66	$15	$66	$68
Autism	$127	$93	$118	$132	$64	$160	$58	$160	$163
Autoimmune disease	$587	$759	$762	$879	$138	$856	$125	$855	$869
Basic behavioral and social science	$1,104	$1,119	$1,149	$1,410	$206	$1,163	$198	$1,163	$1,184
Batten disease	$8	$5	$5	$5	$2	$5	$1	$5	$5
Behavioral and social science	$3,060	$3,157	$3,215	$3,471	$582	$3,526	$603	$3,525	$3,590
Biodefense[a]	$1,735	$1,735	$1,736	$1,755	$213	$1,794	$221	$1,549	$1,853
Bioengineering	$1,469	$2,610	$2,853	$3,155	$569	$3,166	$760	$3,162	$3,225
Biotechnology	$9,814	$5,344	$5,179	$5,619	$1,051	$5,682	$1,203	$5,675	$5,808
Brain cancer	$193	$204	$194	$234	$42	$274	$36	$274	$279
Brain disorders	$4,670	$3,592	$3,729	$3,538	$685	$3,847	$619	$3,845	$3,915
Breast cancer	$707	$729	$726	$722	$111	$763	$61	$763	$778
Burden of illness	$524	$60	$48	$43	$11	$48	$8	$48	$49
Cancer	$5,643	$5,549	$5,570	$5,629	$1,120	$5,823	$803	$5,823	$5,934
Cardiovascular	$2,370	$1,942	$2,027	$2,008	$396	$2,144	$398	$2,143	$2,180
Cerebral palsy	$16	$30	$28	$21	$4	$19	$3	$19	$19
Cervical cancer	$96	$67	$69	$84	$15	$93	$8	$93	$95
Charcot-Marie-Tooth disease	$7	$9	$12	$14	$2	$15	$1	$15	$16
Child abuse and neglect research	$38	$41	$30	$32	$5	$32	$5	$32	$33
Childhood leukemia	$55	$50	$39	$47	$12	$55	$12	$54	$55
Chronic fatigue syndrome (ME/CFS)	$4	$4	$4	$5	$0	$6	$0	$6	$6
Chronic liver disease and cirrhosis	$379	$253	$241	$274	$37	$284	$45	$284	$289
Chronic obstructive pulmonary disease	$91	$72	$75	$96	$18	$118	$15	$118	$120
Climate change	$47	$4	$4	$4	$2	$4	$2	$4	$5
Clinical research	$9,116	$9,862	$9,629	$10,336	$1,854	$10,720	$1,540	$10,707	$10,908
Clinical trials	$2,949	$3,422	$3,562	$2,966	$485	$3,286	$356	$3,282	$3,343
Colo-rectal cancer	$282	$273	$274	$281	$48	$291	$26	$291	$297
Comparative effectiveness research	—	**	+	$194	$246	$558	$320	$558	$568
Complementary and alternative medicine	$299	$426	$430	$513	$70	$521	$55	$521	$531
Conditions affecting unborn children	$110	$81	$81	$95	$8	$98	$21	$98	$99
Contraception/reproduction	$314	$460	$473	$427	$65	$419	$56	$419	$426
Cooley's anemia	$34	$22	$22	$21	$3	$20	$3	$20	$20
Cost effectiveness research	$155	$50	$49	$52	$16	$80	$14	$80	$82

TABLE 7.1

Estimates of funding for various research, conditions, and disease categories, fiscal years 2007–12 [CONTINUED]

Research/disease areas (Dollars in millions and rounded)	Fiscal year 2007 actual NIH historical method[j]	Fiscal year 2007 actual NIH revised method	Fiscal year 2008 actual	Fiscal year 2009 actual (Non-ARRA)	Fiscal year 2009 actual (ARRA)[k]	Fiscal year 2010 actual (Non-ARRA)	Fiscal year 2010 actual (ARRA)[k]	Fiscal year 2011 Estimated	Fiscal year 2012 Estimated
Crohn's disease	$69	$47	$51	$55	$14	$66	$12	$66	$68
Cystic fibrosis	$82	$78	$90	$86	$13	$86	$13	$86	$88
Dental/oral and craniofacial disease	$417	$484	$463	$490	$75	$497	$67	$497	$506
Depression	$345	$398	$402	$402	$48	$420	$50	$420	$428
Diabetes[b]	$1,037	$1,069	$1,080	$1,030	$121	$1,046	$153	$1,044	$1,060
Diagnostic radiology	$694	$1,046	$1,095	$976	$206	$1,073	$280	$1,072	$1,091
Diethylstilbestrol (DES)	$6	$5	$4	$4	$1	$4	$1	$4	$4
Digestive diseases	$1,234	$1,460	$1,426	$1,538	$243	$1,657	$228	$1,656	$1,687
Digestive diseases– (Gallbladder)	$6	$6	$7	$7	$1	$5	$0	$5	$5
Digestive diseases– (Peptic ulcer)	$23	$15	$14	$17	$3	$30	$3	$30	$30
Down syndrome	$16	$16	$17	$18	$4	$22	$6	$22	$22
Drug abuse (NIDA only)[c, m]	$1,001	$1,001	$1,007	$1,040	$135	$1,067	$125	$1,059	$1,080
Duchenne/Becker muscular dystrophy	$23	$23	$22	$27	$6	$33	$5	$33	$34
Dystonia	$16	$18	$15	$16	$2	$14	$1	$14	$14
Eating disorders[d]	—	**	+	$26	$5	$28	$4	$28	$29
Emerging infectious diseases	$1,816	$1,733	$2,098	$2,080	$307	$2,118	$350	$2,117	$2,161
Emphysema	$21	$30	$29	$28	$11	$23	$9	$23	$23
Endometriosis	$12	$12	$15	$15	$2	$15	$1	$15	$15
Epilepsy	$105	$145	$145	$128	$21	$134	$27	$134	$137
Estrogen	$164	$283	$245	$235	$34	$231	$23	$231	$235
Eye disease and disorders of vision	$714	$800	$796	$862	$129	$817	$110	$817	$831
Facioscapulohumeral muscular dystrophy	$4	$3	$3	$3	$2	$5	$1	$5	$5
Fetal alcohol syndrome	$34	$32	$34	$34	$7	$33	$5	$33	$34
Fibroid tumors (uterine)	$14	$20	$16	$18	$2	$12	$2	$12	$12
Fibromyalgia	$9	$11	$12	$11	$2	$9	$0	$9	$9
Food safety	$278	$230	$244	$262	$37	$290	$35	$290	$295
Fragile X syndrome	$27	$22	$26	$27	$5	$25	$4	$25	$26
Frontotemporal Dementia (FTD)	$31	$17	$17	$22	$2	$18	$1	$18	$19
Gene therapy	$325	$250	$249	$221	$28	$248	$32	$248	$252
Gene therapy clinical trials	$31	$12	$16	$11	$0	$14	$0	$14	$14
Genetic testing	$395	$402	$383	$316	$76	$298	$121	$298	$304
Genetics	$4,878	$7,000	$6,872	$7,278	$1,676	$7,473	$1,440	$7,470	$7,614
Global warming climate change	$56	$1	$1	$3	$1	$2	$2	$2	$2
Headaches	—	**	N/A	N/A	N/A	$18	$1	$18	$18
Health disparities[e]	$2,744	$2,744	$2,614	$2,806	$434	$2,728	$351	$2,726	$2,777
Health effects of climate change	$164	$258	$286	$179	$35	$188	$23	$188	$191
Health services	$1,023	$730	$743	$1,102	$316	$1,143	$334	$1,142	$1,185
Heart disease	$2,126	$1,126	$1,217	$1,202	$227	$1,329	$235	$1,328	$1,352
Heart disease-coronary heart disease	$382	$379	$367	$426	$98	$457	$80	$457	$465
Hematology	$1,128	$881	$894	$908	$151	$961	$141	$961	$978
Hepatitis	$174	$176	$180	$178	$23	$204	$25	$204	$208
Hepatitis-A	$2	$6	$6	$4	$0	$4	$0	$4	$4
Hepatitis-B	$42	$53	$53	$51	$6	$66	$4	$66	$67
Hepatitis-C	$108	$100	$93	$97	$12	$100	$12	$100	$102
HIV/AIDS[f, l]	$2,906	$2,906	$2,928	$3,019	$319	$3,085	$322	$3,086	$3,160
Hodgkin's disease	$17	$12	$16	$26	$1	$24	$1	$24	$25
Homelessness	$18	$14	$13	$16	$3	$15	$3	$15	$16
Homicide and legal interventions	$8	$1	*	$2	$1	$1	$0	$1	$1
HPV and/or cervical cancer vaccines	$20	$16	$19	$25	$2	$25	$2	$25	$25
Human fetal tissue[g]	$19	**	$40	$41	$22	$55	$24	$55	$56
Human genome	$1,099	$1,246	$1,259	$1,775	$566	$1,904	$598	$1,903	$1,939
Huntington's disease	$53	$49	$51	$57	$12	$65	$7	$65	$66
Hyperbaric oxygen	$2	$3	$4	$3	$0	$2	$0	$2	$2
Hypertension	$390	$231	$263	$266	$41	$251	$50	$251	$255

(BMI of 23 to 24.9), mild obesity (BMI of 30 to 34.9) decreased disability-free life expectancy by 2.7 years in men and by 3.6 years in women.

THE HIGH COST OF LOSING WEIGHT

According to Jeffrey M. Jones of the Gallup Organization, in *In U.S., More Would Like to Lose Weight Than*

TABLE 7.1

Estimates of funding for various research, conditions, and disease categories, fiscal years 2007–12 [CONTINUED]

Research/disease areas (Dollars in millions and rounded)	Fiscal year 2007 actual NIH historical method[i]	Fiscal year 2007 actual NIH revised method	Fiscal year 2008 actual	Fiscal year 2009 actual (Non-ARRA)	Fiscal year 2009 actual (ARRA)[k]	Fiscal year 2010 actual (Non-ARRA)	Fiscal year 2010 actual (ARRA)[k]	Fiscal year 2011 Estimated	Fiscal year 2012 Estimated
Immunization	$1,342	$1,713	$1,734	$1,773	$191	$1,798	$231	$1,798	$1,835
Infant mortality/(LBW)	$464	$227	$246	$246	$32	$273	$53	$273	$278
Infectious diseases	$3,059	$3,433	$3,575	$3,627	$526	$3,890	$568	$3,888	$3,968
Infertility	$51	$65	$73	$75	$17	$76	$16	$75	$77
Inflammatory bowel disease	$80	$74	$81	$91	$22	$106	$19	$106	$108
Influenza	$271	$280	$204	$316	$46	$308	$88	$308	$315
Injury–childhood injuries	$27	$28	$26	$33	$3	$36	$3	$36	$36
Injury–trauma–(head and spine)	$219	$164	$150	$161	$33	$179	$31	$178	$182
Injury–traumatic brain injury	$82	$73	$59	$71	$15	$85	$9	$85	$86
Injury–unintentional childhood injury	$21	$17	$15	$19	$1	$22	$1	$22	$22
Injury (total) accidents/adverse effects	$403	$299	$299	$340	$58	$372	$46	$372	$379
Interstitial cystitis	$23	$10	$10	$11	$1	$12	$1	$12	$12
Kidney disease	$450	$531	$523	$570	$85	$552	$98	$552	$561
Lead poisoning	$15	$13	$9	$11	$3	$11	$1	$11	$12
Liver cancer	$90	$103	$89	$94	$12	$102	$10	$102	$104
Liver disease	$423	$589	$562	$572	$79	$627	$85	$627	$639
Lung	$1,013	$1,169	$1,211	$1,265	$234	$1,269	$207	$1,269	$1,292
Lung cancer	$249	$164	$169	$178	$36	$201	$22	$201	$205
Lupus	$84	$113	$126	$115	$19	$112	$15	$112	$114
Lyme disease	$22	$26	$22	$25	$5	$24	$5	$24	$25
Lymphoma	$158	$186	$193	$184	$22	$195	$14	$195	$199
Macular degeneration	$70	$135	$135	$85	$8	$104	$9	$104	$106
Malaria	$104	$112	$132	$110	$11	$134	$14	$134	$136
Malaria vaccine	$36	$31	$32	$34	$3	$41	$4	$41	$42
Mental health	$1,853	$2,061	$2,086	$2,129	$382	$2,246	$334	$2,246	$2,287
Mental retardation (Intellectual and Developmental Disabilities (IDD))	$204	$305	$350	$281	$94	$311	$87	$311	$317
Methamphetamine	$45	$66	$67	$69	$13	$73	$14	$73	$74
Migraines	—	**	N/A	N/A	N/A	$15	$0	$15	$15
Mind and body	$133	$571	$567	$494	$90	$549	$81	$548	$558
Minority health[e]	$2,407	$2,407	$2,396	$2,592	$378	$2,526	$312	$2,525	$2,572
Mucopolysaccharidoses (MPS)	$10	$8	$7	$7	$0	$8	$0	$8	$8
Multiple sclerosis	$98	$149	$169	$137	$25	$133	$18	$133	$135
Muscular dystrophy	$47	$58	$56	$66	$17	$74	$12	$74	$75
Myasthenia gravis	$6	$10	$9	$9	$3	$8	$3	$8	$8
Myotonic dystrophy	$8	$9	$9	$9	$4	$10	$2	$10	$10
Nanotechnology[h]	$215	$257	$304	$343	$73	$435	$76	$435	$443
Networking and information technology R&D[h]	$507	$959	$911	$1,174	$168	$647	$248	$646	$663
Neurodegenerative	$1,166	$1,579	$1,621	$1,553	$262	$1,571	$243	$1,571	$1,599
Neurofibromatosis	$13	$12	$14	$17	$2	$24	$1	$24	$24
Neuropathy	$59	$118	$121	$119	$13	$121	$10	$121	$123
Neurosciences	$4,809	$5,102	$5,224	$5,320	$848	$5,515	$794	$5,513	$5,612
Nutrition	$1,075	$1,327	$1,391	$1,400	$205	$1,435	$208	$1,434	$1,460
Obesity	$661	$595	$664	$745	$117	$824	$147	$823	$837
Organ transplantation	$358	$187	$175	$139	$32	$150	$37	$150	$153
Orphan drug	$1,158	$653	$645	$441	$118	$512	$89	$512	$522
Osteogenesis imperfecta	$5	$8	$5	$5	$1	$8	$4	$8	$8
Osteoporosis	$164	$167	$183	$198	$21	$181	$23	$181	$184
Otitis media	$15	$20	$18	$15	$7	$19	$2	$19	$20
Ovarian cancer	$103	$89	$96	$102	$13	$122	$10	$122	$125
Paget's disease	$4	$1	$1	$1	$1	$1	$0	$1	$1
Pain conditions–chronic	$224	$277	$279	$333	$53	$360	$44	$360	$366
Parkinson's disease	$187	$143	$152	$162	$24	$154	$18	$154	$157
Patient safety	—	**	N/A	N/A	N/A	$859	$263	$858	$875
Pediatric	$3,173	$2,622	$2,771	$2,996	$505	$3,286	$479	$3,282	$3,341
Pediatric AIDS[f]	$262	$262	$241	$227	$20	$216	$15	$216	$220
Pediatric research initiative	$171	**	$209	$214	$256	$308	$148	$307	$312
Pelvic inflammatory disease	$3	$4	$3	$3	$1	$4	$1	$4	$4
Perinatal–birth-preterm (LBW)	$351	$181	$197	$177	$23	$183	$47	$183	$186
Perinatal–neonatal respiratory distress syndrome	$9	$23	$18	$31	$5	$31	$3	$31	$32
Perinatal period–conditions originating in perinatal period	$387	$413	$449	$470	$65	$542	$84	$541	$551

TABLE 7.1

Estimates of funding for various research, conditions, and disease categories, fiscal years 2007–12 [CONTINUED]

Research/disease areas (Dollars in millions and rounded)	Fiscal year 2007 actual NIH historical method[j]	Fiscal year 2007 actual NIH revised method	Fiscal year 2008 actual	Fiscal year 2009 actual (Non-ARRA)	Fiscal year 2009 actual (ARRA)[k]	Fiscal year 2010 actual (Non-ARRA)	Fiscal year 2010 actual (ARRA)[k]	Fiscal year 2011 Estimated	Fiscal year 2012 Estimated
Pick's disease	$1	$3	$2	$2	$0	$2	$0	$2	$2
Pneumonia	$132	$105	$93	$108	$15	$93	$17	$93	$95
Pneumonia & influenza	$405	$382	$295	$392	$58	$396	$102	$396	$404
Polycystic kidney disease	$36	$33	$41	$38	$7	$35	$6	$35	$36
Prescription drug abuse	—	**	N/A	N/A	N/A	$29	$7	$29	$29
Prevention	$6,729	$4,596	$4,623	$5,332	$844	$5,983	$849	$5,981	$6,113
Prostate cancer	$345	$295	$290	$310	$47	$331	$31	$331	$337
Psoriasis	$10	$22	$8	$13	$3	$13	$3	$13	$13
Regenerative medicine	$575	$697	$723	$799	$144	$820	$142	$819	$834
Rehabilitation	$344	$379	$403	$404	$75	$458	$93	$458	$466
Rett syndrome	$6	$6	$9	$9	$4	$13	$2	$13	$13
Reye's syndrome	$1	$0	$0	$0	$0	$0	$0	—	—
Rural health	$208	$173	$170	$186	$42	$207	$33	$207	$211
Schizophrenia	$358	$220	$249	$265	$85	$276	$63	$276	$282
Scleroderma	$12	$12	$20	$21	$2	$19	$2	$19	$19
Screening and brief intervention for substance abuse	—	**	N/A	N/A	N/A	$26	$4	$26	$27
Septicemia	$49	$93	$95	$92	$19	$90	$17	$90	$92
Sexually transmitted diseases/herpes	$288	$282	$245	$250	$43	$250	$38	$250	$255
Sickle cell disease	$94	$78	$80	$63	$14	$73	$12	$73	$75
Sleep research	$190	$219	$225	$217	$33	$226	$22	$226	$230
Small pox	$122	$142	$94	$94	$4	$92	$5	$92	$94
Smoking and health	$534	$324	$310	$329	$78	$336	$55	$336	$342
Spina bifida	$9	$14	$15	$14	$3	$12	$6	$12	$12
Spinal cord injury	$64	$90	$80	$80	$14	$87	$16	$87	$88
Spinal muscular atrophy	$11	$11	$10	$11	$3	$16	$3	$16	$17
Stem cell research	$657	$968	$938	$1,044	$187	$1,099	$187	$1,098	$1,118
Stem cell research–embryonic-human	$42	$74	$88	$120	$23	$126	$40	$125	$128
Stem cell research–embryonic-non-human	$106	$120	$150	$148	$29	$175	$20	$175	$178
Stem cell research–nonembryonic-human	$203	$226	$297	$339	$58	$341	$74	$341	$347
Stem cell research–nonembryonic-non-human	$306	$400	$497	$550	$88	$570	$74	$569	$580
Stem cell research–umbilical cord blood/placenta	$22	$44	$46	$49	$10	$42	$8	$42	$42
Stem cell research–umbilical cord blood/placenta–human	$19	$38	$38	$42	$9	$40	$7	$40	$40
Stem cell research–umbilical cord blood/placenta–non-human	$2	$9	$9	$10	$1	$5	$1	$5	$5
Stroke	$340	$288	$296	$329	$54	$337	$54	$337	$343
Substance abuse[l]	$1,523	$1,636	$1,763	$1,653	$245	$1,674	$216	$1,666	$1,697
Substance abuse prevention	—	**	N/A	N/A	N/A	$43	$10	$43	$44
Sudden infant death syndrome	$81	$25	$29	$22	$6	$25	$2	$25	$26
Suicide	$43	$52	$39	$36	$15	$36	$4	$36	$37
Suicide prevention	—	**	N/A	N/A	N/A	$17	$2	$17	$18
Teenage pregnancy	$16	$24	$21	$23	$5	$22	$5	$22	$23
Temporomandibular Muscle/Joint Disorder (TMJD)	$15	$18	$19	$15	$1	$16	$1	$16	$16
Tobacco	$536	$325	$311	$331	$78	$339	$55	$339	$345
Topical microbicides	$99	$92	$102	$92	$7	$84	$5	$84	$86
Tourette syndrome	$11	$9	$8	$7	$3	$7	$0	$7	$7
Transmissible Spongiform Encephalopathy (TSE)	$43	$50	$44	$43	$4	$48	$3	$48	$49
Transplantation	$534	$544	$519	$571	$94	$574	$109	$574	$584
Tuberculosis	$166	$188	$142	$189	$27	$189	$35	$189	$192
Tuberculosis vaccine	$17	$23	$18	$15	$3	$13	$3	$13	$14
Tuberous sclerosis	$12	$20	$20	$20	$3	$20	$2	$20	$20
Underage drinking	—	**	N/A	N/A	N/A	$75	$5	$75	$76
Underage drinking–prevention & treatment (NIAAA only)[n]	—	**	N/A	N/A	N/A	$56	$2	$55	$56
Urologic diseases	$526	$535	$534	$578	$81	$563	$56	$562	$573
Uterine cancer	$22	$24	$16	$25	$4	$26	$4	$26	$26
Vaccine related	$1,358	$1,659	$1,632	$1,593	$185	$1,737	$222	$1,736	$1,771

TABLE 7.1

Estimates of funding for various research, conditions, and disease categories, fiscal years 2007–12 [CONTINUED]

Research/disease areas (Dollars in millions and rounded)	Fiscal year 2007 actual NIH historical method[j]	Fiscal year 2007 actual NIH revised method	Fiscal year 2008 actual	Fiscal year 2009 actual (Non-ARRA)	Fiscal year 2009 actual (ARRA)[k]	Fiscal year 2010 actual (Non-ARRA)	Fiscal year 2010 actual (ARRA)[k]	Fiscal year 2011 Estimated	Fiscal year 2012 Estimated
Vaccine related (AIDS)[f]	$597	$597	$556	$561	$35	$535	$27	$535	$546
Vector-borne diseases	$424	$478	$417	$401	$66	$426	$68	$426	$435
Violence against women	$24	$49	$45	$39	$2	$36	$2	$36	$37
Violence research	$106	$190	$183	$182	$21	$174	$19	$174	$177
Vulvodynia	—	**	+	$1	$1	$2	$1	$2	$2
West Nile virus	$69	$81	$39	$59	$7	$46	$6	$45	$46
Women's health[e]	$3,470	$3,470	$3,514	$3,725	$506	$3,691	$449	$3,689	$3,757
Youth violence	$60	$123	$115	$111	$12	$102	$10	$102	$104
Youth violence prevention	—	**	N/A	N/A	N/A	$32	$2	$32	$33

*The minimum reporting threshold for a specific disease/condition is $500,000. Reporting of $0 does not indicate that no research is being conducted.

**No methodology was identified for RCDC in 2007; therefore there is no data available under the "Fiscal year 2007" column.

' Indicates a new category. Funding support data not available prior to the actual fiscal year 2009 or fiscal year 2010 level reported.

[a]Reporting for this category does not follow the standard RCDC process. The total amount reported is consistent with reporting requirements for this category to the U.S. Office of Management & Budget (OMB). The project listing does not include non-project or other support costs associated with the annual total for this category.

[b]Includes research funded from the Type 1 diabetes appropriation of $150,000,000. These are project listings only.

[c]Reporting for this category does not follow the standard RCDC process. Spending is reported consistent with U.S. Office of National Drug Control Policy (ONDCP) requirements (Only NIDA).

[d]Reported total for this category encompasses research for anorexia, bulimia nervosa, binge eating disorders, and eating disorders not otherwise specified.

[e]Reporting for this category does not follow the standard RCDC process. This category assigns project funding according to populations tracked by gender or ethnicity. The databases used to track gender/ethnicity are complex and not currently compatible with the RCDC system.

[f]Reporting for this category does not follow the standard RCDC process. These are project listings only and non-project or other support costs associated with the annual total for the category are not included.

[g]Reporting for this category does not follow the standard RCDC process. This category uses a non-standard approach involving subject matter expert reviews of manually collected project listings.

[h]The data provided reflects funding amounts reported by the NIH RCDC process for this category. Actual and estimate levels presented on this site supersede fiscal years 2010–2012 amounts detailed in OMB MAX DE application tables that were based on preliminary fiscal year 2010 funding support information.

[i]Reporting for this category does not follow the standard RCDC process. This category includes all spending reported under the Drug Abuse category as well as projects categorized under the broader area of Substance Abuse. These are project listings only.

[j]To illustrate the effect of the RCDC methodology change, the table shows a side-by-side comparison of fiscal year 2007 levels produced with the prior method ("NIH Historical Method") compared with levels that would have resulted if the new methodology had been implemented ("NIH Revised Method"). "NIH Historical Method" figures are considered the official "Actual" for fiscal year 2007. The "NIH Revised Method" levels provide for comparability to fiscal year 2008 RCDC actuals.

[k]Separate columns are used to distinguish fiscal year 2009 and fiscal year 2010 actual support funded from American Recovery & Reinvestment Act (ARRA) accounts from projects funded by regular annual NIH appropriations.

[l]The fiscal year 2011 column estimate does not reflect the legislative impact of funding levels provided in Public Law 111-117 and Public Law 112-10. The current estimate of HIV/AIDS funding in fiscal year 2011 is $3,059,277,000.

[m]The fiscal year 2011 column estimate does not reflect the legislative impact of funding levels provided in Public Law 111-117 and Public Law 112-10. The current estimate of funding in fiscal year 2011 is $1,050,542,000.

[n]The fiscal year 2011 column estimate does not reflect the legislative impact of funding levels provided in Public Law 111-117 and Public Law 112-10. The current estimate of funding in fiscal year 2011 is $55,030,000.

Note: ARRA = two separate columns fiscal year 2009 and fiscal year 2010 actual support funded from American Recovery & Reinvestment Act (ARRA) accounts from projects funded by regular NIH appropriations.

RCDC = Research, Condition, and Disease Categories. NIH = National Institutes of Health.

SOURCE: "Estimates of Funding for Various Research, Condition, and Disease Categories (RCDC)," U.S. Department of Health and Human Services, National Institutes of Health, March 2011, http://report.nih.gov/rcdc/categories/PFSummaryTable.aspx (accessed November 7, 2011)

Are Trying To (November 20, 2009, http://www.gallup.com/poll/124448/In-U.S.-More-Lose-Weight-Than-Trying-To.aspx), in 2009 approximately 27% of Americans were seriously trying to lose weight. Gabriel I. Uwaifo et al. indicate in "Obesity" (November 8, 2011, http://emedicine.medscape.com/article/123702-overview) that Americans spend about $33 billion per year to lose or prevent weight gain. The market research firm Marketdata Enterprises Inc. forecasts in *U.S. Weight Loss and Diet Control Market* (May 2011, http://www.marketresearch.com/Marketdata-Enterprises-Inc-v416/Weight-Loss-Diet-Control-11th-6314539/) that the U.S. weight-loss industry produced revenues in excess of $60 billion in 2010, up 3.2% from $58.6 billion in 2008.

Along with commercial weight-loss centers, medically supervised weight-loss programs, and prescription diet drugs, products such as diet books, audio and video programs, web-based diet and nutrition services, low-calorie and low-carbohydrate food products, meal replacements, and over-the-counter (nonprescription) appetite suppressants compete for consumer dollars. Marketdata Enterprises indicates that the commercial weight-loss center market had $3.1 billion in revenues in 2010, with Weight Watchers being the clear front-runner in both 2009 and 2010.

Between 2009 and 2010 over-the-counter diet pills and meal replacement sales declined by 2%, to $2.7

billion. However, Marketdata Enterprises predicts annual gains of 3.3% in this market segment, yielding a $3 billion market in 2014. Even though hospital-based weight-loss programs continue to attract dieters, more growth occurred in the medical clinic sector. One medical clinic chain, the Centers for Medical Weight Loss, grew from 60 centers in 2007 to more than 450 in 2011. A franchised clinic program, Medi-Weightloss, also expanded during this same period.

Weight Watchers was the leader in the online dieting arena as well, with more than 1 million paid subscribers and revenues of $238 million in 2010. In general, online diet programs were down 17% from 2009; however, Marketdata Enterprises anticipates 8% annual growth through 2014. Because most paid sites have not been profitable, many are shifting to an advertising-based revenue model that enables users free access to the sites.

According to Marketdata Enterprises, the most affluent dieters are purchasing home-delivered diet foods, which accounted for $924 million of the weight-loss market in 2010. NutriSystem owns about 55% of this market—other firms including Jenny Direct, Medifast, Diet to Go, 5 Squares, BistroMD, Atkins at Home, eDiets Meal Delivery, Chefs Diet, Freshology, Sunfare, Seattle Sutton's Healthy Eating, HMR at Home, In the Zone, and Personal Chef to Go also cater to this market. The cost averages $726 per month for home-delivered diet food, and dieters can spend as much as $1,200 per month.

Medical and Behavioral Treatments

The greatest proportion of outlays for weight loss are for food products and commercial weight-loss programs. However, in "Screening and Interventions for Obesity in Adults: Summary of the Evidence for the U.S. Preventive Services Task Force" (*Annals of Internal Medicine*, vol. 139, no. 11, December 2, 2003), one of the first analyses of the costs that are associated with behavioral interventions for weight loss, Kathleen M. McTigue et al. observe that medical and behavioral treatment options for obesity also involve considerable cost. The researchers state, "Intensive counseling programs require a large amount of time and a substantial staffing commitment. Based on average wholesale price, 1-year supplies of orlistat (120 mg 3 times daily) and sibutramine (15 mg daily) cost $1445.40 and $1464.78 U.S., respectively." It is important to note that consumers generally purchase prescription drugs at retail rather than at wholesale prices, so their costs are considerably higher than those reported by McTigue et al.

In "Economic Evaluation of an Internet-Based Weight Management Program" (*American Journal of Managed Care*, vol. 16, no. 4, April 1, 2010), Rafia S. Rasu et al. compare the cost of a behavioral treatment program delivered via the Internet with usual care (a face-to-face nutrition-based weight management and physical fitness program, an annual fitness assessment, and a yearly preventive health checkup with a health care provider) in a sample of overweight adults serving in the U.S. Air Force. The costs associated with the Internet intervention included distribution materials and letterhead; the cost of the training sessions; the costs of educational materials, equipment, supplies, and other items (e.g., website and computer costs); and the costs for employees (project staff) while they worked on the training sessions as well as on the baseline and follow-up appointments to measure weight. The Internet intervention involved 227 participants and the total cost per participant was $49.24, which was $15.09 lower than the per participant cost of usual treatment. Rasu et al. find that even though an Internet intervention has higher initial costs, it becomes more cost effective over time, and conclude that it "is a cost-effective choice for weight management."

According to William E. Encinosa et al., in "Recent Improvements in Bariatric Surgery Outcomes" (*Medical Care*, vol. 47, no. 5, May 2009), weight-loss surgery costs declined between 2002 and 2006, from $29,563 to $27,905 for patients without complications and from $41,807 to $38,175 for patients who experienced complications. Even hospital payments for those readmitted because of complications decreased from $80,001 to $69,960. Some of the decline in costs may be related to volume—between 2001 and 2005 weight-loss surgeries grew by 115%. Encinosa et al. opine that the decrease in cost was also due to a move to the less invasive laparoscopic technique, which requires shorter hospital stays, and to an increase in procedures that use gastric banding without bypass.

Long-Term Savings

Even though surgical treatment of obesity is a relatively recent phenomenon, research reveals that its costs are offset by a reduction in future utilization of health care services and a resultant reduction in health care costs. In "The Clinical Effectiveness and Cost-Effectiveness of Bariatric (Weight Loss) Surgery for Obesity: A Systematic Review and Economic Evaluation" (*Health Technology Assessment*, vol. 13, no. 41, September 2009), a review of research assessing the clinical effectiveness and cost effectiveness of bariatric surgery for obesity, Julien Picot et al. conclude that, overall, bariatric surgery is cost effective in comparison to nonsurgical treatment for people with moderate to severe obesity. However, the researchers do observe that nearly all the studies they reviewed suffered from methodological problems that may compromise the extent to which their result can be generalized to the entire population of obese adults. For example, some studies included one-year postsurgery models and others used five-year postsurgery economic models, and some did not consider the probabilities of developing or reversing obesity-related diseases with or without the surgical intervention.

Pierre-Yves Cremieux et al. evaluate in "A Study on the Economic Impact of Bariatric Surgery" (*American Journal of Managed Care*, vol. 14, no. 9, September 2008) the third-party payer's return on investment for weight-loss surgery. The researchers matched 3,651 bariatric surgery patients to control subjects with clinically severe obesity who did not undergo the surgery and compared their health care costs. The mean (average) weight-loss surgery cost the payer between $17,000 and $26,000, and Cremieux et al. estimate that "all costs [were] recouped within 2 years for laparoscopic surgery patients and within 4 years for open surgery patients." The study also reveals that the bariatric surgery costs were recouped more quickly in 2005 than they were in 2002. In 2005 it took six years to recoup the costs of open bariatric surgery, compared with just two years for laparoscopic bariatric surgery. Cremieux et al. attribute this improvement to "surgical experience, improved technology, and dedicated facilities."

Even community-based weight-loss programs have the potential to save money. Kenneth E. Thorpe and Zhou Yang estimate in "Enrolling People with Prediabetes Ages 60–64 in a Proven Weight Loss Program Could Save Medicare $7 Billion or More" (*Health Affairs*, vol. 30, no. 9, September 2011) the net savings to Medicare over a 10-year period by enrolling two groups of people—people aged 60 to 64 years who have prediabetes and a BMI higher than 24 and people with the same BMI who are at risk for cardiovascular disease (high blood pressure or elevated cholesterol) independent of whether they have prediabetes—in a community-based weight-loss program that was developed by the Centers for Disease Control and Prevention, the YMCA, and the UnitedHealth Group. This program, which features trained lifestyle coaches who help people make healthier food choices and increase physical activity, has demonstrated the ability to help people aged 60 years and older lose weight and reduce their risk of developing diabetes by as much as 71%. By enrolling the two at-risk groups, Thorpe and Yang project Medicare savings of as much as $3.7 billion over the next 10 years and as much as $15.1 billion over the course of the participants' lifetime. Thorpe and Yang assert, "Our results show the potential savings to Medicare if a proven community-based approach to reducing obesity and related chronic disease were to be made available, nationwide, to high-risk individuals soon to become Medicare beneficiaries. In doing so, they also present a potential business case for the federal government to partner with the private sector in order to encourage broad enrollment in effective weight loss programs."

CATERING TO AN EXPANDING MARKET

Along with increased costs, many businesses have discovered that they must literally expand their products and services to meet the needs of overweight and obese consumers. Scott Mayerowitz describes in "Living Large: Products for the Obese" (ABC News, January 5, 2009) a wide array of products—from heavy-duty weight scales, portable chairs, and seatbelt extenders, to super-sized robes and towels—that are designed to meet the needs of obese Americans.

According to the Franklin Furniture Institute of Mississippi State University, in *Tipping the Scales: Weighing the Bariatric Furniture Market* (October 2009, http://www.ffi.msstate.edu/pdf/bariatric_furniture.pdf), the market for furniture that can accommodate extra weight is an unmet need and is estimated to be as great as $400 million per year. The institute describes adults aged 40 to 59 years with BMIs of 30 or greater as the target market for seating, beds, and furniture frames that can withstand additional weight and pressure.

According to Amy Wilson, in "Plus-Sized Women: It's Our Turn for Fine Fashion" (CNN.com, June 21, 2011), the market research firm NPD Group reports that between April 2010 and April 2011 sales of plus-sized women's apparel accounted for 17% of the market and $17.5 billion in sales. In the article "Demand for Plus-Size Girls' Apparel Expanding" (Reuters, October 9, 2007), Marshal Cohen, an analyst with the NPD Group, opines that the children's plus-sized market could eventually grow to 18% of the total children's apparel market of more than $35 billion. The article "Expanding Plus-Size and Big-and-Tall Clothing Market Estimated to Reach $107 Billion by 2012" (PRNewswire, June 26, 2007) notes that another market research firm, Packaged Facts, predicts that the plus-sized clothing market will grow by 41% between 2006 and 2012, with commensurate growth in sales, from $47.1 billion in 2006 to almost $65 billion in 2012.

Hot Topic, a California-based company that specializes in clothing for teenagers and young women, launched a chain of six stores in 2001 called Torrid that offer fashion-forward plus-sized clothing for young women. Hot Topic (2011, http://investorrelations.hottopic.com/phoenix.zhtml?c=120007&p=irol-homeProfile&t=&id=&) notes that in FY 2008 it had 159 Torrid stores in 36 states that offered an array of clothing and lingerie for young women. The press release "Hot Topic, Inc. Reports July Comp Store Sales up 7.3%" (August 3, 2011, http://online.wsj.com/article/PR-CO-20110803-910754.html) indicates that Torrid's sales increased nearly 10% from 2010 to 2011.

In "Plus-Size Revelation: Bigger Women Have Cash, Too" (*New York Times*, June 18, 2010), Stephanie Clifford reports that the clothing chain Forever 21 launched Faith 21, its plus-sized line, in 2010 and that this line's sales exceeded expectations. That same year Target introduced a plus-sized line called Pure Energy aimed at younger women, as did the high-fashion designer Elie Tahari. However, Clifford also notes that some stores, such as Ann Taylor and Old Navy, and designers, such as Liz Claiborne, have limited or discontinued plus-sized clothing. Industry observers speculate that one reason for discontinuing to offer plus-sized clothing may be that the use of wider bolts of fabric and specialized machinery increase the costs of production and decrease profit margins in comparison with regular-sized clothing.

Demand for larger, sturdier hospital beds and stretchers to accommodate extremely heavy patients, special imaging equipment such as computed tomography and magnetic resonance imaging to accommodate obese patients, bigger blood pressure cuffs, recliners constructed to hold 350 pounds (159 kg), automobiles that comfortably seat obese drivers and passengers, and devices that enable people who cannot bend over to put on their socks and shoes have prompted the design and manufacture of these and other specialty products.

Even morticians have observed and responded to the obesity epidemic. According to Mikaela Conley, in "Obesity Epidemic Spurs Demand for Oversized Caskets" (ABC News, January 4, 2011), caskets, mortuary lifts, grave openings, and vaults are growing in capacity to accommodate larger bodies. Conley notes that the Goliath Casket Company has also continued to increase the size of its offerings. Besides offering a 29-inch (74-cm) coffin, it makes caskets that are up to 52 inches (132 cm) wide. The 52-inch caskets are constructed with extra supports that are intended for body weights of between 800 and 1,000 pounds (363 and 454 kg).

CHAPTER 8

POLITICAL, LEGAL, AND SOCIAL ISSUES
OF OVERWEIGHT AND OBESITY

The Healthy, Hunger-Free Kids Act makes the most significant investment in the National School Lunch program in more than 30 years. I look forward to continuing to work with the First Lady and Secretary [Tom] Vilsack to combat our national childhood obesity epidemic and increase students' access to the nutritional food they need to help them learn.

—Kathleen Sebelius, U.S. Secretary of Health and Human Services, at the signing of the Healthy, Hunger-Free Kids Act of 2010 (December 13, 2010)

THE GLOBAL POLITICS OF OBESITY

At the international level, the World Health Organization (WHO) has developed an aggressive strategy to combat an escalating global epidemic of overweight and obesity throughout the world. In *Global Strategy on Diet, Physical Activity, and Health* (October 2005, http://www.who.int/dietphysicalactivity/strategy/eb11344/strategy_english_web.pdf), the WHO exhorts individuals and populations to:

- Achieve energy balance and a healthy weight

- Limit energy intake from total fats and shift fat consumption away from saturated fats to unsaturated fats and toward the elimination of trans fatty acids

- Increase consumption of fruits and vegetables and legumes, whole grains and nuts

- Limit the intake of free sugars

- Limit salt (sodium) consumption from all sources and ensure that salt is iodized

- Engage in at least 30 minutes of regular, moderate-intensity physical activity on most days

The WHO asserts that "government is crucial in achieving lasting change in public health" and believes that governments should take the lead in initiating and developing the strategy and ensuring that it is implemented. The WHO also recommends sharply limiting the marketing of food to children and using tax and pricing policies to influence food consumption. According to the WHO, these measures are necessary to reverse the rising rates of obesity-related illnesses (heart disease, diabetes, and cancer), which are forecast to account for nearly three-quarters of deaths worldwide by 2020.

The WHO strategy was developed by an international team of experts using the latest scientific evidence available and has been commended by public health officials throughout the world. It is not, however, favored by some food manufacturers because among its proposals are restrictions on advertising unhealthful foods to children and the imposition of taxes and farm subsidy changes aimed at increasing prices of sugary and high-fat foods. For example, the International Sugar Organization strenuously objects to the recommendation that sugar amounts to no more than 10% of food and drink calories consumed per day, calling instead for a 25% cap. Table 8.1 shows that the total U.S. consumption of caloric sweeteners spiked in 1999, 2000, 2002, and 2005, but that the overall use of caloric sweeteners has not varied significantly between 1997 and 2010.

U.S. opposition to the WHO strategy has been criticized as a clear effort to appease U.S. food and sugar suppliers. Some WHO scientists and consumer advocacy groups suggest the U.S. objections—specifically those about the recommendations to limit sugar consumption and to reconsider food advertising aimed at young children—aim to protect industries that have recently been under attack rather than to improve public health. However, the food industry itself publicly pledged to support the WHO strategy. For example, the Grocery Manufacturers of America, the world's largest association of food and drink companies, which includes PepsiCo Inc. and Hershey Foods Corp., said it was committed to working with the WHO to combat obesity.

TABLE 8.1

Total estimated deliveries of caloric sweeteners for domestic food and beverage use, by calendar year, 1966–2010[a]

Calendar year	Sugar[b]		Corn sweeteners				Honey	Other edible syrups	Total caloric sweeteners[c]
	Raw value	Refined basis	High fructose corn sweetner/syrup	Glucose syrup	Dextrose	Total			
				1,000 short tons, dry basis					
1966	10,235	9,565	0	952	415	1,367	98	69	11,099
1967	10,474	9,789	3	984	428	1,415	89	50	11,342
1968	10,656	9,959	15	1,031	444	1,489	90	70	11,608
1969	10,950	10,234	33	1,061	459	1,553	101	61	11,949
1970	11,163	10,433	56	1,102	471	1,629	103	51	12,216
1971	11,345	10,603	86	1,163	482	1,731	93	52	12,478
1972	11,487	10,736	121	1,257	485	1,863	105	52	12,756
1973	11,429	10,681	218	1,384	489	2,092	95	53	12,922
1974	10,945	10,229	295	1,480	486	2,262	75	43	12,609
1975	10,302	9,628	527	1,515	473	2,515	108	43	12,294
1976	10,893	10,180	782	1,514	452	2,748	100	44	13,072
1977	11,099	10,373	1,057	1,517	429	3,003	100	44	13,519
1978	10,889	10,177	1,198	1,551	410	3,159	120	45	13,501
1979	10,756	10,052	1,660	1,519	399	3,578	117	44	13,791
1980	10,189	9,522	2,158	1,472	393	4,024	94	50	13,690
1981	9,769	9,130	2,626	1,486	390	4,501	96	46	13,773
1982	9,153	8,554	3,090	1,479	392	4,961	104	46	13,665
1983	8,812	8,236	3,655	1,523	398	5,577	116	47	13,975
1984	8,428	7,877	4,399	1,552	408	6,359	108	47	14,391
1985	8,003	7,479	5,386	1,607	418	7,411	104	48	15,043
1986	7,731	7,225	5,498	1,632	430	7,561	121	50	14,957
1987	8,103	7,573	5,792	1,679	441	7,912	104	55	15,644
1988	8,136	7,604	5,998	1,747	452	8,197	100	54	15,955
1989	8,304	7,761	5,960	1,587	438	7,985	95	53	15,894
1990	8,615	8,051	6,202	1,700	455	8,358	103	53	16,565
1991	8,622	8,058	6,376	1,776	463	8,615	116	53	16,842
1992	8,826	8,249	6,652	1,943	461	9,056	126	53	17,483
1993	8,886	8,305	7,086	2,050	481	9,617	135	56	18,112
1994	9,072	8,478	7,398	2,093	502	9,993	126	54	18,651
1995	9,258	8,652	7,676	2,176	528	10,380	120	57	19,209
1996	9,381	8,767	7,788	2,216	537	10,541	131	57	19,496
1997	9,473	8,853	8,240	2,364	511	11,116	129	58	20,156
1998	9,592	8,964	8,552	2,358	502	11,411	130	59	20,564
1999	9,905	9,257	8,897	2,281	488	11,666	147	60	21,131
2000	9,899	9,252	8,845	2,230	476	11,551	157	60	21,020
2001	9,839	9,195	8,920	2,205	469	11,595	134	61	20,985
2002	9,742	9,105	9,045	2,224	473	11,741	153	62	21,061
2003	9,468	8,848	8,849	2,209	449	11,507	146	63	20,564
2004	9,661	9,029	8,779	2,292	487	11,558	130	64	20,781
2005	9,977	9,324	8,756	2,261	481	11,497	156	66	21,043
2006	9,936	9,286	8,702	2,053	463	11,218	174	66	20,745
2007	9,876	9,230	8,479	2,067	448	10,994	141	67	20,432
2008	10,605	9,911	8,080	2,036	419	10,535	151	69	20,666
2009	10,422	9,740	7,698	1,991	417	10,105	141	69	20,056
2010	10,910	10,196	7,555	1,956	450	9,961	160	72	20,389

NA = Not available.

[a]Per capita deliveries of sweeteners by U.S. processors and refiners and direct-consumption imports to food manufacturers, retailers, and other end users represent the per capita supply of caloric sweeteners. The data exclude deliveries to manufacturers of alcoholic beverages. Actual human intake of caloric sweeteners is lower because of uneaten food, spoilage, and other losses.

[b]Based on U.S. sugar deliveries for domestic food and beverage use.

[c]Total includes sugar, refined basis.

SOURCE: "Table 49. U.S. Total Estimated Deliveries of Caloric Sweeteners for Domestic Food and Beverage Use, by Calendar Year," in *Sugar and Sweeteners: Recommended Data*, U.S. Department of Agriculture, Economic Research Service, May 24, 2011, http://www.ers.usda.gov/Briefing/Sugar/Data.htm (accessed November 9, 2011)

The WHO strategy did not become official until it was endorsed by member states at the United Nations (UN) summit in May 2004. The strategy is not binding, but it is considered a guiding document for public health efforts on the issue worldwide. The strategy provides member states with a range of policy options to address two of the major risks responsible for the growing burden of chronic diseases that are attributable to unhealthy diet and physical inactivity. It explains how healthier diets and physical activity can help prevent and control these diseases. The strategy describes the roles of WHO member states, UN agencies, civil society, educators, and the private sector to help reduce the occurrence of obesity. It recommends obesity-prevention measures, including effective food and agriculture policies, fiscal policies, surveillance systems, consumer education, and nutrition labeling. The strategy also emphasizes the need for countries to develop national strategies with a long-term, sustainable perspective on making healthy choices at both the individual and community levels.

At the 63rd World Health Assembly in May 2010, WHO member states endorsed guidelines for the marketing of foods and beverages to children. The WHO recommendations, which were published in *Set of Recommendations on the Marketing of Foods and Non-alcoholic Beverages to Children* (2010, http://whqlibdoc.who.int/publications/2010/9789241500210_eng.pdf), aim to create new policies and strengthen existing policies on food marketing to children "in order to reduce the impact on children of marketing of foods high in saturated fats, trans-fatty acids, free sugars, or salt." Among the recommendations is an admonition against the marketing of low-nutritional-value foods in schools, specifically, "Settings where children gather should be free from all forms of marketing of foods high in saturated fats, trans-fatty acids, free sugars, or salt. Such settings include, but are not limited to, nurseries, schools, school grounds and pre-school centres, playgrounds, family and child clinics and paediatric services and during any sporting and cultural activities that are held on these premises." The WHO also called for government policies to enforce the recommendations, advising "clear definitions of sanctions" and "a system for reporting complaints."

Is Sugar the New Tobacco?

The WHO named sugar as one of the chief culprits in the current epidemic of obesity and obesity-related diseases, diabetes, and cardiovascular heart disease. The WHO approach to food is not, however, comparable to its strategy to combat tobacco use. The food strategy aims to provide member states and other interested stakeholders with a range of recommendations and policy options to promote healthier diets and more physical activity. It is up to member states to decide how these should be further developed and implemented at the national level. Because the strategy was endorsed at the World Health Assembly, member states are responsible for determining which specific policy options are appropriate to their circumstances. The WHO will then provide technical support for the implementation of programs, as requested by member states.

AMERICANS CRAVE SUGAR

The United States remains the world leader in sweetener consumption and is among the top sugar producers and importers. Stephen Haley of the U.S. Department of Agriculture (USDA) estimates in *Sugar and Sweeteners Outlook* (October 2011, http://www.ers.usda.gov/Publications/SSS/2011/10Oct/SSSM278.pdf) that the demand for sugar remained strong in 2011. Table 8.2 shows monthly estimates of the U.S. sugar supply and use during fiscal year 2011. Sugar is the most subsidized U.S. crop. At a rate of nearly $500 per acre annually, U.S. sugar producers receive

$1.4 billion in federal subsidies each year. U.S. sugar prices are artificially inflated because of import restrictions that protect producers from foreign competition. According to Bill Straub, in "Lugar Again Sets Sights on Sugar Subsidies" (*Evansville [IN] Courier and Press*, April 3, 2011), U.S. sugar prices were at a record high in 2011. Americans paid 20 cents more per pound of refined sugar than consumers in other countries.

Sugar (sucrose, dextrose, fructose, corn syrup, or maltodextrin) is a key ingredient of many processed food products. Table 8.3 lists the names of added sugars that may be the principal ingredients of processed foods. Gary Taubes reports in "Is Sugar Toxic?" (*New York Times*, April 13, 2011) that Americans' consumption of sugar has been increasing since the 1980s. The average American consumes about 90 pounds (41 kg) of added sugar (consumption in addition to naturally occurring sugar in fruit and vegetables) per year, which translates to about 400 calories per day from added sugars.

The health food industry has been warning the public about the perils of the overconsumption of refined sugars for more than 30 years, and mainstream nutritionists and public health professionals have joined the ranks of those calling for reduced sugar consumption. Along with ending sugar subsidies, they want to sharply limit the advertising of sugary products to children, ban the sale of soft drinks in schools, and conduct widespread community public health education programs to inform Americans about the health risks of consuming excessive amounts of refined sugars.

According to Rachel K. Johnson et al., in "Dietary Sugars Intake and Cardiovascular Health: A Scientific Statement from the American Heart Association" (*Circulation*, vol. 120, no. 11, September 2009), the American Heart Association issued a statement in September 2009 that offers guidance about limiting the consumption of added sugars and describes the relationship between excess sugar consumption and metabolic abnormalities, health problems, and shortfalls in essential nutrients. The statement indicates that most women should consume no more than 100 calories (about 25 grams or 6 teaspoons) of added sugars per day. Most men should consume no more than 150 calories (about 37.5 grams or 9 teaspoons) each day.

THE U.S. WAR ON OBESITY GAINS MOMENTUM

Besides generating international debate, the issue of obesity is receiving considerable attention from lawmakers, public health officials, and politicians throughout the United States. In *A Time for Action: Policy Recommendations from PHAI's Fifth Conference on Public Health, Law, and Obesity* (November 21, 2008, http://phaionline.org/wp-content/uploads/2008/10/phai_obesity_recommendations.pdf), the Public Health Advocacy

TABLE 8.2

Monthly estimates of fiscal year 2012 sugar supply and use, May–October 2011

	May 2011	June 2011	July 2011	August 2011	September 2011	October 2011
	1,000 short tons, raw value					
Beginning stocks*	1,611	1,607	1,527	1,785	1,745	1,418
Total production	**8,190**	**8,190**	**8,190**	**8,110**	**7,935**	**7,935**
Beet sugar	4,800	4,800	4,800	4,750	4,575	4,575
Cane sugar	3,390	3,390	3,390	3,360	3,360	3,360
Florida	1,630	1,630	1,630	1,630	1,630	1,630
Louisiana	1,440	1,440	1,440	1,400	1,400	1,400
Texas	150	150	150	160	160	160
Hawaii	170	170	170	170	170	170
Puerto Rico	0	0	0	0	0	0
Total imports	**2,599**	**2,774**	**3,072**	**2,962**	**2,962**	**3,151**
Tariff-rate quota imports	1,259	1,259	1,259	1,384	1,384	1,636
Other program imports	350	350	350	350	350	350
Non-program imports	990	1,165	1,463	1,228	1,228	1,165
Mexico	980	1,155	1,453	1,218	1,218	1,155
Total supply	**12,400**	**12,571**	**12,789**	**12,857**	**12,642**	**12,504**
Exports	200	200	200	200	200	200
Adjustments	0	0	0	0	0	100
Total deliveries	**11,315**	**11,315**	**11,315**	**11,315**	**11,315**	**11,315**
Domestic food and beverage	11,125	11,125	11,125	11,125	11,125	11,125
Other use	190	190	190	190	190	190
Total use	**11,515**	**11,515**	**11,515**	**11,515**	**11,515**	**11,615**
Ending stocks	885	1,056	1,274	1,342	1,127	889
Stocks/use ratio	7.69	9.17	11.06	11.66	9.79	7.65

*As of May 2004, includes all stocks held by processors, millers, and refiners, including stocks held for others.
NA = Not available.

SOURCE: "Table 26. Monthly Estimates of Fiscal 2012 U.S. Sugar Supply and Use," in *Sugar and Sweeteners: Recommended Data*, U.S. Department of Agriculture, Economic Research Service, October 14, 2011, http://www.ers.usda.gov/Briefing/Sugar/Data.htm (accessed November 9, 2009)

TABLE 8.3

Names for added sugars that appear on food labels

A food is likely to be high in sugars if one of these names appears first or second in the ingredient list or if several names are listed.

Brown sugar	Invert sugar
Corn sweetener	Lactose
Corn syrup	Malt syrup
Dextrose	Maltose
Fructose	Molasses
Fruit juice concentrate	Raw sugar
Glucose	Sucrose
High-fructose corn syrup	Syrup
Honey	Table sugar

SOURCE: "Box 21. Names for Added Sugars That Appear on Food Labels," in *Nutrition and Your Health: Dietary Guidelines for Americans*, 5th ed., U.S. Department of Health and Human Services and U.S. Department of Agriculture, 2000, http://www.health.gov/dietaryguidelines/dga2000/document/choose.htm (accessed November 9, 2009)

Institute (PHAI), a nonprofit legal research center that focuses on public health law, offers 47 recommendations for the administration of President Barack Obama (1961–) to combat obesity. The recommendations include:

- Develop and support an array of federal policies to increase access to healthy food at the state and local levels, including an Innovations Fund to support grocery store development, new cooperatives, local entrepreneurship, and requirements for electronic payment access in all retail food environments, including farmers markets

- Impose federal taxes (sales or excise) on purchases of unhealthy foods and beverages and earmark the revenue for obesity programs

- Promote and fund innovative farm-to-school and farm-to-community programs across the nation to support local farmers and increase access to locally grown food

- Eliminate all "competitive foods" from schools; restrict food sold and served in schools to the National School Lunch and School Breakfast Programs

- Establish and implement financial incentives for schools to improve and promote enhanced nutrition standards in the National School Lunch and School Breakfast Programs, and the Child and Adult Care Food Program

- Require federal food programs to align with the U.S. dietary guidelines and provide the necessary federal resources (i.e., reimbursement, commodities, and incentives) to achieve alignment

- Establish strict federal regulations limiting food and beverage advertising to children, including the Internet

- Provide federal support in the form of funding, technical assistance, and public and food industry education to implement and evaluate state and local menu labeling laws

- Increase federal National Institutes of Health funding for nutrition research

- Encourage states and localities to continue to develop and test innovative strategies to prevent and reverse the obesity epidemic; hence avoid including preemption provisions in federal laws that could impact the obesity epidemic

Skirmishes in the war on obesity do not center on whether there is a problem, but on how best to address it. Participants on one side characterize the food industry, advertisers, and the media as complicit, in that they entice consumers with seductive advertising and sugary, high-calorie treats. Their opponents believe consumers should exercise personal responsibility and make their own choices about food and exercise.

In "Tackling the Politics of Obesity" (*Atlantic*, July 27, 2009), Marc Ambinder asserts that even though the food industry has conditioned Americans to crave unhealthy, inexpensive foods, obesity researchers are unwilling to confront the industry about this practice. Ambinder observes that part of this resistance may stem from the fact that it is difficult to "demonize the food industry for lowering their prices, making the food supply safer than it ever was, and feeding more people." He further notes that even if it were possible to dramatically alter Americans' food choices, the United States would have to "roughly double the production of fruits and vegetables to keep up with demand."

The PHAI contends that food industry processing and marketing practices have encouraged excessive food consumption. The PHAI Obesity Project considers the existing state of regulation, legislation, and litigation related to the food industry's contribution to obesity and the potential for new legal strategies to effectively reduce this contribution.

Jennifer L. Pomeranz and Kelly D. Brownell of Yale University assert in "Advancing Public Health Obesity Policy through State Attorneys General" (*American Journal of Public Health*, vol. 101, no. 3, March 2011) that the war on obesity requires "government action at multiple levels and across disciplines." The researchers call on state attorneys general to assume lead roles to champion nutrition policy and to protect consumers, especially children, from misleading marketing and advertising practices. Attorneys general can also reach across state lines to tackle issues such as food marketing

in schools and web-tracking and analytics that target food marketing to individual Internet users, including children. They can advocate consumer education and can issue formal written opinions about issues such as the legality of taxing sugar-sweetened beverages. Pomeranz and Brownell aver that "there is much room for greater attorney general involvement in formulating and championing solutions to this public health problem. Obesity may not be on the radar of every attorney general as a topic for their attention, so state and local advocates should contact and work with their attorneys general to support public health measures at every level."

The Nutrition Facts Label: How Accurate Is It?

Despite the requirement for accurate food labeling, U.S. Food and Drug Administration (FDA) oversight has not been entirely successful in its efforts to prevent inaccurate or misleading information on food labels. The U.S. Government Accountability Office (GAO) finds in *Food Labeling: FDA Needs to Better Leverage Resources, Improve Oversight, and Effectively Use Available Data to Help Consumers Select Healthy Foods* (September 2008, http://www.gao.gov/new.items/d08597.pdf) that the FDA has not been able to track, monitor, and conduct label reviews on even a small fraction of the thousands of foods entering the United States from foreign countries. The GAO concludes that the FDA's oversight and enforcement efforts are not adequate to address the increasing numbers of domestic or imported food products. In addition, FDA efforts to ensure that companies correct labeling violations are also lacking.

In "Front-of-Package Food and Beverage Labeling: New Directions for Research and Regulation" (*American Journal of Public Health*, vol. 40, no. 3, March 2011), Jennifer L. Pomeranz of Yale University explains that the use of a wide variety of icons and claims on packaged food and research finding misleading and confusing claims as well as messages that imply healthfulness for products that do not meet objective nutrition standards have prompted several government agencies to reassess food labeling regulations in an effort to ensure that consumers obtain accurate information. Responding to consumer complaints, the FDA announced in October 2009 that it would draft criteria for front-of-package labeling, conduct consumer research to determine the best method to communicate information, and work with the food industry to develop a single front-of-package symbol to help consumers make informed and nutritious choices. In October 2010 the FDA suggested that front-of-package labels should display calories, serving sizes, saturated fat, trans fat, and sodium. Pomeranz reports that the following month the Grocery Manufacturers Association announced plans to develop its own front-of-package labeling guidelines. Because adherence with the FDA guidelines is voluntary, the food industry is free to design its own schema for labeling. Pomeranz suggests that the FDA should mandate adherence to its guidelines if the industry fails to adopt science-based criteria.

Kelly D. Brownell and Jeffrey P. Koplan worry in "Front-of-Package Nutrition Labeling—An Abuse of Trust by the Food Industry?" (*New England Journal of Medicine*, vol. 364, no. 25, June 23, 2011) that the Nutrition Keys, the new, voluntary nutrition-labeling system food and beverage companies plan to use on the front of packages to "help busy consumers make informed choices," may not achieve its stated goals. Even though the Nutrition Keys will list the amount and percentage of the recommended daily value for calories, saturated fat, sodium, and sugars, Brownell and Koplan think the system may confuse consumers because it incorporates many symbols and the food company is free to vary the nutrients listed on the package. They also speculate that that food companies may fortify foods of questionable nutritional value to give them more favorable labels. Finally, because the Institute of Medicine (IOM) is performing a rigorous scientific evaluation of front-of-label packaging, Brownell and Koplan are dismayed that the food industry is advocating its untested and somewhat inconsistent approach rather than waiting for the IOM recommendations.

Can and Should Laws Change Americans' Diets?

The American legal professor John F. Banzhaf III (1940–), who campaigned against tobacco, advocates using the legal system to create change in Americans' diets. He exhorts attorneys to bring lawsuits against fast-food purveyors and junk-food manufacturers to increase consumer awareness of the role the food industry plays in promoting obesity. Banzhaf was interviewed in Morgan Spurlock's (1970–) documentary film *Super Size Me* (2004), which focuses on the fast-food industry's promotion of unhealthy eating and the director's experience subsisting on a diet of fast food for 30 days.

The Center for Consumer Freedom is an advocacy group that is supported by restaurant and food companies and that represents major corporations such as RJR Nabisco. The center marshals lawyers, publicists, and lobbyists to respond to antiobesity crusaders and derides lawsuits and legislation aimed at limiting consumers' rights to choose the foods they want to consume. It also pokes fun at the self-appointed "food police" (legislators, public health officials, and others) that is intent on modifying Americans' diets and at mandates by the Center for Science in the Public Interest (CSPI; a nonprofit advocacy group for nutrition, food safety, health, and other issues) to offer consumers nutritional data. It is credited with helping defeat a measure that would have required chain restaurants to offer nutritional data about their products. In "Sugar Cops Sour on Cereal" (October 11, 2011, http://

www.consumerfreedom.com/news_detail.cfm/h/4539-sugar-cops-sour-on-cereal), the Center for Consumer Freedom staunchly opposes banning or restricting food advertising to children. It asserts that physical inactivity as opposed to the overconsumption of foods high in sugar, fat, and calories is the primary cause of childhood obesity. Furthermore, the center opines in "Food Cops Target Soda (Again? Really?)" (September 1, 2011, http://www.consumerfreedom.com/news_detail.cfm/h/4515-food-cops-target-soda-again-really) that soda and sweet drinks do not disproportionately contribute to obesity and argues against a proposed tax on these beverages.

The Obesity Society Action Plan

In its position statement, the Obesity Society (formerly the American Obesity Association; June 24, 2010, http://www.obesity.org/images/pdf/Obesity2010/TOS_Washington_Times_Eradicating.pdf) provides an ambitious agenda for the government and private sector that enumerates specific funding priorities, programs, and services to prevent, treat, and educate Americans. It calls for:

- A "war on obesity, not the obese." The Obesity Society asserts that this war will not be waged or won by further stigmatizing obese people and calls for efforts to end discrimination and eliminate the social stigma associated with obesity.

- Educating the public to improve awareness of obesity as "a complex disease involving genes, behavior and environment" rather than as a moral weakness.

- Informing the public about obesity, its causes, and consequences and engaging in "a national debate on obesity, similar to past campaigns in smoking and cholesterol."

- Expanding access to professional treatment of obesity so that its medical, social, and economic consequences can be averted.

- Ensuring reimbursement for medical treatment for obesity, including drugs and surgery.

- Including nutrition education, lifestyle counseling, and obesity diagnosis and management into medical school curricula and other health professionals' training.

- Revising national policies, such as farm policies promoting the production of energy-dense foods with low nutritional value, that exacerbate the problem.

- Preventing excess weight gain in children and adults, teaching healthy behaviors and lifestyles early in life, and providing healthy school lunches.

- Building environments that encourage healthier behaviors such as walking and more physical activity at work.

- Recognizing the economic impact of obesity on medical expenditures and lost wages.

- Supporting research to address the problem by doubling funding from federal agencies including the National Institutes of Health, the USDA, and the Centers for Disease Control and Prevention (CDC).

The Healthy, Hunger-Free Kids Act

In December 2010 President Obama signed the Healthy, Hunger-Free Kids Act into law. That same year First Lady Michelle Obama (1964–) launched Let's Move!, an ambitious campaign that is aimed at improving children's nutrition and increasing their physical activity. According to the White House, in the press release "Remarks by the President and First Lady at the Signing of the Healthy, Hunger-Free Kids Act" (December 13, 2010, http://www.whitehouse.gov/the-press-office/2010/12/13/remarks-president-and-first-lady-signing-healthy-hunger-free-kids-act), the first lady attended the bill-signing ceremony at Harriet Tubman Elementary School in Washington, D.C. She praised the bipartisan support for the bill in Congress, saying, "While we may sometimes have our differences, we can all agree that in the United States of America, no child should go to school hungry. We can all agree that in the wealthiest nation on earth, all children should have the basic nutrition they need to learn and grow and to pursue their dreams."

The Healthy, Hunger-Free Kids Act authorizes funding for federal school meal and child nutrition programs and increases access to healthy food for low-income children. The bill reauthorizes child nutrition programs for five years and includes $4.5 billion in new funding for these programs over 10 years. Furthermore, it:

- Authorizes the USDA to establish nutritional standards for all foods that are sold in schools during the school day, including vending machines, lunch lines, and school stores

- Provides increased reimbursement to schools that meet updated nutritional standards for federally subsidized lunches

- Assists communities to establish local farm-to-school networks, create school gardens, and use more local foods in schools

- Improves access to drinking water in schools

- Establishes standards for school wellness policies, including goals for nutrition promotion and education and physical activity

- Promotes nutrition and wellness in child care settings through the federally subsidized Child and Adult Care Food Program

- Supports breastfeeding through the Women, Infants, and Children program

Table 8.4 compares elementary school lunch menus before and after enactment of the Healthy, Hunger-Free Kids Act. Ron Nixon reports in "School Lunch Proposals Set off a Dispute" (*New York Times*, November 1, 2011) that the changes to the school lunch program intended to help combat childhood obesity was met with opposition from many in the food industry. For example, the National Potato Council said the move to reduce starch in children's diets by offering fewer weekly servings of potatoes in favor of other vegetables and fruits was "overly restrictive." However, Margo G. Wootan, the director of nutrition policy at the CSPI, countered industry objections by asserting, "This whole fight obscures the fact that the U.S.D.A.'s proposal is about helping kids eat a wide variety of vegetables and make lunches overall healthier."

Jeffrey Levi et al. find in *F as in Fat: How Obesity Threatens America's Future, 2011* (July 2011, http://healthyamericans.org/assets/files/TFAH2011FasInFat10.pdf) that in 2011, 26 states and the District of Columbia had established farm-to-school programs that improve students' diets by bringing fresh local produce to schools. In 2011 the USDA proposed a new rule to update meals that were served through the National School Lunch and School Breakfast Programs based on the recommendations made by the IOM in *School Meals: Building Blocks for Healthy Children* (2010, http://books.nap.edu/openbook.php?record_id=12751). The overarching goal is to enable students to select from a variety of appealing, healthful options, which in turn will result in their consumption of foods that promote their health.

OVERWEIGHT, OBESITY, AND THE LAW

Health care coverage and the availability of services to prevent or treat obesity vary widely. The economic recession that lasted from late 2007 to mid-2009 (but whose effects were still felt in 2012) further compromised access to health care services. The many people who had been laid off lost their health insurance because they could not afford to continue paying for it, and the growing ranks of the uninsured were straining the already strapped Medicaid (a federal and state health care program for people below the poverty level) and other safety net programs. Levi et al. aver that the Patient Protection and Affordable Care Act (PPACA), which was signed into law in March 2010, has the potential to significantly enhance obesity-prevention efforts. The law authorizes new resources and initiatives such as coverage for a range of preventive services, including screening for obesity, diet counseling for adults who are at risk for chronic diseases, and referral to intensive behavioral interventions that are intended to reduce obesity.

The PPACA also funds the Childhood Obesity Demonstration Project, which was established through the

TABLE 8.4

Revised elementary school lunch menus, December 2010

Monday	Tuesday	Wednesday	Thursday	Friday
Before	**Before**	**Before**	**Before**	**Before**
Bean and cheese burrito (5.3 oz) with mozzarella cheese (1 oz) Applesauce (1/4 cup) Orange Juice (4 oz) 2% Milk (8 oz)	Hot dog on bun (3 oz) with ketchup (4 T) Canned Pears (1/4 cup) Raw Celery and Carrots (1/8 cup each) with ranch dressing (1.75 T) Low-fat (1%) Chocolate Milk (8 oz)	Pizza sticks (3.8 oz) with marinara sauce (1.4 cup) Banana Raisins (1 oz) Whole Milk (8 oz)	Breaded beef patty (4 oz) with ketchup (2 T) Wheat roll (2 oz) Frozen Fruit Juice Bar (2.4 oz) 2% Milk (8 oz)	Cheese pizza (4.8 oz) Canned Pineapple (1/4 cup) Tater Tots (1/2 cup) with ketchup (2 T) Low-fat (1%) Chocolate Milk (8 oz)
After	**After**	**After**	**After**	**After**
Submarine Sandwich (1 oz turkey, 0.5 oz low-fat cheese) on Whole Wheat Roll Refried Beans (1/2 cup) Jicama (1/4 cup) Green Pepper Strips (1/4 cup) Cantaloupe wedges, raw (1/2 cup) Skim Milk (8 oz) Mustard (9 grams) Reduced fat mayonnaise (1 oz) Low Fat Ranch Dip (1 oz)	Whole Wheat Spaghetti with Meat Sauce (1/2 cup) and Whole Wheat Roll Green Beans, cooked (1/2 cup) Broccoli (1/2 cup) Cauliflower (1/2 cup) Kiwi Halves, raw (1/2 cup) Low-fat (1%) Milk (8 oz) Low Fat Ranch Dip (1 oz) Soft Margarine (5 g)	Chef Salad (1 cup romaine, 0.5 oz low-fat mozzarella, 1.5 oz grilled chicken) with Whole Wheat Soft Pretzel (2.5 oz) Corn, cooked (1/2 cup) Baby Carrots, raw (1/4 cup) Banana Skim Chocolate Milk (8 oz) Low Fat Ranch Dressing (1.5 oz) Low Fat Italian Dressing (1.5 oz)	Oven-Baked Fish nuggets (2 oz) with Whole Wheat Roll Mashed Potatoes (1/2 cup) Steamed Broccoli (1/2 cup) Peaches (canned, packed in juice–1/2 cup) Skim Milk (8 oz) Tarter Sauce (1.5 oz) Soft Margarine (5 g)	Whole Wheat Cheese Pizza (1 slice) Baked Sweet Potato Fries (1/2 cup) Grape tomatoes, raw (1/4 cup) Applesauce (1/2 cup) Low-fat (1%) Milk (8 oz) Low Fat Ranch Dip (1 oz)

Note: Comparison of current National School Lunch Program (NSLP) elementary meals vs. proposed elementary meals.

SOURCE: "Before/After Elementary School Lunch Menu," in "President Obama Signs Healthy, Hunger-Free Kids Act of 2010 into Law," The White House, Office of the Press Secretary, December 13, 2010, http://www.whitehouse.gov/sites/default/files/cnr_chart.pdf (accessed November 10, 2011)

Children's Health Insurance Program Reauthorization Act of 2009. The demonstration project funds programs that are aimed at children aged two to 12 years who are covered by the Children's Health Insurance Program, which provides low-cost health insurance to over 7 million children of working families. The CDC observes in the press release "CDC Takes New Steps to Combat Childhood Obesity" (September 29, 2011, http://www.cdc.gov/media/releases/2011/p0929_combat_child_obesity.html) that minority children and those in low-income communities are at higher risk for obesity and its consequences.

The PPACA requires chain restaurants and food establishments to disclose calorie counts and other nutritional information (fat, saturated fat, cholesterol, sodium, total carbohydrates, sugars, fiber, and total protein) for standard menu items. Vending machine operators with 20 or more machines must also disclose calorie content for many items. Even though this requirement was effective following the enactment of the PPACA, the FDA began enforcing this rule in April 2011.

Levi et al. report that in 2011 the majority of states (34 states and the District of Columbia) had imposed a tax on soda and sugar-sweetened beverages. Even though research indicates that such taxes do deter consumers, to date, there is little evidence that they appreciably affect weight loss. For example, Roland Sturm et al. find in "Soda Taxes, Soft Drink Consumption, and Children's Body Mass Index" (*Health Affairs*, vol. 29, no. 5, May 2010) that soda taxes do reduce soda consumption among

subgroups of at-risk children—those who are overweight, are African-American, are from low-income families, watch television more than most, or attend schools that permit soda sales to students.

In "Is a Tax on Junk Food Moving a Step Closer?" (*European Heart Journal*, vol. 32, no. 15, August 2011), Lois Rogers observes that cost is acknowledged as the "single biggest factor in reducing smoking rates in the West," so it may be expected to exert a comparable effect on food purchases. Rogers reports that in 2010 Denmark become the first nation in the world to tax sugar and New Zealand launched a research project to evaluate the social, economic, and health impacts of selectively taxing foods with little or no nutritional value at a higher rate.

Lawsuits Attack Food Service Industry

A number of individuals and advocacy groups have brought lawsuits against the food service industry. Some claim they deserve compensation for the damage that fattening foods have done to their health. Others focus on advertising and marketing that they feel is deceptive and misleads people into eating unhealthy products. Many attorneys and public health professionals believe such lawsuits can serve as vehicles that reverse the obesity epidemic, in part because the media attention generated by such lawsuits motivates food companies to produce healthier products and to reconsider marketing and advertising practices.

The first class-action suit was the widely publicized case of Caesar Barber, a 56-year-old New Yorker weighing 270 pounds (122 kg), who claimed that four fast-food restaurants (McDonald's, Burger King, Wendy's, and KFC) jeopardized his health by promoting high-calorie, high-fat, and salty menu items. In "Whopper of a Lawsuit: Fast-Food Chains Blamed for Obesity, Illnesses" (ABC News, July 26, 2002), Geraldine Sealey reports that Barber filed the lawsuit in the New York State Supreme Court "on behalf of an unspecified number of other obese and ill New Yorkers who also feast on fast food." According to Sealey, Barber's suit alleged that the fast-food restaurants, where he ate "four or five times a week even after suffering a heart attack, did not properly disclose the ingredients of their food and the risks of eating too much." Barber's suit was dismissed, so he filed for a second time. His second suit was also dismissed, and he was barred from filing for a third time. By 2005 a number of cases that were similar Barber's had been filed.

Legislation Protects Food Industry Interests

The food industry and others argue that Americans choose what they eat and should not be able to blame the food industry if their personal choices have unhealthy consequences. State and federal legislators who agree with this viewpoint have enacted or attempted to enact laws that protect the food industry from weight-related lawsuits.

In October 2005 the U.S. House of Representatives passed a bill that would prevent most obesity or weight-related claims against the food industry and make it harder for consumers to sue restaurants and food retailers for serving fattening fare. By a vote of 307 to 119 lawmakers endorsed the Personal Responsibility in Food Consumption Act, which informed consumers that if they gain weight as a result of eating high-fat, high-calorie, and sugar-laden food, they have only themselves to blame. However, the legislation did not receive a vote in the U.S. Senate, so it did not become law. The act was reintroduced three times, but as of January 2012 it had not become law.

The restaurant and food-processing industries have also championed state measures such as the Idaho Commonsense Consumption Act, signed into law in April 2004, which bans civil lawsuits for obesity and obesity-related health problems. That same year Arizona (2004, http://azleg.state.az.us/alispdfs/46leg/2R/House/SummaryJUD.pdf) enacted legislation affirming that "there is no duty to warn a consumer that a non-defective food product may cause health problems if consumed excessively and provides an affirmative defense."

According to Pomeranz, in "Efforts to Immunize Food Manufacturers from Obesity-Related Lawsuits: A Challenge for Public Health" (August 17, 2011, http://

www.corporationsandhealth.org/), as of 2011, 24 states had passed legislation to limit obesity liability to provide some measure of protection or even immunity for food companies that were threatened by obesity lawsuits. Advocates in favor of this legislation contend that the central issue is "common sense and personal responsibility" and generally subscribe to the opinion that obesity is an individual health issue as opposed to a larger societal and public health problem. Opponents of legislation limiting liability suggest that it is unrealistic to expect consumers to assume personal responsibility when food companies do not disclose relevant information about their products such as the number of calories and fat content.

THE FOOD INDUSTRY RESPONDS TO PUBLIC OUTCRY

Mounting pressure on the food industry to change its marketing practices and offer healthier products has had some success. For example, in March 2004 McDonald's responded to growing attention to the relationship between portion size and obesity by announcing that it would discontinue its supersized products—french fries and soft drinks—in an effort to simplify its menu and appeal to consumers' heightened awareness about obesity. McDonald's also piloted a new "Go Active" meal for adults that included a salad, a pedometer to count steps, and a bottle of water in several test markets throughout the country. Industry observers applauded these moves, citing the corporation's shift from the "value" aspect of fast food—providing more food for less money—to more health-conscious salads and reasonable portion sizes that emphasize nutrition rather than value. They also expressed the hope that other fast-food chains would follow suit and offer more nutritional information and low-calorie fare.

In another effort to counter charges that its food is unhealthy and contributes to obesity, McDonald's began displaying nutrition facts on the packaging of its menu items in 2006. Customers of the world's largest restaurant company can learn the amount of calories and fat, among other information, in a McDonald's product by looking at the wrapper instead of having to go to the corporation's website or ask for nutrition information at the counter.

Jeffrey P. Koplan and Kelly D. Brownell opine in "Response of the Food and Beverage Industry to the Obesity Threat" (*Journal of the American Medical Association*, vol. 304, no. 13, October 6, 2010) that even though industry self-regulation can be effective and public-private partnerships can promote health, some common food industry practices undermine public health. For example, the food industry has attempted to offset the marketing of calorie-dense, low-nutrient foods such as sugary cereals by using packaging with images of children playing outside or athletes to suggest that these foods support health and fitness. The food industry also reframes dietary issues by emphasizing "balance," "calories out," and physical activity. Koplan and Brownell observe that the physical activity needed to "balance" a supersized burger meal containing more than 2,300 calories would be running a marathon.

Despite widespread consensus among health professionals that consumption of sweetened beverages and fast food should markedly decrease and that consumption of fruits and vegetables should increase, the food industry persists in promoting the notion that there are no bad foods and that only total consumption counts. Koplan and Brownell note that all calories are not equal: 100 calories of broccoli, 100 calories of french fries, and 100 calories of soda have markedly different nutrient content.

The food industry does not accept responsibility for the obesity epidemic; instead, it blames consumers and their inability to be aware of what and how much they eat and drink. According to Koplan and Brownell, the food industry assumes seemingly contradictory positions: it does not object to government policies such as corn subsidies that support beef production and enable the industry to sweeten foods at low cost with high-fructose corn syrup, but it does oppose government interventions to reduce obesity such as taxes on low-nutrient foods, which it views as encroaching on personal freedom.

FOOD INDUSTRY LAUNCHES ANTIOBESITY INITIATIVE

Even though Koplan and Brownell exhort the food industry to make more concerted efforts to promote healthier foods, they concede that the "industry has endorsed the Let's Move! campaign launched by the White House. Other recent positive actions include the availability of smaller portion sizes and nutritional labeling."

In "The Role and Challenges of the Food Industry in Addressing Chronic Disease" (*Global Health*, vol. 6, May 28, 2010), Derek Yach, the senior vice president of global health policy for PepsiCo, and his colleagues state that the food industry is doing much to reduce the burden of overweight and obesity-related diseases. Yach et al. cite as examples "global public commitments to address food reformulation, consumer information, responsible marketing, promotion of healthy lifestyles, and public-private partnerships." They also present PepsiCo's pledge to increase the amount of whole grains, fruits, vegetables, nuts, seeds, and low-fat dairy in its product portfolio and to increase the range of foods and beverages that offer solutions for managing calories.

PepsiCo states in *2010 Annual Report* (2011, http://www.pepsico.com/annual10/performance/performance.html?nav=human) that by 2012 it will display calorie count and key nutrients on food and beverage pack-

aging, will advertise to children under the age of 12 years "only products that meet our global science-based nutrition standards," and will eliminate the direct sale of sugary soft drinks in schools. The company will work to develop affordable, nutritious food products for underserved and low-income communities and will enhance efforts to promote healthier communities. PepsiCo also pledges that by 2015 it will reduce the average amount of sodium per serving by 25%. By 2020 it will reduce the average amount of saturated fat per serving in key global food brands by 15% and the average amount of added sugar per serving in beverages by 25%.

THE HEALTHY WEIGHT COMMITMENT FOUNDATION AND CHILDHOOD OBESITY

In October 2009 a group of 41 retailers, nongovernmental organizations, and food and beverage manufacturers launched the Healthy Weight Commitment Foundation (HWCF), a national initiative intended to reduce the rate of obesity, especially among children and adolescents. In the press release "Retailers, NGOs, and Food and Beverage Industry Launch National Initiative to Help Reduce Obesity" (2009, http://www.prnewswire.com/), the HWCF explains that members of the foundation, which include the Campbell Soup Co., General Mills Inc., Kellogg Co., Nestlé USA, Ralston Foods/Post Foods, and PepsiCo, have invested $20 million in the initiative. The initiative targets three key audiences—markets, the workplace, and schools—and will conduct a nationwide public education campaign that focuses on ways to help people reach and maintain a healthy weight by balancing calories consumed with calories expended through physical activity.

By 2012 the HWCF (http://www.healthyweightcommit.org/about/overview/) had a membership of more than 190 retailers, food and beverage manufacturers, restaurants, sporting goods and insurance companies, trade associations, nongovernmental organizations, and professional sports organizations. In May 2011 the HWCF launched Together Counts, a national campaign that encourages families to eat meals and participate in physical activities together to help prevent obesity and promote good health. The Together Counts website (http://www.togethercounts.com/) provides families with tools to track their progress and compare them with the results in their community and across the United States. The site also offers tips and advice to promote participation and a mobile application that enables participants to log and track their progress.

WEIGHT-BASED DISCRIMINATION

Nearly everyone who is overweight or obese has suffered some form of bias, from disapproving glances and unsolicited advice about how to lose weight to the seemingly unending stream of "fat jokes" and the unflattering and even humiliating portrayal of overweight people in the media. Despite the pervasive anti-fat bias in American culture, until recently there were anecdotal reports, but little evidence, demonstrating that negative attitudes toward obese individuals resulted in stigmatization and clear instances of discrimination.

In "The Stigma of Obesity: A Review and Update" (*Obesity*, vol. 17, no. 5, May 2009), Rebecca M. Puhl and Chelsea A. Heuer of Yale University find that the prevalence of weight discrimination increased by 66% between 1995 and 2006 and describe it as comparable to rates of racial discrimination. The researchers review data revealing that systematic discrimination against obese individuals occurs in at least three areas: education, employment, and health care. They also acknowledge that evidence points to discrimination in adoption proceedings, jury selection, and housing.

Puhl and Heuer observe that obese people suffer discrimination in many aspects of life. For example, in the workplace they may be "the target of derogatory humor and pejorative comments from co-workers and supervisors," and in educational settings obese students often experience teasing, taunts, derogatory comments, and derision from peers. Health care professionals and educators have been found to hold and promote negative stereotypes about people who are obese, and the media, especially television and film, continue to stigmatize overweight and obese characters. Puhl and Heuer assert that overweight people "remain one of the last acceptable targets of humor and ridicule in North American television and film." Even the news media participates by blaming obese people for contributing to "rising fuel prices, global warming, and causing weight gain in their friends."

Several studies find distinct anti-fat bias in children as young as age three and increasingly negative stereotypic attitudes as children age. Puhl and Heuer observe that an analysis of 25 popular videos and 20 popular books for young children attributed many "desirable traits such as sociability, kindness, happiness, and success" to thin female characters, whereas overweight characters were "commonly depicted as evil, unattractive, unfriendly, and cruel."

Overweight and obese job applicants and workers may be subjected to weight-based discrimination in employment. Many studies document discrimination in hiring practices, especially when the positions sought involved public contact, such as sales or direct customer service. Obese workers face inequities in wages, benefits, and promotions, and several studies confirm that the economic penalties are greater for women than for men. Overweight women earn less doing the same work as their normal-weight counterparts and have dimmer pros-

pects for promotion. The courts have considered cases in which workers contended that their job terminations were weight-related. The outcomes of these cases indicate that termination can occur because of employer prejudice and arbitrary weight standards.

According to Leila Azarbad and Linda Gonder-Frederick, in "Obesity in Women" (*Psychiatric Clinics of North America*, vol. 33, no. 2, June 2010), overweight and obese women seem to be more prone to obesity-related stigma and discrimination than men, ostensibly because there is greater societal pressure on women to strive for beauty and thinness. Research shows a reluctance to hire obese applicants of both genders, but this bias is stronger against women than men. Obesity is associated not only with social and occupational bias but also with economic burdens for women. Obese women tend to have lower socioeconomic status and earnings than their healthy-weight peers. Even though some of the economic burden may be attributable to obesity-related health problems and physical disability, stigma, bias, and negative attitudes toward overweight people also contribute. Azarbad and Gonder-Frederick cite research documenting the presence of negative responses to obese people in children as young as three years old, who view larger body shapes less favorably than normal-weight or thin figures. Surprisingly, this bias persists among obese people themselves, who hold negative attitudes toward others who are overweight or obese.

Weight Bias among Health Professionals

Azarbad and Gonder-Frederick report that many health care professionals, even those who specialize in obesity treatment, also harbor negative attitudes and stereotype people who are overweight or obese. Anti-fat bias among health care professionals may discourage obese people from seeking medical care and compromise the care they receive. Even though research indicates that obese patients often delay or cancel medical appointments for a variety of reasons, including fear about being weighed or undressing in front of health professionals, speculation exists that presumed or real prejudice on the part of health professionals may also deter them from seeking medical care.

In "Weight Bias among Health Professionals Specializing in Obesity" (*Obesity Research*, vol. 11, no. 9, September 2003), the first study to assess the attitudes of health professionals who work with people who are obese, Marlene B. Schwartz et al. administered a standardized test that measured bias to 389 health professionals (physicians, researchers, dieticians, nurses, psychologists, and others) who attended an international obesity conference in Quebec, Canada, in 2001. Bias was assessed using the Implicit Associations Test (IAT), a timed test that analyzes the automatic associations respondents make about particular attributes. For example, the IAT helped identify whether test takers held negative attitudes and stereotypical views about obese people, such as considering them to be lazy, unmotivated, sluggish, or worthless.

Schwartz et al. find that the health professionals they tested—one-third of whom provided direct clinical care to obese patients—exhibited significant anti-fat bias. They linked the stereotypes lazy, stupid, and worthless with obese people, with younger health professionals displaying more anti-fat bias than older health professionals. Schwartz et al. hypothesize that younger health professionals may be more strongly imprinted with societal pressures to be thin, which have intensified in recent decades. Another explanation may be that older health professionals, who have more maturity and experience, may have overcome some of their negative attitudes about obese patients. Despite the presence of bias, the researchers concede that even though it is intuitively appealing to assume that bias has an influence on treatment, their research does not demonstrate that bias resulted in poorer treatment of obese patients.

OBESE AMERICANS RECEIVE FEWER PREVENTIVE HEALTH SERVICES. Ironically, people who are obese and usually receive more medical care for chronic diseases related to obesity may also receive fewer preventive services. Does bias contribute to this disparity in preventive care? Truls Østbye et al. examine in "Associations between Obesity and Receipt of Screening Mammography, Papanicolaou Tests, and Influenza Vaccination: Results from the Health and Retirement Study (HRS) and the Asset and Health Dynamics among the Oldest Old (AHEAD) Study" (*American Journal of Public Health*, vol. 95, no. 9, September 2005) the association between body mass index (BMI; body weight in kilograms divided by height in meters squared) and receipt of screening mammography and Papanicolaou tests (screening for cervical cancer) among middle-aged women and the association between BMI and receipt of influenza (flu) vaccination among older adults.

Østbye et al. find significant differences in how often obese women were given mammograms and Pap smears to screen for cancer. They also note that obese men and women were less likely to receive flu shots. Seventy-one percent of the obese women studied reported having mammograms, compared with 78% of those who were not obese. Similarly, 54% of the obese women reported having Pap smears, compared with 73% of the nonobese women. In addition, 57% of the obese men and women whose records were reviewed reported receiving flu shots, compared with 78% of normal-weight people. Østbye et al. pose several potential explanations for the disparity in preventive services: obese patients' reluc-

tance to undress for cancer screening tests, practitioners' difficulties in performing screening tests on obese women, and obese patients may require so many medical care services for chronic diseases that preventive care may be overlooked.

Airlines Weigh Their Options

In June 2002 Southwest Airlines became the center of a fiery debate when the airline decided to strengthen its enforcement of a policy established in 1980 of requesting and requiring passengers who, because of excessive girth, must occupy two airplane seats to purchase both seats. The policy allows passengers to be reimbursed for the additional seat if their flight is not full. The National Association to Advance Fat Acceptance, an advocacy group, and other consumer groups called the move discriminatory. Regardless, Southwest Airlines is not the only airline with this policy; Continental, Northwest, and other commercial carriers also require large-sized passengers to pay for two seats.

In 2003 the Federal Aviation Administration (FAA) proposed requiring all passengers on small airlines to be weighed in along with their luggage. The FAA asserted that before takeoff, the pilot must calculate the weight of the aircraft as well as that of its passengers, luggage, and crew to determine which seats passengers should occupy to ensure proper balance. For this reason it is vital to know exact passenger and luggage weights on small planes, where several people with a few extra pounds can tilt the plane away from its center of gravity. Even though operators of smaller commuter airlines acknowledged the safety issue, they were reluctant to support the FAA recommendation because they feared that weighing people would discourage them from using commuter airlines, many of which were already strapped financially.

In May 2003 the FAA ruled that airlines must assume that passengers weigh between 190 and 195 pounds (86 and 88 kg), depending on the season. At the same time, checked bags on domestic flights were adjusted from an estimated 25 pounds (11 kg) to 30 pounds (14 kg). The 30-pound estimate for checked bags on international flights remained unchanged. The requirement followed shortly after the crash of a commuter plane that killed all 21 people aboard. Investigators suspect the propeller plane was slightly above its maximum weight on takeoff, with most of the weight toward the tail. The weight distribution problem was compounded by a maintenance error that made it difficult to lower the nose with the control column. After the 19-seat plane rose above the ground, its nose pointed dangerously skyward; the pilots were unable to level it off, and the plane spun to the ground.

Andrew L. Dannenberg, Deron C. Burton, and Richard J. Jackson estimate in "Economic and Environmental

Costs of Obesity: The Impact on Airlines" (*American Journal of Preventive Medicine*, vol. 27, no. 3, October 2004) that the average American gained 10 pounds (4.5 kg) during the 1990s. The extra weight required an additional 350 million gallons (1.3 billion L) of fuel used by airlines in 2000. This extra weight translated into about $275 million in excess costs in 2000 alone. The extra fuel represented 2.4% of the total volume of jet fuel used domestically that year, and along with the monetary cost, there was the environmental impact of burning all that extra jet fuel to transport what Dannenberg, Burton, and Jackson call "this additional adiposity." The article "Gov't Study: Obese Passengers Pushing up Cost of Flights" (Associated Press, November 4, 2004) notes that Jack Evans, the spokesperson for the Air Transport Association of America, which represents major U.S. airlines, agreed that weight is a real issue. He explained that weight considerations and fuel prices have prompted airlines to replace metal forks and spoons with plastic utensils and to forgo bulky magazines: "We're dealing in a world of small numbers—even though it has a very incremental impact. When you consider airlines are flying millions of miles, it adds up over time."

In "Airline Policies Juggle Larger Passengers" (CNN.com, June 26, 2009), Stephanie Chen reports that an increasing number of airlines are forcing obese passengers to pay more than normal-weight passengers. In April 2009 United Airlines established the policy that "passengers who are unable to safely fit into one seat must pay full price for a second seat. They may receive it free if the plane has vacant seats. Flight attendants on the airlines are responsible for making sure passengers are fitting in their seats and may ask heavier passengers requiring two seats to pay extra." Chen observes that "some larger passengers don't mind paying for the second seat. Other heavier fliers argue while tall passengers pay a fee for legroom, the fees are only a fraction of the price of an entire seat."

In 2011 Southwest Airlines had another weight-related skirmish with two passengers. The article "Another Too-Fat-to-Fly Controversy Hits Southwest Airlines" (CBS News, May 18, 2011) reports that on a return trip from Dallas, Texas, to New York City, Kenlie Tiggeman and her mother were questioned about their weight and clothing sizes in front of a gate filled with airline passengers and then informed by the gate agent that each would have to purchase an additional seat. Southwest Airlines policy states that when a passenger "cannot fit in a seat with the armrests down, a second seat must be purchased. If the flight is not full, that added charge will be refunded." However, Tiggeman, who in the past had purchased two seats but lost more than 100 pounds (45 kg), said she did fit in the airline seat. Southwest Airlines not only apologized for the incident but

also refunded the fees for the return flight for Tiggeman and her mother and issued them vouchers good for purchasing air travel on Southwest.

San Francisco Bans Weight-Based Discrimination and Hears Landmark Cases

The San Francisco Human Rights Commission reports in "Compliance Guidelines to Prohibit Weight and Height Discrimination" (http://www.sf-hrc.org/Modules/ShowDocument.aspx?documentid=159) that on July 26, 2001, it unanimously approved historic guidelines for implementing a height-weight antidiscrimination law, and the city became the first jurisdiction in the United States to offer guidelines on how to prevent discrimination based on weight or height. Santa Cruz, California; Seattle, Washington; Washington, D.C.; and Michigan have similar laws that ban discrimination based on height or weight.

The strength of the ordinance was tested in 2003, when Jennifer Portnick, a 240-pound (109-kg) aerobics instructor, was refused a job at Jazzercise Inc., an international dance-fitness organization based in Carlsbad, California, and brought her case before the San Francisco Human Rights Commission. She eventually reached an agreement with the company to drop a requirement about the appearance of instructors. It was the first case settled under the San Francisco ordinance, which has become known as the "Fat and Short Law."

Patricia Leigh Brown reports in "240 Pounds, Persistent, and Jazzercise's Equal" (*New York Times*, May 8, 2002) that Portnick's attorney, Sondra Solovay, the author of *Tipping the Scales of Justice: Fighting Weight-Based Discrimination* (2000), said Portnick was "geographically lucky" to have filed her case in one of just four jurisdictions in the country that outlawed weight-based discrimination.

Weight Bias Influences Adoption Decision

Grant Slater reports in "Man Resorts to Surgery to Adopt Child" (Associated Press, August 25, 2007) the case of Gary Stocklaufer, a man weighing 558 pounds (253 kg) who was prevented from adopting a child because of his weight. Stocklaufer and his wife were ordered by a Missouri judge to give the four-month-old boy, a relative of the couple, whom they had raised since he was one week old, to another couple for possible adoption. Because the Stocklaufers served as licensed foster parents and already had one adopted child, they and adoption activists alleged that weight was the deciding factor. In a desperate attempt to regain the child, Stocklaufer dieted to 480 pounds (218 kg) before he underwent bariatric surgery, which eventually reduced his weight to 308 pounds (140 kg). According to the article "Judge Rules in Baby Max Custody Case" (KMBC.com, January 7, 2008), in January 2008 the

Stocklaufers were awarded custody of the then eight-month-old baby boy. The presiding judge ruled that "in the child's best interest [the Stocklaufers will] be permitted to adopt him." Adoption experts consider this a landmark case because it is the first one in which a couple seeking to adopt has resorted to surgery to surmount the increasingly prevalent practice of denying adoptions on the basis of weight.

The Origins of Stigma and Bias

Rebecca M. Puhl and Kelly D. Brownell of Yale University observe in the landmark study "Psychosocial Origins of Obesity Stigma: Toward Changing a Powerful and Pervasive Bias" (*Obesity Reviews*, vol. 4, no. 4, November 2003) that many people intensely dread the possibility of becoming obese. In one survey 24% of women and 17% of men said they would sacrifice three or more years of their life to be thin. There are reports of women who choose not to become pregnant because they fear gaining weight and becoming fat. Others smoke cigarettes in an effort to remain thin or reject the advice that they quit smoking because they fear they will gain weight should they quit. This powerful fear of fat, coupled with widespread perceptions that overweight people lack competence, self-control, ambition, intelligence, and attractiveness, create a culture in which it is socially acceptable to hold negative stereotypes about obese individuals and to discriminate against them.

One explanation of the origin of weight stigma is that traditionally Americans believe in self-determination and individualism—people get what they deserve and are responsible for their circumstances. In this context, when overweight is viewed as resulting from controllable behaviors, it is easy to understand that if an individual believes overweight people are to blame for their weight, then they should be stigmatized. Other research findings—that many Americans view life as predictable, with effort and ability inevitably producing the desired outcomes, and that attractive people are deemed good and believed to embody many positive qualities—support this theory. Interestingly, researchers find that in other countries the best predictors of anti-fat attitudes were cultural values that held both negative views about fatness and the belief that people are responsible for their life outcome.

Several other theories about the origins of weight stigma have been proposed. Conflict theory suggests that prejudice arises from conflicts of interest between groups and struggles to acquire or retain resources or power. Social identity theory posits that groups develop their social identities by comparing themselves to other groups and designating other groups as inferior. Integrated threat theory proposes that stigmatized groups are perceived as a threat. Proponents of this theory suggest that overweight and obese people threaten deeply held cultural

values of self-discipline, self-control, moderation, and thinness. Another theory, evolved dispositions theory, proposes that members of a group will be stigmatized if they threaten or undermine group functioning. This evolutionary adaptation may predispose people to shun obese individuals because they are at increased health risk and may not be able to make sufficient contributions to the group's welfare because of weight-related illness or disability.

Reducing Weight Bias and Stigma

In the landmark study "Demonstrations of Implicit Anti-fat Bias: The Impact of Providing Causal Information and Evoking Empathy" (*Health Psychology*, vol. 22, no. 1, January 2003), Bethany A. Teachman et al. wondered if anti-fat bias would be reduced when people were told that an individual's obesity resulted largely from genetic factors rather than from overeating and lack of exercise. The researchers assigned study participants to one of three groups. The first group received no information about the cause of obesity; the second group was given an article asserting that the principal cause of obesity was genetic; and the third group was given an article that attributed most obesity to overeating and lack of physical activity. As the researchers anticipated, the group told that obesity was controllable—resulting from overeating and inactivity—revealed the greatest amount of bias. However, to their surprise, Teachman et al. find that the group informed that obesity was primarily genetic in origin did not have significantly lower levels of bias than either the control group that had received no prior information or the group informed that obesity was caused by overeating and inactivity.

Teachman et al. also wanted to find out whether eliciting empathy for obese people would significantly reduce negative attitudes. The researchers hypothesized that by sharing written stories about weight-based discrimination with study participants they would feel empathy with the subjects in the stories, which they would then generalize to the entire population of obese people. Even though some study participants in the group that read the stories displayed lower bias, the majority did not have lower bias than the control group that had not read the stories of discrimination. The researchers speculate that the stories describing negative evaluations of an obese person might actually have served to reinforce rather than diminish bias.

Puhl and Brownell note that the increasing prevalence of obesity has not acted to reduce weight bias. They also refute the notion that stigma is necessary to motivate overweight and obese people to lose weight. They reiterate that dieting is not associated with long-term weight loss, regardless of the individual's motivation. Furthermore, they indicate that stigma can lead to discrimination and exert a harmful influence on health and quality of life. Puhl and Brownell assert that unless stigma is reduced, obese people will continue to contend with prejudice and discrimination.

Even though few studies have evaluated the effectiveness of strategies to reduce weight stigma, a variety of initiatives have produced varying degrees of attitudinal change. These approaches include:

- Educating participants about external uncontrollable causes such as the biological and genetic factors that contribute to obesity.

- Teaching and encouraging young children to practice size acceptance.

- Improving attitudes by combining efforts to elicit empathy with education about the uncontrollable causes of obesity.

- Encouraging direct personal contact with overweight and obese individuals to dispel negative stereotypes.

- Changing individuals' beliefs by exposing them to opposing attitudes and values held by a group that they consider important. This approach, which is called social consensus theory, relies on the observation that after learning that a group does not share the individuals' beliefs, they are more likely to modify their beliefs to be similar to those expressed by the group they respect or wish to join.

Puhl and Brownell describe the results of their experiments using social consensus theory to modify attitudes toward obese people. They conducted experiments with university students in which participants reported their attitudes toward obese people before and after the researchers offered them varying consensus opinions of other students. In one experiment, participants who were told that other students held more favorable attitudes about obese people reported significantly fewer negative attitudes and more positive attitudes about obese people than they had before they learned about the opinions of other students. Furthermore, they also changed their ideas about the causes of obesity, favoring the uncontrollable causes after they were told the other students believed obesity was attributable to these causes.

A second experiment confirmed that the power to alter the participants' beliefs depended on whether the source of the opposing beliefs was an in-group or out-group. Not surprisingly, participants' attitudes toward obese people were more likely to change when the information they were given came from a source they valued—an in-group. In a third experiment the researchers compared attitudinal change produced by social consensus with other methods to reduce stigma, including one in which participants were given written material about the controllable or uncontrollable causes of obesity. Puhl and Brownell find that social consensus theory was as effective as or more effective than any of the other methods they applied. They state that social consensus theory also offers an explanation about why obese individuals themselves express negative stereotypes—they want to belong to the valued social group and choose to accept negative stereotypes to align themselves with current culture. Furthermore, by accepting prevailing cultural values and beliefs, they not only resemble the in-group more closely but also distance themselves from the out-group, where identity and membership are defined by being overweight or obese.

Even though Puhl and Brownell consider social consensus a promising approach to reducing weight bias and stigma, they caution that there are many unanswered questions about its widespread utility and effectiveness. They conclude that "an ideal and comprehensive theory of obesity stigma would identify the origins of weight bias, explain why stigma is elicited by obese body types, account for the association between certain negative traits and obesity, and suggest methods for reducing bias. Existing theories do not yet meet all these criteria."

Weight Bias in the Media

Puhl and Heuer describe how the media takes a dim view of people who are obese, often casting them as "targets of humor and ridicule." The researchers point out that in recent years news reports have attributed a host of ills to people who are obese, ranging from playing a role in rising fuel prices and global warming to causing weight gain among their friends. Children's entertainment also consistently presents thin characters in a positive light and overweight characters negatively. Because most American adults are overweight or obese, it would be helpful to see overweight and obese people in lead roles and cast in a flattering light, as opposed to being in television reality shows, "where the entire cast is trying desperately to become thin."

In "Pros, Cons of Reality TV's Approach to Weight Loss" (*Los Angeles Times*, January 31, 2011), Brendan Borrell asserts that the only media outlets that are not averse to overweight and obesity are reality television shows—*The Biggest Loser, Losing It with Jillian, I Used to Be Fat*, and *Heavy*—that focus on weight loss. Supporters of these shows believe they are inspiring, because they prompt viewers to improve their diet and become more physically active. Detractors are concerned that these shows perpetuate stereotypes and that their emphasis on competition and dramatic weight loss may promote fasting, eating disorders, and other dangerous behaviors. For example, Borrell points out that contestants on *The Biggest Loser* have admitted to using dangerous methods to lose weight and at least two have been hospitalized. Lynn Grefe of the National Eating Disorders Association worries about viewers' attempts to duplicate the exercise regimens that are featured on the shows. She observes that the people "on these television programs clearly are obese, but they are afforded medical supervision. The person viewing at home who says, 'I'll do those jumping jacks and turn my life around' could have a heart attack."

Advocacy Groups Promote Size and Weight Acceptance

Our vision [is] a society in which people of every size are accepted with dignity and equality in all aspects of life. Our mission [is] to eliminate discrimination based on body size and provide fat people with the tools for self-empowerment though public education, advocacy, and support.

—National Association to Advance Fat Acceptance (2011)

There is a robust social movement that advocates size and weight acceptance with the overarching goal of assisting people to have a positive body image at any weight and to achieve health at any size. Nearly all the organizations that champion size acceptance characterize the preoccupation with dieting and weight loss as unhealthy and unproductive, citing statistics about diet failures, the dangers of weight cycling (the repeated loss and regain of body weight), and low self-esteem. The size acceptance movement proposes that it is possible to be fit and fat and that health and beauty are attainable at all weights. It also works to reduce "fat phobia," anti-fat bias, and weight-based discrimination.

The International Size Acceptance Association (ISAA) promotes size acceptance and aims to end size discrimination throughout the world by means of advocacy and visible, lawful actions. The ISAA asserts that people of all sizes can become more fit and is committed to helping people of all sizes strive for higher levels of fitness and improvement in their overall quality of life. Similarly, the ISAA observes that everyone can benefit from healthier food choices and is committed to helping inform the public about healthy nutrition.

The Council on Size and Weight Discrimination, a nonprofit advocacy organization working to end "sizism," bigotry, and discrimination against people who are heavier than average, focuses its advocacy efforts on affecting changes in medical treatment, job discrimination, and media images. The council's basic principles were derived from the "Tenets of the Nondiet Approach" (Karin Kratina, Dayle Hayes, and Nancy King, *Moving away from Diets: Healing Eating Problems and Exercise Resistance*, 2003) and focus on:

- Total health enhancement and well-being, rather than on weight loss or achieving a specific "ideal weight"

- Self-acceptance and respect for the diversity of bodies that come in a wide variety of shapes and sizes, rather than on the pursuit of an idealized weight at all costs

- The pleasure of eating well, based on internal cues of hunger and satiety (the feeling of fullness or satisfaction after eating), rather than on external food plans or diets

- The joy of movement, encouraging all physical activities, rather than on prescribing a specific routine of regimented exercise

The National Association to Advance Fat Acceptance (NAAFA; 2011, http://www.naafaonline.com/dev2/about/index.html) is a nonprofit human rights organization dedicated to eliminating discrimination based on body size and providing people with the "tools for self-empowerment through advocacy, public education, and support." Founded in 1969, the NAAFA has assumed a proactive role in protesting social prejudice, bias, and discrimination and in working with the Federal Trade Commission to stop diet fraud. The organization also seeks to improve legal protection for people who are overweight and obese by educating lawmakers and serving as a national legal clearinghouse for attorneys challenging size discrimination.

In an ongoing effort to counter discrimination, the organization has issued statements that are aimed at preventing overweight and obese children from suffering from bullying in school. Furthermore, in October 2011 the NAAFA (http://issuu.com/naafa/docs/) released guidelines for health care providers who treat people who are overweight and obese. The guidelines detail respectful treatment of overweight and obese patients and advise health care providers to:

- Weigh patients in a private setting

- Ensure that patients have access to waiting room seating, examination room facilities, and durable medical equipment that comfortably accommodates them

- Not assume that all the patient's health problems are caused by excess weight

- Not assume that patients want weight-loss counseling or information

CHAPTER 9
DIET AND WEIGHT-LOSS LORE, MYTHS, AND CONTROVERSIES

One of the challenges facing public health professionals as they seek to combat obesity among Americans is helping consumers to distinguish myths, lore, legends, and outright fraud from accurate, usable information about nutrition, diet, exercise, and weight loss. Some of these inaccuracies are so long-standing and deeply rooted in American culture that even the most educated consumers unquestioningly accept them as facts. Others began with a kernel of truth but have been so wildly distorted or misinterpreted that they are confusing, misleading, or entirely erroneous. The rapid influx and dissemination of information about the origins of overweight and obesity and the conflicting accounts of how best to treat these problems compound the challenge. With media reports and advertisements trumpeting different diets nearly every week, it is no wonder that Americans are confused about diet and weight loss.

The fiction that people who are overweight or obese are lazy and weak-willed is among the most harmful myths because it serves to promote stigma, bias, and discrimination. Another common misconception is that it is equally easy or difficult for all people to lose weight. There are biological and behavioral factors that affect an individual's body weight, and people vary in terms of genetic propensity to become overweight, basal metabolic rate (BMR), and the number of fat cells. BMR, often referred to simply as the metabolic rate, is the number of calories an individual expends at rest to maintain normal body functions. BMR changes with age, weight, height, diet, and exercise habits (and varies based on gender) and has been found to vary by as much as 1,000 calories per day. Differences in metabolic rate explain, in part, why not all people who adhere to the same diet achieve the same results in terms of pounds lost or rate of weight loss. Another factor that produces variation in weight loss is the number of fat cells in the dieter's body. Even though fat cells do not determine body weight, they are affected by weight gain and act to limit weight loss because their number cannot be decreased. For example, a normal-weight person has about 40 billion fat cells, whereas an individual who weighs 250 pounds (113 kg) with a body mass index (BMI; body weight in kilograms divided by height in meters squared) of 40 may have as many as 100 billion fat cells. Weight loss causes fat cells to shrink in size but does not decrease their number. As a result, individuals with twice as many fat cells as normal-weight people may be able to shrink their fat cells to a normal size but even when they have attained a healthy weight they will still have twice as many fat cells.

DIET AND WEIGHT-LOSS MYTHS

It is impossible to recount all the fantastic and improbable claims that have been made in recent years. This section considers some of the most persistent myths about diet, exercise, and weight loss.

Low-Carbohydrate Diets

MYTH. A low-carbohydrate diet is the fastest, healthiest, and best way to lose weight.

FACT. Low-carbohydrate diets may initially produce more rapid weight loss than other diets; however, most of the loss is water weight rather than fat. The water loss occurs as the kidneys flush out the excess waste products resulting from the digestion of protein and fat. Many low-carbohydrate diets encourage the consumption of high-fat foods, such as butter, heavy cream, bacon, and cheese. Long-term, high-fat diets may raise blood cholesterol levels. In addition, low-carbohydrate, high-protein diets produce a state of ketosis (the accumulation of ketones from partly digested fats as a result of inadequate carbohydrate intake), which may increase the risk of gout (a severe arthritis attack that occurs in one joint—typically the big toe, ankle, or knee—and is caused by defects in uric acid metabolism) and kidney stones. Furthermore, most nutritionists and researchers concur that nearly all diets can affect weight loss, and no compelling evidence exists to proclaim that one diet is vastly superior to another. A key factor in the success of any weight-loss diet is adherence (whether dieters can remain faithful to the regimen they have chosen), and as of January 2012, low-carbohydrate diets had not demonstrated superiority in terms of adherence. Boredom and frustration with a low-carbohydrate regimen may occur when dieters crave the carbohydrates that they are forbidden or can eat only in small amounts.

Still, there is one unanswered question about diet and weigh loss: Why do some dieters successfully lose weight using a low-carbohydrate or low-fat diet, whereas others on the same diet are unsuccessful? Cara B. Ebbeling et al. of the Children's Hospital Boston in Boston, Massachusetts, assert in "Effects of a Low-Glycemic Load vs Low-Fat Diet in Obese Young Adults" (*Journal of the American Medical Association*, vol. 297, no. 19, May 16, 2007) that which diet will be the most effective for each individual depends in part on the dieter's hormonal profile—specifically on differences in insulin secretion as measured by the serum insulin concentration. The researchers compared 73 subjects following a low-glycemic load (a ranking system for carbohydrate content in food based on its glycemic index [a measure of a food's ability to raise blood glucose] and the portion size) diet or a low-fat diet and measured their body weight, body fat, and insulin concentration before and after six months of dieting and during a 12-month follow-up period. During the six months of dieting high insulin secretors lost more weight (2.2 pounds [1 kg] per month) on the low-glycemic load diet than on the low-fat diet (0.9 pound [0.4 kg] per month). After 18 months the high insulin secretors had lost a total of 12.8 pounds (5.8 kg) on the low-glycemic load diet, compared with just 2.6 pounds (1.2 kg) on the low-fat diet. The low-glycemic load dieters also lost more body fat than the low-fat dieters and were more successful at maintaining their weight loss. In contrast, dieters who were considered low insulin secretors fared equally well on both diets. Ebbeling et al. also observe that independent of insulin secretion status, the low-glycemic load diet had beneficial effects: high-density lipoprotein increased and triglycerides decreased. Subjects on the low-fat diet did not realize these benefits, but they did experience reductions in low-density lipoprotein.

Calorie Reduction

MYTH. The dieter needs to cut calories drastically to lose weight.

FACT. Weight loss may be accomplished with modest reductions in calorie consumption. Low-calorie diets often result in metabolic adaptations, such as a significant reduction in the resting metabolic rate, which may produce weight maintenance or even weight gain rather than the desired weight loss. Many nutritionists and diet plans advise simultaneously reducing total caloric intake and modifying the balance of macronutrients (nutrients that the body uses in relatively large amounts: carbohydrates, fats, and proteins)—some weight-loss diets reduce fat intake, others reduce carbohydrates.

Negative-Calorie Foods

MYTH. It takes more calories to eat and digest some foods such as celery or cabbage than these foods contain, so eating them causes or speeds weight loss.

FACT. There are no foods, including celery and cabbage, that when eaten cause weight loss. However, foods containing caffeine may temporarily boost metabolism but they do not cause weight loss. In addition, some evidence suggests that eating grapefruit or drinking grapefruit juice may help people who are obese to lose weight. Ken Fujioka et al. of the Scripps Clinic in San Diego, California, compare weight loss over a 12-week period among 91 obese individuals. One-third of the subjects ate half a grapefruit before each meal three times per day and another third drank a glass of grapefruit juice before every meal. The third group did not include grapefruit in their meals. In "The Effects of Grapefruit on Weight and Insulin Resistance: Relationship to the Metabolic Syndrome" (*Journal of Medicinal Food*, vol. 9, no. 1, Spring 2006), Fujioka et al. report that after 12 weeks subjects who ate grapefruit lost an average of 3.6 pounds (1.6 kg) and those who drank grapefruit juice lost an average of 3.3 pounds (1.5 kg), whereas those in the control group who consumed no grapefruit lost an average of 0.6 of a pound (0.3 kg). Fujioka et al. attribute the weight loss not to the direct eating of grapefruit but to lowered levels of insulin, which were confirmed by measurements of blood glucose and insulin levels. They posit that the more efficiently sugar is metabolized, the less likely it is to be stored as fat. Furthermore, lowering insulin levels reduces feelings of hunger—elevated insulin levels stimulate the brain's hypothalamus, producing feelings of hunger.

Similarly, a review of 11 studies about the effects of green tea on weight loss and weight maintenance finds some evidence that green tea may help regulate body weight. Rick Hursel, Wolfgang Viechtbauer, and Margriet S. Westerterp-Plantenga of Maastricht University report in "The Effects of Green Tea on Weight Loss and Weight Maintenance: A Meta-Analysis" (*International Journal of Obesity*, vol. 33, no. 9, September 2009) that "catechins [phytochemical compounds] or an epigallocatechin gallate (EGCG [the most abundant catechin in tea]) caffeine mixture have a small positive effect on [weight loss] and [weight management]."

Eating at Night

MYTH. Eating after 8:00 p.m. causes weight gain.

FACT. Weight gain or loss does not depend on the time of day food is consumed—excess calories will be stored as fat whether they are consumed midmorning or just before bedtime. In general, weight is governed by the amount of food consumed (measured in total calorie count) and the amount of physical activity expended during the day.

However, there is evidence that eating early in the day and eating breakfast are habits associated with maintaining a healthy weight. In the editorial "Make It an Early Bird" (*New York Times*, November 21, 2007), Jennifer Ackerman indicates that research reveals that people who eat breakfast tend to consume fewer calories throughout the day, compared with those who make dinner their biggest meal. This may be because the system in the brain that signals satiety (the feeling of fullness or satisfaction after eating) is more effective early in the day—at night an individual may be more prone to succumb to overeating.

Natural Weight-Loss Products

MYTH. Organic, natural, or herbal weight-loss products are safer than synthetic (produced in the laboratory) over-the-counter (nonprescription) or prescription drugs.

FACT. Simply because products are organic or naturally occurring does not necessarily mean they are effective, risk-free, or safe. For example, Katherine Zeratsky of the Mayo Clinic in Rochester, Minnesota, explains in "Is Bitter Orange Safe and Effective for Weight Loss?" (November 25, 2009, http://mayoclinic.com/health/bitter-orange/AN01218) that bitter orange (*Citrus aurantium*) may help promote weight loss, but it can also cause side effects comparable to those of ephedra, such as rapid heart rate, increased blood pressure, and increased risk of fainting and developing migraines. It may even increase the risk for heart attack or stroke, especially when consumed in conjunction with other stimulants such as caffeine. Furthermore, bitter orange may interfere with the absorption and action of prescription medications, which in turn can cause or exacerbate a health problem.

In "An Evidence-Based Review of Fat Modifying Supplemental Weight Loss Products" (*Journal of Obesity*, October 2011), Amy M. Egras et al. explain that a 2008 survey found that more than one-third of adults who tried to lose weight had used a dietary supplement to assist their weight loss. Even though dietary supplements are widely used, there are very little data on the safety and efficacy of these products. Dietary supplements are considered food and not drugs, so the U.S. Food and Drug Administration (FDA) does not regulate them as it does prescription medications. When a dietary supplement is found to be unsafe after being marketed, the FDA can then determine whether to remove it from the market. The first time the FDA withdrew a dietary supplement for weight loss from the market was in 2004, when serious health risks were associated with the use of ephedra.

Egras et al. analyze studies that tested dietary supplements for weight loss and find evidence that some supplements such as conjugated linoleic acid (an unsaturated fatty acid in the milk and meat of cows, sheep, and goats), pyruvate (a substance that naturally occurs in apples, beer, and red wine that helps to produce energy), and *Irvingia gabonensis* (a supplement derived from the African mango) have demonstrated some potential benefit for weight loss. The researchers conclude that more research is necessary "to draw any definitive conclusions on the use of dietary supplements for weight loss."

Low-Fat and Low-Carbohydrate Foods

MYTH. Low fat, nonfat, and low carbohydrate mean few or no calories.

FACT. A low-fat or nonfat food is usually lower in calories than the same sized portion (as measured by weight) of the full-fat food; however, a food product can contain zero grams of fat and still have a high calorie content. Many fat-free foods replace the fat with sugar and contain just as many or more calories as full-fat versions. Even though most fruits and vegetables are naturally low in fat and calories, processed low-fat or nonfat foods may be high in calories because extra sugar, flour, or starch thickeners have been added to enhance the low-fat foods' taste or texture.

Similarly, low-carbohydrate foods are often higher in calories than their "regular" counterparts because their fat content is higher. Many foods that are naturally low in carbohydrates such as meat, butter, and cheese are also calorie-dense. Many nutritionists suggest limiting the consumption of low-carbohydrate versions of foods, such as low-carbohydrate frozen desserts, because they not only contain as many or more calories per serving than regular frozen desserts but also are often sweetened with artificial sweeteners that lack any nutrients.

Eliminating Starchy Foods

MYTH. Pasta, potatoes, and bread are fattening foods and should be eliminated or sharply limited when trying to lose weight.

FACT. Potatoes, rice, pasta, bread, beans, and some starchy vegetables such as squash, yams, sweet potatoes, turnips, beets, and carrots are not innately fattening. (They are often fattening only due to the "extras" that are put on them, such as butter, sour cream, margarine, or cheese.) They are rich in complex carbohydrates, which are important sources of energy. Furthermore, foods that are high in complex carbohydrates are often low in fat and calories because carbohydrates contain only 4 calories per gram, compared with the 9 calories per gram contained by fats. In "A Randomized Trial of a Low-Carbohydrate Diet vs Orlistat Plus a Low-Fat Diet for Weight Loss" (*Archives of Internal Medicine*, vol. 170, no. 2, January 25, 2010), William S. Yancy Jr. et al. report the results of a study in which dieters on a low-carbohydrate diet lost the same amount of weight as dieters on a low-fat, high-carbohydrate diet. The 146 overweight or obese subjects were randomly assigned to one of the two diets and the diet drug orlistat, and after 48 weeks both diets helped subjects lose about 10% of their initial, pre-diet weight. The diets were comparable in terms of adherence, and both groups decreased their calorie consumption by about 29% from the baseline.

Genetic Destiny

MYTH. People from families where many members are overweight or obese are destined to become overweight.

FACT. It is true that studies of families find similarities in body weight and that immediate relatives of obese people are at an increased risk for overweight and obesity, compared with people with normal-weight family members. Even though it is generally accepted that genetic susceptibility or predisposition to overweight or obesity is a factor, researchers believe environmental and behavioral factors make equally strong, if not stronger, contributions to the development of obesity. As a result, people from overweight or obese families may have to make a concerted effort to maintain healthy body weight and prevent weight gain, but they are not destined to become overweight or obese simply by virtue of the genes they inherited.

Exercise Alone

MYTH. Exercise is a better way to lose weight than dieting.

FACT. Even though there are many health benefits from exercise, weight loss is not generally considered a direct benefit. Research consistently demonstrates that for weight loss, diet trumps exercise because it is simpler to reduce caloric intake significantly through diet than to increase caloric expenditure significantly through exercise. For example, if a 155-pound (70-kg) person wants to reduce his or her consumption by 400 calories per day, it might be achieved by simply eliminating dessert and reducing portion sizes. In contrast, expending 400 calories per day requires considerable effort. To burn 400 calories a 155-pound person has to spend an hour bicycling 10 miles per hour (16 km/hr), ice skating at 9 miles

per hour (14.5 km/hr), or water skiing or walking uphill at about 3.5 miles per hour (5.6 km/hr). However, many studies demonstrate that exercise is an important way to prevent overweight and maintain weight loss.

D. Enette Larson-Meyer et al. combined calorie restriction with exercise and reported their findings in "Caloric Restriction with or without Exercise: The Fitness versus Fatness Debate" (*Medicine and Science in Sports and Exercise*, vol. 42, no. 1, January 2010). The researchers randomly assigned 36 otherwise healthy overweight adults to a 25% caloric restricted diet alone or to a 25% energy deficit regime produced equally by calorie restriction and exercise—12.5% by decreasing food intake and 12.5% by increasing energy expended through regular aerobic exercise.

Subjects in both groups lost about the same amount of weight and visceral fat; however, the calorie restriction and exercise group had improved insulin sensitivity, low-density lipoprotein and cholesterol levels, and diastolic blood pressure. Larson-Meyer et al. conclude that "results of the current study suggest that beyond changes in fatness, combining caloric restriction with exercise is important for increasing aerobic fitness and optimizing improvements in risk factors for diabetes and cardiovascular disease."

Eating Disorders

MYTH. Eating disorders occur exclusively among middle- and upper-class white females.

FACT. Like many myths about diet, weight, and nutrition, this one is based on fact: an estimated 90% of people with anorexia nervosa or bulimia nervosa are female. However, according to Susan Z. Yanovski of the National Institutes of Health, in the landmark study "Eating Disorders, Race, and Mythology" (*Archives of Family Medicine*, vol. 9, no. 1, January 2000), binge-eating disorder occurs in both genders and across all socioeconomic classes. Yanovski attributes the myth that eating disorders are limited to middle- and upper-class white women to the fact that many studies were conducted on college campuses where few minority students were enrolled, and other research looked at people seeking treatment, often at referral centers. Yanovski observes that "studies done on such populations, which may be more likely to be white and of higher socioeconomic status, have limited generalizability." She also cites research that finds that minorities are substantially affected by eating disorders—one study found that African-American women were as likely as white women to report binge eating. Another revealed that the prevalence of binge eating was comparable among Hispanic, non-Hispanic white, and African-American women, but that binge-eating symptoms were more severe among the Hispanic group. Yanovski concludes that the "recognition that eating disorders are color-blind can ensure that appropriate recognition and treatment are available to all patients at risk."

In "Why Men Should Be Included in Research on Binge Eating: Results from a Comparison of Psychosocial Impairment in Men and Women" (*International Journal of Eating Disorders*, October 26, 2011), Ruth H. Striegel et al. report that even though binge beating disorder has been associated with women, a significant number of men suffer from this disorder. The researchers estimate that among the 4 million Americans with an eating disorder, between 5% and 10% of men and about 11% of women are binge eaters. Because more men than previously thought are affected, Striegel et al. call for efforts "to raise awareness of the clinical significance of binge eating in men so that this group can receive appropriate screening and treatment services."

Freshmen in College Gain Weight

MYTH. College freshmen gain an average of 15 pounds (6.8 kg) during their first year of school.

FACT. Historically, college students were warned about the "freshman 15," the 15 pounds that students supposedly gain during their first year of college, presumably because freed from the constraints of healthy eating at home, they subsist on a diet of unhealthy food. However, Jay L. Zagorsky and Patricia K. Smith dispel in "The Freshman 15: A Critical Time for Obesity Intervention or Media Myth?" (*Social Science Quarterly*, vol. 92, no. 5, December 2011) the myth of freshman weight gain. The researchers analyze data from 7,418 college freshmen and find that first-year students, both male and female, gained an average of 2.5 to 3.5 pounds (1.1 to 1.6 kg) during their first year in college.

WHY DIETS FAIL

Historically, diets have been considered to have "failed" when lost weight is regained. Many nutritionists and obesity researchers believe diets fail because most are not sustainable. The more restrictive the diet, the less likely an individual will be to remain faithful to it because, in general, people cannot endure extended periods of hunger and deprivation. Diets may also fail because they neglect to teach dieters new eating habits to assist them to maintain their weight loss. Most overweight people gained their excess weight by consuming more calories per day than they needed. Dieting creates a temporary deficit of calories or specific macronutrients such as carbohydrates or fat. Because the weight-loss diet is viewed as a temporary measure with a beginning and an end, at its conclusion most dieters return to their previous eating habits and often regain the lost weight or even more weight. Many nutritionists and dieticians who work with people who are overweight or obese assert that diets do not fail; instead, dieters fail to learn how to eat properly to prevent weight regain.

Consumers are not the only ones who believe that diets are doomed to fail. Many health professionals and researchers cite the statistic that 95% of diets fail. This oft-cited statistic has been attributed to Albert James Stunkard (1922–), the director emeritus of the Obesity Society (formerly the American Obesity Association). Stunkard put forth the 95% failure rate based on research he performed in 1959, which involved advising 100 overweight patients to diet, with no follow-up or support to increase their adherence to the diet. In "Whether Obesity Should Be Treated?" (*Health Psychology*, vol. 12, no. 5, September 1993), Kelly D. Brownell of Yale University observes that this statistic has been widely applied even though it is quite dated, was not confirmed by subsequent studies, and involved only subjects in university-based research programs.

The article "New Diet Winners: We Rate the Diet Books and Plans" (*Consumer Reports*, vol. 72, no. 6, June 2007) observes that only recently have successful dieters been studied to learn from their successes and incorporate them into more effective, and ideally sustainable, weight-loss plans. It cites as an example the new emphasis on achieving satiety without consuming too many calories by consuming low-density foods. This article may help dispel the myth that dieters are doomed to fail.

Improving Long-Term Weight Loss

More recent research demonstrates that dieters find it challenging to maintain weight loss; however, it refutes the 95% failure rate. In "One-Year Weight Maintenance after Significant Weight Loss in Healthy Overweight and Obese Subjects: Does Diet Composition Matter?" (*American Journal of Clinical Nutrition*, vol. 90, no. 5, November 2009), Elizabeth A. Delbridge et al. observe that "for many people, maintenance of weight loss is elusive." The researchers also find that the protein or carbohydrate composition of the diet used for weight loss had no effect on successful weight maintenance.

Kelly S. Dale et al. compare in "Determining Optimal Approaches for Weight Maintenance: A Randomized Controlled Trial" (*Canadian Medical Association Journal*, vol. 180, no. 10, May 12, 2009) the effectiveness of two support programs—one providing intensive support from nutrition and activity specialists and the other consisting of weigh-ins and encouragement from a relatively inexperienced nurse—and two diets—a high-fat diet and a high-carbohydrate diet—intended to promote long-term weight maintenance. The study subjects were 200 women aged 25 to 70 years who had intentionally lost at least 5% of their initial body weight in the previous six months and had a BMI of 27 or greater.

The researchers find that over the course of two years subjects assigned to either of the diets had reduced weight, BMI, waist circumference, and blood pressure, with no significant differences between the two diets. Similarly, subjects who received intensive and relatively costly support from highly trained health professionals fared no better than those who received less intensive support from a less experienced nurse. Dale et al. conclude, "We have shown that women who are sufficiently motivated to join a 2-year study can maintain their weight and, in many instances, further reduce their weight, waist circumference and body fat mass with a simple, inexpensive nurse-support program."

Nutrigenetics (using genetic information to custom-tailor a weight-loss diet) may help improve the success of weight-loss and weight-maintenance efforts. In "Improved Weight Management Using Genetic Information to Personalize a Calorie Controlled Diet" (*Nutrition Journal*, vol. 6, October 18, 2007), Ioannis Arkadianos et al. indicate that they offered nutrigenetic testing and developed individual diets for people who historically had failed to lose weight. They compare the results these dieters achieved to a control group that did not receive nutrigenetic screening or a personalized diet and find that subjects in the nutrigenetic group fared better in terms of adherence to their diet, weight loss and maintenance, and improvements in blood glucose levels.

Approaches to enhance motivation focus on two areas: improved social supports and tangible financial incentives. Strategies to improve social supports emphasize including spouses or significant others in the weight-loss process to teach them to provide social support for their partner's weight-loss efforts. Such strategies demonstrate modest success as do contracts in which groups agree to aim for individual or group weight loss.

According to Eric A. Finkelstein et al., in "A Pilot Study Testing the Effect of Different Levels of Financial Incentives on Weight Loss among Overweight Employees" (*Journal of Occupational and Environmental Medicine*, vol. 49, no. 9, September 2007), financial incentives may be effective inducements to lose weight. The researchers followed 200 overweight workers in North Carolina, who were randomly assigned to one of three groups. One group received no incentives, whereas the other two groups received either $7 or $14 for each percentage point of weight lost. For example, a 200-pound (91-kg) subject in the group received $7 for each percentage point of weight lost. The subject lost 10 pounds (4.5 kg), or 5% of his or her weight, and received $35. Finkelstein et al. find that workers who received the most money and other incentives such as time off lost the most weight. At three months, subjects with no financial incentive lost 2 pounds (0.9 kg), those in the $7 group

lost approximately 3 pounds (1.4 kg), and those in the $14 group lost 4.7 pounds (2.1 kg).

Financial incentives may encourage people to lose weight, but they do not appear to prevent weight regain. In "Financial Incentives for Extended Weight Loss: A Randomized, Controlled Trial" (*Journal of General Internal Medicine*, vol. 26, no. 6, June 2011), Leslie K. John et al. analyze data from a 32-week-long weight-loss program—24 weeks of weight loss followed by eight weeks of weight maintenance. Sixty-six program participants were given the goal of losing 1 pound (0.5 kg) per week and received a financial incentive for achieving this weight loss. To assess longer-term maintenance following the 32-week intervention, participants returned for a weigh-in approximately 36 weeks after they completed the 32-week program. The researchers find that the incentive did promote weight loss and maintenance through the 32-week program; however, after the program ended there was significant weight regain. John et al. conclude that "future research is needed to devise techniques that promote sustained weight loss over longer periods of time."

Teaching patients skills that are useful for weight maintenance as opposed to weight loss emphasizes that there are two distinctly different sets of strategies: one set focuses on weight loss and the other set focuses on maintaining a stable energy balance around a lower weight. The most commonly used model for teaching maintenance-specific skills is relapse prevention, which involves teaching people to identify situations in which lapses in behavioral adherence are likely to occur, to plan strategies in advance to prevent lapses, and to get back on track should they occur. Relapse prevention is based on the idea that breaking the so-called rules in terms of remaining faithful to diet and exercise programs may often lead to negative psychological reactions that in turn prompt reversion to pre-weight-loss behaviors.

Brent Van Dorsten and Emily M. Lindley of the University of Colorado, Denver, review in "Cognitive and Behavioral Approaches in the Treatment of Obesity" (*Medical Clinics of North America*, vol. 95, no. 5, September 2011) research about long-term weight maintenance following weight loss using relapse prevention strategies. The researchers report that long-term contact with treatment providers is an important factor in successful weight maintenance. Long-term follow-up contacts may be face-to-face, via telephone, Internet, or e-mail. Even though the optimal frequency of contacts to support weight maintenance is not yet known, the frequency of weighing is another factor identified by successful weight-loss maintainers. The use of personal trainers and monetary incentives for weight loss as well as group worksite competitions also demonstrate the capacity to promote long-term engagement with, and adherence to, weight-loss programs.

WEIGHT-LOSS SCHEMES DEFRAUD CONSUMERS

There is a long history of marketing so-called fat-burning pills, potions, and products to Americans seeking effortless weight loss. Peter N. Stearns, in *Fat History: Bodies and Beauty in the Modern West* (1997), and Laura Fraser, in *Losing It: False Hopes and Fat Profits in the Diet Industry* (1998), offer detailed histories of magical cures and weight-loss fads. At the beginning of the 20th century products such as obesity belts and chairs that delivered electrical stimulation, as well as corsets, tonics, and mineral waters, claimed to cause weight loss.

Diet pills appeared in 1910 with the introduction of weight-loss tablets that contained arsenic (a poisonous metallic element), strychnine (a plant toxin formerly used as a stimulant), caffeine, and pokeberries (formerly used as a laxative). During the 1920s cigarette makers promoted their product as a diet aid, urging Americans to smoke rather than eat. During the 1930s diet pills containing dinitrophenol, a chemical used to manufacture explosives, dyes, and insecticides, enjoyed brief popularity after it was observed that factory workers making munitions lost weight. Their popularity was short lived, as cases of temporary blindness and death were attributed to their use.

The second half of the 20th century saw the proliferation of questionable, and often entirely worthless, weight-loss devices and gimmicks, including inflatable suits to "sweat off pounds," diet drinks and cookies, and slimming creams, patches, shoe inserts, and wraps to reduce fat thighs and abdomens. Even though the claims made for many of these products sounded too good to be true, unsuspecting Americans spent billions of dollars in the hope of achieving quick, easy, and permanent weight loss.

The promotion of dubious and potentially dangerous weight-loss products continued during the second decade of the 21st century. As of January 2012, the FDA had recalled more than 40 products marketed for weight loss that contained potentially harmful ingredients and issued consumer alerts about dozens of others. The agency has also issued warning letters, seized products, and criminally prosecuted people responsible for these illegal diet products. For example, in "Beware of Fraudulent Weight-Loss 'Dietary Supplements'" (March 15, 2011, http://www.fda.gov/ForConsumers/ConsumerUpdates/ucm 246742.htm), Michael Levy, the director of the FDA Division of New Drugs and Labeling Compliance, explains that many dietary supplements marketed as weight-loss aids are "actually very powerful drugs masquerading as 'all-natural' or 'herbal' supplements, and they carry significant risks to unsuspecting consumers." The FDA finds that many of these supplements contain dangerous combinations of "seizure medications, blood pressure medications, and other drugs not approved in the U.S." Levy cautions, "Make no mistake—they can kill you."

Weighing the Claims

In May 2000 the Partnership for Healthy Weight Management, a coalition of scientific, academic, health care, government, commercial, and public interest representatives, initiated consumer and media education programs that aimed not only to increase public awareness of the obesity epidemic in the United States but also to promote responsible marketing of weight-loss products and programs. The partnership also published the consumer guide *Finding a Weight Loss Plan That Works for You* (December 28, 2009, http://www.ftc.gov/bcp/edu/pubs/consumer/health/hea05.pdf), which was designed to help overweight and obese consumers find weight-loss solutions to meet their needs. The guide contains a checklist that enables consumers to compare weight-loss plans based on a variety of criteria. (See Table 9.1.) It also advises consumers about how to select weight-loss programs and services based on specific information from potential providers.

In November 2002 the Federal Trade Commission (FTC) convened a workshop attended by researchers, scholars, media experts, and medical professionals from the government, academia, and private industry that aimed to evaluate claims and develop new and more effective ways to combat false and deceitful weight-loss advertising claims. The FTC summarized the workshop proceedings, including attendees' assessments of eight broad categories of advertising claims, in *Deception in Weight-Loss Advertising Workshop: Seizing Opportunities and Building Partnerships to Stop Weight-Loss Fraud* (December 2003, http://www.ftc.gov/os/2003/12/031209weightlossrpt.pdf). The following section considers the advertising claims and summarizes the attendees' assessments of these claims. It also draws on an analysis of the FTC report by Stephen Barrett in "Impossible Weight-Loss Claims: Summary of an FTC Report" (December 16, 2003, http://www.quackwatch.org/01QuackeryRelated Topics/PhonyAds/weightlossfraud.html).

No Diet or Exercise Required

CLAIM. The advertised product causes substantial weight loss without exercise or diet.

EXAMPLES. "U.S. patent reveals weight loss of as much as 28 pounds in 4 weeks…. Eat all your favorite foods and still lose weight. The pill does all the work," and "Lose up to 2 pounds daily without diet or exercise." Table 9.2 contains other examples of comparable claims.

TABLE 9.1

Checklist for evaluating weight loss products and services

Use this checklist to gather and compare information from all weight loss programs you're considering.

Make several copies of the blank form so you can fill out one for each program. A provider's willingness to give you this information is an important factor in choosing a program. If you need help to evaluate the information you gather, talk with your primary health care provider or a registered dietitian.

Program name _____
Address _____
Phone number _____

In this program, my daily caloric intake will be: _____

My daily caloric intake is determined by: _____
I   will   will not be evaluated initially by program staff.

The evaluation will be made by (check all that apply):
   Physician   Nurse   Registered dietitian   Other company-trained employee

My progress is supervised by (check all that apply):
   Physician   Nurse   Licensed psychologist
   Registered dietitian   Company-trained employee

I will   will not be evaluated by a physician during the course of my treatment.

During the first month, my progress will be monitored:
   Weekly   Biweekly   Monthly   Other _____

After the first month, my progress will be monitored:
   Weekly   Biweekly   Monthly   Other _____

My weight loss plan includes (check all that apply):
   Nutrition information about healthy eating   At least 1,200 calories/day for women or 1,400 calories/day for men
   Suggested menus and recipes   Keeping food diaries or other monitoring activities
   Portion control   Liquid meal replacements
   Prepackaged meals   Dietary supplements (vitamins, minerals, botanicals, herbals)
   Prescription weight loss drugs   Help with weight maintenance and lifestyle changes
   Surgery

My plan includes regular physical activity that is (check both if both apply):
   Supervised (at the program site)   _____ times per week, _____ minutes per session.
   Unsupervised (on my own time)   _____ times per week, _____ minutes per session.

The physical activity includes (check all that apply):
   Walking   Swimming   Stationary cycling
   Strength training   Aerobic dancing   Other _____

The weight loss plan includes (check all that apply):
   Family counseling   Group support   Lifestyle modification advice
   Weight maintenance advice   Weight maintenance counseling
   The staff explained the risks associated with this weight loss progam. They are:
_____
_____

   The staff explained the costs of this program. (Check all that apply and fill in the blanks.)
   I will be charged a one-time entry fee of $ ___.
   I will be charged $ ___ per visit.
   Food replacements will cost about $ ___ per month.
   Prescription weight loss drugs will cost about $ ___ per month.
   Vitamins and other dietary supplements will cost about $ ___ per month.
   Diagnostic tests are required and will cost about $ ___ .
   Other costs include _____ at $ ___.

Total cost for this program $____

The program gave me information about:
   The health risks of being overweight.   The difficulty many people have maintaining weight loss.
   The health benefits of weight loss.   How to improve my chances at maintaining my weight.

Other information to ask for:
   Participants in this program have lost an average of ___ lbs. over ___ months/years.
   Participants in this program have kept off ___ % of their weight loss for ___ years.

This information is based on the following (check one):
   All participants.
   Participants who completed the program.
   Other _____

Notes: _____
_____

SOURCE: "Checklist for Evaluating Weight Loss Products and Services," in *Finding a Weight Loss Program That Works for You*, Federal Trade Commission, The Partnership for Healthy Weight Management, December 28, 2009, http://www.ftc.gov/bcp/edu/pubs/consumer/health/hea05.pdf (accessed November 16, 2011)

ASSESSMENT. The consensus was that products purporting to cause weight loss without diet or exercise would either need to cause malabsorption (impair the absorption) of calories or to increase metabolism. Because the number of calories that can be malabsorbed is limited to 1,200 to 1,300 calories per week, or about

TABLE 9.2

Examples of claims that promise weight loss without diet or exercise

"Awesome attack on bulging fatty deposits ... has virtually eliminated the need to diet." (Konjac root pill)

"They said it was impossible, but tests prove [that] my astounding diet-free discovery melts away. . . 5, 6, even 7 pounds of fat a day." (ingredients not disclosed)

"The most powerful diet pill ever discovered! No diet or workout required. The secret weight-loss pill behind Fitness models, Show Biz and Entertainment professionals! No prescription required to order." (ingredients not disclosed)

"Lose up to 30 lbs . . . No impossible exercise! No missed meals! No boring foods or small portions!" (plant extract fucus vesiculosus)

"Lose up to 8 to 10 pounds per week ... [n]o dieting, no strenuous exercise." (elixir purportedly containing 16 plant extracts)

"My 52 lbs of unwanted fat relaxed away without dieting or grueling exercise." (hypnosis seminar)

"No exercise ... [a]nd eat as much as you want—the more you eat, the more you lose, we'll show you how." (meal replacement)

SOURCE: Richard L. Cleland et al., "Table 5. Lose Weight without Diet or Exercise Claims," in *Weight-Loss Advertising: An Analysis of Current Trends*, Federal Trade Commission, September 2002, http://www.ftc.gov/bcp/reports/weightloss.pdf (accessed November 16, 2011)

0.3 of a pound (0.1 kg) per week, malabsorption alone is unlikely to lead to substantial weight loss. Similarly, there is no thermogenic (heat-producing) agent, such as ephedrine combined with caffeine, able to boost metabolism enough to produce weight loss without diet or exercise. In fact, the mechanism by which ephedrine products appear to assist weight loss is by suppressing appetite rather than by speeding metabolism. Furthermore, even though green tea extract was found to increase metabolism, it was by a scant 4%.

No Restrictions on Eating

CLAIM. Users can lose weight while still enjoying unlimited amounts of high-calorie foods.

EXAMPLE. "Eat All the Foods You Love and Still Lose Weight (Pill Does All the Work)."

ASSESSMENT. This claim was viewed as a variation of the assertion that dieters can lose weight without reducing caloric intake or increasing exercise, because this claim states that users not only can lose weight without reducing caloric intake but also may increase caloric intake and still lose weight. The assembled experts concurred that if this claim was true, it would defy the laws of physics.

Permanent Weight Loss

CLAIM. The advertised product causes permanent weight loss.

EXAMPLES. "Take it off and keep it off. You won't gain the weight back afterwards because your weight will have reached an equilibrium," and "People who use this product say that even when they stop using the product, their weight does not jump up again."

ASSESSMENT. Even if a product caused weight loss through a reduction of calories, appetite suppression, or malabsorption, weight would be regained once use of the product stopped and calorie consumption returned to previous levels. Researchers and health professionals have repeatedly observed that dieters tend to regain weight lost over time once the diet, intervention, or other treatment ends. According to the Food and Nutrition Board of the National Academy of Sciences, "Many programs and services exist to help individuals achieve weight control. But the limited studies paint a grim picture: those who complete weight-loss programs lose approximately 10 percent of their body weight only to regain two-thirds of it back within 1 year and almost all of it back within 5 years." Furthermore, there are no published scientific studies supporting the claim that a nonprescription drug, dietary supplement, cream, wrap, device, or patch can cause permanent weight loss.

Fat Blockers

CLAIM. The advertised product causes substantial weight loss through the blockage or absorption of fat or calories.

EXAMPLES. "[The named ingredient] can ingest up to 900 times its own weight in fat, that's why it's a fantastic fat blocker," and "The Super Fat Fighting Formula inhibits fats, sugars and starches from being absorbed in the intestines and turning into excess weight, so that you can lose pounds and inches easily."

ASSESSMENT. Science does not support the possibility that sufficient malabsorption of fat or calories can occur to cause substantial weight loss. To lose even 1 pound (0.5 kg) per week requires malabsorption of about 500 calories per day or about 55 grams of fat. To lose 2 pounds (0.9 kg) per day, as promised in some advertisements, would require the malabsorption of 7,000 calories per day, which is impossible given that it is several times the total calories that most people consume daily, let alone the number of calories consumed from fat. The FTC has challenged deceptive fat-blocker claims for some of the most popular diet products on the market. The evidence supports the position that consumers cannot lose substantial weight through the blockage of absorption of fat. It is not scientifically feasible for a nonprescription drug, dietary supplement, cream, wrap, device, or patch to cause substantial weight loss through the blockage of absorption of fat or calories.

Quick Weight Loss

CLAIM. The user of the advertised product can safely lose more than 3 pounds (1.4 kg) per week for time

TABLE 9.3

Examples of claims that promise fast results

"This combination of plant extracts constitutes a weight-loss plan that facilitates what is probably the fastest weight loss ever observed from an entirely natural treatment." (elixir purportedly containing 16 plant extracts)

"Just fast and easy, effective weight loss!" (fucus vesiculosus)

"Lose 10 lbs. in 8 Days!" (apple cider vinegar)

"Rapid weight loss in 28 days!" (ephedra)

"Knock off your unwanted weight and fat deposits at warp speeds! You can lose 18 pounds in one week!" (ingredients not disclosed)

"Clinically proven to cause rapid loss of excess body fat." (phosphosterine)

"Two clinically proven fat burning formulations that are guaranteed to get you there fast or it costs you absolutely nothing." (ingredients not disclosed)

SOURCE: Richard L. Cleland et al., "Table 4. Representative Claims That Promise Fast Results," in *Weight Loss Advertising: An Analysis of Current Trends*, Federal Trade Commission, September 2002, http://www.ftc.gov/bcp/reports/weightloss.pdf (accessed November 16, 2011)

periods exceeding four weeks. Table 9.3 shows claims that promise unbelievably rapid results.

EXAMPLE. "Lose three pounds per week, naturally and without side effects."

ASSESSMENT. Significant health risks are associated with medically unsupervised, rapid weight loss over extended periods of time. Basically, "the more restrictive the diet, the greater are the risks of adverse effects associated with weight loss." One documented risk is the increased incidence of gallstones. The claim that consumers using products such as these can safely lose more than 3 pounds per week for a period of more than four weeks is not scientifically feasible.

Weight-Loss Creams and Patches

CLAIM. The advertised product that is worn on the body or rubbed into the skin causes substantial weight loss.

EXAMPLES. "Lose two to four pounds daily with the Diet Patch," and "Thigh Cream drops pounds and inches from your thighs."

ASSESSMENT. Diet patches and creams that are worn or applied to the skin have not been proven to be safe or effective. Furthermore, their alleged mechanisms of action are not scientifically credible.

Guaranteed Success

CLAIM. The advertised product causes substantial weight loss for all users.

EXAMPLE. "Lose excess body fat. No willpower required. Works for everyone no matter how many times you've tried and failed before."

ASSESSMENT. This claim assumes that overweight and obesity arise from a single cause or are amenable to

a single solution. Because the causes of overweight and obesity are thought to be genetic factors and environmental conditions, and contributing factors such as diet, metabolic rate, level of physical activity, and adherence to weight-loss treatment vary, it is unlikely that one product will be effective for all users. Even FDA-approved prescription drugs for weight loss have a high level of nonresponders, and surgical treatment for obesity is not successful 100% of the time. The claim that a nonprescription drug, dietary supplement, cream, wrap, device, or patch will cause substantial weight loss for all users is not scientifically feasible.

Targeted Weight-Loss Products

CLAIM. Users of the advertised product can lose weight from only those parts of the body where they wish to lose weight.

EXAMPLE. "And it has taken off quite some inches from my butt (5 inches) and thighs (4 inches), my hips now measure 35 inches. I still wear the same bra size though. The fat has disappeared from exactly the right places."

ASSESSMENT. Small published studies of aminophylline cream indicate that its use may cause the redistribution of fat from the thighs to other fat stores; however, it has not been shown to cause fat loss. Even if some products were capable of causing more weight loss from certain areas of the body, no part would be spared completely—fat is lost from all fat stores throughout the body.

Red Flag Campaign and Other Initiatives Target Phony Weight-Loss Claims

Another outcome of the November 2002 workshop was the design of an education initiative to assist the media to voluntarily screen weight-loss product ads containing claims that are "too good to be true." The media were targeted for intensive education not only because broad-based public education has proven largely inadequate to protect consumers from persuasive messages trumpeting easy weight loss but also to acknowledge the media's powerful ability to reduce weight-loss fraud by sharply limiting the dissemination of obviously false weight-loss advertising. In December 2003 the FTC launched its Red Flag campaign to assist the media to reduce deceptive weight-loss advertising and promote positive, reliable advertising messages about weight loss. The FTC (2012, http://www.ftc.gov/bcp/edu/microsites/redflag/falseclaims.html) defines Red Flag claims as those that promise to:

- Cause weight loss of two pounds or more a week for a month or more without dieting or exercise

- Cause substantial weight loss no matter what or how much the consumer eats

- Cause permanent weight loss (even when the consumer stops using product)

- Block the absorption of fat or calories to enable consumers to lose substantial weight

- Safely enable consumers to lose more than three pounds per week for more than four weeks

- Cause substantial weight loss for all users

- Cause substantial weight loss by wearing it on the body or rubbing it into the skin

In April 2004 the FTC filed claims against seven companies for making false weight-loss claims, and in November 2004 the FTC announced six new cases against advertisers using bogus weight-loss claims. In each of these cases the FTC sought to stop the bogus ads and to secure reparation for consumers. The FTC also launched a website (http://wemarket4u.net/fatfoe/) to help consumers identify false weight-loss claims.

In 2011 the FTC continued to file actions to stop false and unsupported weight-loss claims. For example, the FTC reports in "FTC Seeks to Halt 10 Operators of Fake News Sites from Making Deceptive Claims about Acai Berry Weight Loss Products" (April 19, 2011, http://www.ftc.gov/opa/2011/04/fakenews.shtm) that actions were taken against 10 companies marketing açaí berry weight-loss products. The FTC indicates that the companies made false and unsupported claims that açaí berry supplements cause rapid and substantial weight loss. The FTC also charged the companies with fabricating news reports and testimonials that were intended to defraud consumers.

In "FTC Settlement Prohibits Marketer from Claiming that Nivea Skin Cream Can Help Consumers Slim Down" (June 29, 2011, http://www.ftc.gov/opa/2011/06/beiersdorf.shtm), the FTC notes that it stopped Beiersdorf, Inc., the maker of Nivea skin creams, from claiming that regular use of its Nivea My Silhouette! skin cream could significantly reduce consumers' body size, tone their stomachs, thin their waists, and help them slim down. To settle the FTC claim that it made false statements about of one of its skin creams, Beiersdorf agreed to pay $900,000. The FTC chairman Jon Leibowitz (1958–) commented, "The real skinny on weight loss is that no cream is going to help you fit into your jeans."

Despite FTC actions, purveyors of weight-loss products continue to make unsubstantiated claims. For example, in "NonSensa" (*Nutrition Action*, December 2011), the Center for Science in the Public Interest (CSPI) weighs the claims of a product called Sensa, which when sprinkled on food supposedly changes its scent, which in turn sends a satiety signal to the brain. A one-month supply of the flavored granules helps dieters "lose 30+ pounds without dieting" and costs $60. According to the CSPI, the premise that "enhancing the sensory properties of food" will cause weight loss is unproven and the research supporting the product's claims has not been published.

DO VERY-LOW-CALORIE DIETS INCREASE LONGEVITY?

Even though many Americans are overweight, some people are experimenting with very-low-calorie diets in the hope that by remaining extremely thin they will stave off disease and live longer. Advocates of extreme caloric restriction (CR) contend that sharply reducing caloric intake creates biochemical changes that slow the aging process, which theoretically should increase life expectancy.

Most people would find it impossible to adhere to semistarvation diets, but there is sound scientific evidence—such as Luigi Fontana and Samuel Klein's "Aging, Adiposity, and Calorie Restriction" (*Journal of the American Medical Association*, vol. 297, no. 9, March 7, 2007) and Arthur V. Everitt and David G. Le Couteur's "Life Extension by Calorie Restriction in Humans" (*Annals of the New York Academy of Sciences*, vol. 1114, October 2007)—that subsistence diets increase the life span of fruit flies, worms, spiders, guppies, mice, and hamsters by between 10% and 40%. In theory, semi-starvation prolongs life by reducing metabolism (how quickly glucose is used for energy) in an evolutionary adaptation to conserve calories during periods of famine. Dieters are familiar with this process—they know from experience that as they eat less, their metabolic rate drops, which makes losing weight increasingly more difficult. CR adherents experience comparable drops in metabolic rate—one study found that their body temperature dropped by a full degree. Proponents of CR assert that even though metabolism is vital for life, it is also destructive because it produces unstable molecules known as free radicals that can damage cells through a process called oxidation.

In "A Low Dose of Dietary Resveratrol Partially Mimics Caloric Restriction and Retards Aging Parameters in Mice" (*PLoS One*, vol. 3, no. 6, June 4, 2008), Jamie L. Barger et al. indicate that CR inhibits gene expression profiles that are associated with heart and skeletal muscle aging and prevents age-related heart problems.

CR adherents report immediate health benefits including increased mental acuity, reduced need for sleep, sharply reduced cholesterol and fasting blood sugar levels, weight loss, and reduced blood pressure. The regimen is clearly not easy, and even its staunchest advocates, such as members of the Caloric Restriction

Society, concede that many people who practice CR experience constant hunger, obsessions with food, mood disorders such as irritability and depression, and lowered libido (sex drive). CR can also cause people to feel cold, and even with adequate vitamin and mineral supplementation it can cause some people to suffer from osteoporosis (decreased bone mass) and hair loss. Jon Gertner reports in "The Calorie-Restriction Experiment" (*New York Times*, October 7, 2009) that the majority of subjects in the Calerie study achieved their weight-loss goals and were maintaining their weight loss by sticking to their diet. However, he notes that CR is a challenging undertaking and one that most Americans would forgo. Gertner opines that "living a life of less in a culture of more—is extremely difficult to achieve and even more difficult to maintain. Americans' seemingly inexorable slide toward obesity tends to indicate as much: for the majority of us, the desire to eat can easily overwhelm personal willpower and (so far) any messages from public-health campaigns."

In "Why Dietary Restriction Substantially Increases Longevity in Animal Models but Won't in Humans" (*Ageing Research Reviews*, vol. 4, no. 3, August 2005), John P. Phelan and Michael R. Rose challenge the notion that CR will increase longevity. The researchers conclude that severely restricting calories over decades may add a few years to a human life span, but will not enable humans to live to 125 years or more. Phelan and Rose developed a mathematical model based on the known effects of calorie intake and life span that shows that people who consume the most calories have a shorter life span. It also shows that if people severely restrict their calories over their lifetime, their life span increases by between 3% and 7%, which is far less than the 20-plus years some hoped could be achieved by drastic CR. The researchers suggest that "longevity is not a trait that exists in isolation; it evolves as part of a complex life history, with a wide range of underpinning physiological mechanisms involving, among other things, chronic disease processes." They advise Americans to "try to maintain a healthy body weight, but don't deprive yourself of all pleasure. Moderation appears to be a more sensible solution."

Everitt and Le Couteur confirm that even though short-term CR does improve specific markers that are associated with longevity, such as deep body temperature and plasma insulin levels, CR is unlikely to offer markedly increased longevity. The researchers cite as evidence the Okinawans, the longest-lived people on the earth, who consume 40% fewer calories than the average American and live just four years longer. Everitt and Le Couteur surmise that "the effects of CR on human life extension are probably much smaller than those achieved by medical and public health interventions, which have extended life by about 30 years in developed countries in the 20th century, by greatly reducing deaths from infections, accidents, and cardiovascular disease."

The long-term effects of CR are not yet known. Nicholas Wade reports in "Quest for a Long Life Gains Scientific Respect" (*New York Times*, September 28, 2009) that in September 2009 CR adherents attended a conference on aging that was held at Harvard Medical School. Wade notes that at least one researcher, Cynthia Kenyon of the University of California, San Francisco, was inspired to modify her diet based on her laboratory findings that food with a scant 2% sugar decreased the life span of laboratory roundworms. Kenyon said she started a low-carbohydrate diet in 2002 and that "I try to steer clear of desserts and starches, though I do eat chocolate."

Even though model organism and animal studies consistently demonstrate positive responses to CR, it is not yet known whether CR will extend the human life span. Daniel L. Smith Jr., Tim R. Nagy, and David B. Allison of the University of Alabama, Birmingham, observe in "Calorie Restriction: What Recent Results Suggest for the Future of Ageing Research" (*European Journal of Clinical Investigation*, vol. 40, no. 5, May 2010) that preliminary data from a seven-year study confirm many of the metabolic and physiologic responses that have been observed in animals. These responses include reductions in body weight, subcutaneous fat, visceral fat, lean muscle mass, insulin, energy expenditure, and core body temperature and improved lipid profiles. Smith, Nagy, and Allison opine that independent of whether CR confers longevity benefits, it is likely to play a role in disease prevention and healthy aging.

CHAPTER 10
PREVENTING OVERWEIGHT AND OBESITY

Americans will be more likely to change their behavior if they have a meaningful reward—something more than just reaching a certain weight or dress size. The real reward is invigorating, energizing, joyous health. It is a level of health that allows people to embrace each day and live their lives to the fullest without disease or disability.

—Regina Benjamin, U.S. Surgeon General, "HHS Secretary and Surgeon General Join First Lady to Announce Plans to Combat Overweight and Obesity and Support Healthy Choices" (January 28, 2010)

Many obesity researchers and health professionals believe the most effective way to win the war on obesity is to intensify efforts to prevent overweight and obesity among children, adolescents, and adults. They assert that over time prevention is far more cost effective than the expenditures that are associated with weight-loss efforts and medical treatment of obesity-related diseases. They also observe that prevention is a preferable strategy because there is no universally effective long-term treatment that consistently produces and maintains weight loss.

The landmark report *Surgeon General's Call to Action to Prevent and Decrease Overweight and Obesity, 2001* (2001, http://www.surgeongeneral.gov/topics/obesity/calltoaction/CalltoAction.pdf) calls for the design and implementation of interventions to prevent and decrease overweight and obesity, both individually and collectively. It asserts that effective actions must occur at many levels and acknowledges that—even though individual behavioral change is at the core of all strategies to reduce overweight and obesity—to be optimally effective, efforts must not be limited to individual behavioral change.

The report recommends actions to modify group influences by initiating prevention programs that target families, communities, employers and workers, the health care delivery system, and the media, as well as changes

in public policy. Furthermore, the report calls for concerted efforts and predicts that actions to prevent and reduce overweight and obesity will fail unless changes are made at every level of American society. Characterizing these problems as societal rather than as individual, the report observes that individual behavioral change is possible only in "a supportive environment with accessible and affordable healthy food choices and opportunities for regular physical activity." The report also warns that actions aimed exclusively at individual behavioral change that do not consider social, cultural, economic, and environmental influences will be counterproductive, serving only to reinforce negative stereotypes, bias, and stigmatization of people who are overweight or obese.

Many public health professionals believe environmental and policy interventions are the most promising strategies for generating and maintaining healthy nutrition and physical activity behaviors in Americans. Environmental interventions are those actions that modify availability of, access to, pricing of, or education about foods at the places where they are purchased. Policy interventions legislate, regulate, or, through formal or informal rules, serve to guide individual and collective behavior. Examples of environmental and policy initiatives that have met with success include:

- Increasing the availability of fruits and vegetables at school and workplace cafeterias and adding fresh fruit to refrigerated vending machines

- Replacing soft drinks in school vending machines with fruit juices and water

- Instituting daily physical education requirements for students

- Providing point-of-purchase nutrition information at restaurants and grocery stores to encourage healthy food choices

- Allowing workers adequate break time and a location where nursing mothers can express milk so their babies can continue to accrue the health benefits of breastfeeding even after their mother returns to work

In 2010 the U.S. surgeon general Regina Benjamin (1956–) announced plans to help Americans lead healthier lives through better nutrition and regular physical activity and issued the report *The Surgeon General's Vision for a Healthy and Fit Nation, 2010* (January 2010, http://www.surgeongeneral.gov/library/obesity vision/obesityvision2010.pdf). The report includes the following key actions:

- Encouraging Americans to reduce consumption of sodas and juices with added sugars; increase consumption of fruits, vegetables, whole grains, lean proteins, and water; choose low-fat or nonfat dairy products; limit television time to no more than two hours per day; and be more physically active

- Improving child care settings by increasing physical activity, limiting screen time, and practicing good nutrition and healthy sleep practices

- Emphasizing health in schools by teaching students how to develop lifelong healthy habits and offering appealing healthy food options, including fresh fruits and vegetables, whole grains, water, and low-fat or nonfat beverages; schools should require daily physical education—150 minutes per week for elementary students and 225 minutes per week for high school students

- Creating healthy work sites by offering healthy food choices in cafeterias, promoting physical activity through group classes, and incentivizing employees to participate

- Enhancing medical community involvement in promoting healthy lifestyles, explaining the connection between body mass index (BMI; body weight in kilograms divided by height in meters squared) and increased risk for disease, and, when appropriate, referring patients to resources that will help them meet their physical, nutritional, and psychological needs

- Increasing community efforts to improve access to outdoor recreational facilities, limit advertising of less healthful foods and beverages, build and support more walking and bicycle routes, and improve neighborhood safety to enable outdoor physical activity

PREVENTION EFFORTS TARGET FAMILIES, COMMUNITIES, WORK SITES, AND SCHOOLS

Public health education, communication, and other programs aimed at families and communities are identified as the cornerstone of prevention efforts. The *Surgeon General's Vision for a Healthy and Fit Nation* report puts forth communication strategies and corresponding actions to promote awareness about the effects of overweight on health and to support healthy eating and physical activity. For example, the goal of encouraging breastfeeding, which protects against the development of obesity, is translated into the action of creating work sites that "support employees who want to breastfeed by providing written policies and designated private, clean spaces for breastfeeding or expressing milk." (The Centers for Disease Control and Prevention [CDC] notes in *Does Breastfeeding Reduce the Risk of Pediatric Overweight?* [July 2007, http://www.cdc.gov/nccdphp/dnpa/nutrition/pdf/breastfeeding_r2p.pdf] that children who are breastfed for nine months are 30% less likely to become overweight.) Similarly, the goal of increasing opportunities for outdoor physical activity is translated into the recommendations that communities "improve access to outdoor recreational facilities; build or enhance infrastructures to support more walking and bicycling; support locating schools within easy walking distance of residential areas; [and] enhance personal and traffic safety in areas where people are or could be physically active."

In the community, schools offer ideal settings and multiple opportunities for preventing overweight and obesity by educating children about, and engaging them in, healthy eating and physical activity. To reinforce their messages concerning the importance of school physical activity and nutrition programs, schools can ensure that breakfast and lunch programs meet nutrition standards and provide food options that are low in fat, calories, and added sugars. Other ways to improve student health and nutrition include offering healthy snacks in vending machines and school stores and providing all students with quality daily physical education to cultivate the knowledge, attitudes, skills, behaviors, and confidence needed to be physically active for life.

One way to consider how Americans relate to food and physical activity and how to improve diet and activity levels is to use a social-ecological model that looks at the population demographics, environments, organizations, values, and culture that influence nutrition and physical-activity decisions. Public health officials use this model to show how all elements of society combine to shape an individual's food and physical activity choices, which in turn influence calorie balance and risk for overweight and obesity. Figure 10.1 displays the myriad influences on an individual's food and physical activity decisions.

Community Strategies to Prevent Obesity

In "Recommended Community Strategies and Measurements to Prevent Obesity in the United States"

FIGURE 10.1

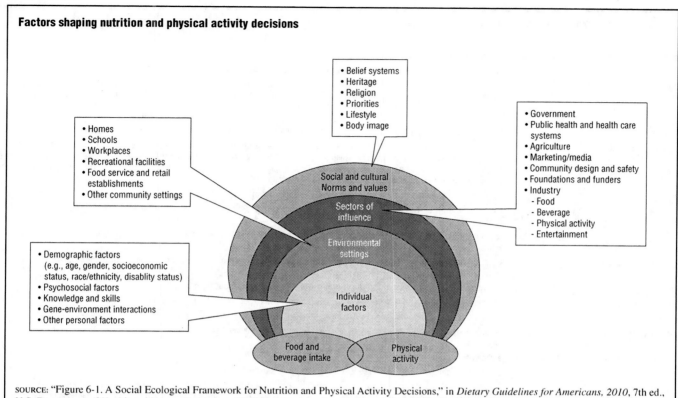

Factors shaping nutrition and physical activity decisions

- Belief systems
- Heritage
- Religion
- Priorities
- Lifestyle
- Body image

- Government
- Public health and health care systems
- Agriculture
- Marketing/media
- Community design and safety
- Foundations and funders
- Industry
  - Food
  - Beverage
  - Physical activity
  - Entertainment

- Homes
- Schools
- Workplaces
- Recreational facilities
- Food service and retail establishments
- Other community settings

Social and cultural Norms and values

Sectors of influence

Environmental settings

- Demographic factors (e.g., age, gender, socioeconomic status, race/ethnicity, disablity status)
- Psychosocial factors
- Knowledge and skills
- Gene-environment interactions
- Other personal factors

Individual factors

Food and beverage intake

Physical activity

SOURCE: "Figure 6-1. A Social Ecological Framework for Nutrition and Physical Activity Decisions," in *Dietary Guidelines for Americans, 2010*, 7th ed., U.S. Department of Health and Human Services and U.S. Department of Agriculture, December 2010, http://health.gov/dietaryguidelines/dga2010/dietaryguidelines2010.pdf (accessed October 21, 2011).

(*Morbidity and Mortality Weekly Report*, vol. 58, no. RR07, July 24, 2009), Laura Kettel Khan et al. of the CDC review studies of population-based interventions targeting communities and identify 24 environmental- and policy-level strategies that communities and local governments can use to plan and monitor changes to help prevent obesity.

Table 10.1 enumerates the 24 recommended strategies and the suggested measurements to monitor their effectiveness. The strategies fall into six broad categories and aim to:

1. Promote the availability of affordable healthy food and beverages

2. Support healthy food and beverage choices

3. Encourage breastfeeding

4. Encourage physical activity or limit sedentary activity among children and youth

5. Create safe communities that support physical activity

6. Encourage communities to organize for change

Federally Funded National Nutrition Education

Together, the U.S. Department of Agriculture (USDA) and the U.S. Department of Health and Human Services (HHS) update *Nutrition and Your Health: Dietary Guidelines for Americans* every five years. First published in 1980, the guidelines serve as the basis for federal food and nutrition education programs. Historically, some public health professionals believed that the USDA food pyramid was flawed because its composition was unduly influenced by pressure from the food industry, whose members knew that even subtle changes to the guidelines affected a food manufacturer's sales. Furthermore, these public health professionals asserted that the guidelines should not be expected to represent objective scientific evidence because they were developed by the U.S. government agency responsible for agriculture, rather than for health.

In December 2010 the seventh version of the dietary guidelines, *Dietary Guidelines for Americans, 2010* (http://health.gov/dietaryguidelines/dga2010/DietaryGuidelines2010.pdf), was released. According to the USDA and the HHS, in the press release "USDA and HHS Announce New Dietary Guidelines to Help Americans Make Healthier Food Choices and Confront Obesity Epidemic" (January 31, 2011, http://www.cnpp.usda.gov/Publications/DietaryGuidelines/2010/PolicyDoc/PressRelease.pdf), the new dietary guidelines emphasize reducing calorie consumption and increasing physical activity in an effort to prevent and reverse the nation's obesity epidemic. They urge Americans to consume

TABLE 10.1

Community strategies and measurements to prevent obesity

Strategies to promote the availability of affordable healthy food and beverages

Strategy 1	Communities should increase availability of healthier food and beverage choices in public service venues.
Suggested measurement	A policy exists to apply nutrition standards that are consistent with the dietary guidelines for Americans (US Department of Health and Human Services, US Department of Agriculture. Dietary guidelines for Americans. 6th ed. Washington, DC: U.S. Government Printing Office; 2005.) to all food sold (e.g., meal menus and vending machines) within local government facilities in a local jurisdiction or on public school campuses during the school day within the largest school district in a local jurisdiction.
Strategy 2	Communities should improve availability of affordable healthier food and beverage choices in public service venues.
Suggested measurement	A policy exists to affect the cost of healthier foods and beverages (as defined by the Institute of Medicine [IOM] [Institute of Medicine. Preventing childhood obesity: health in the balance. Washington, DC: The National Academies Press; 2005]) relative to the cost of less healthy foods and beverages sold within local government facilities in a local jurisdiction or on public school campuses during the school day within the largest school district in a local jurisdiction.
Strategy 3	Communities should improve geographic availability of supermarkets in underserved areas.
Suggested measurement	The number of full-service grocery stores and supermarkets per 10,000 residents located within the three largest underserved census tracts within a local jurisdiction.
Strategy 4	Communities should provide incentives to food retailers to locate in and/or offer healthier food and beverage choices in underserved areas.
Suggested measurement	Local government offers at least one incentive to new and/or existing food retailers to offer healthier food and beverage choices in underserved areas.
Strategy 5	Communities should improve availability of mechanisms for purchasing foods from farms.
Suggested measurement	The total annual number of farmer-days at farmers' markets per 10,000 residents within a local jurisdiction.
Strategy 6	Communities should provide incentives for the production, distribution, and procurement of foods from local farms.
Suggested measurement	Local government has a policy that encourages the production, distribution, or procurement of food from local farms in the local jurisdiction.

Strategies to support healthy food and beverage choices

Strategy 7	Communities should restrict availability of less healthy foods and beverages in public service venues.
Suggested measurement	A policy exists that prohibits the sale of less healthy foods and beverages (as defined by IOM [Institute of Medicine. Preventing childhood obesity: health in the balance. Washington, DC: The National Academies Press; 2005]) within local government facilities in a local jurisdiction or on public school campuses during the school day within the largest school district in a local jurisdiction.
Strategy 8	Communities should institute smaller portion size options in public service venues.
Suggested measurement	Local government has a policy to limit the portion size of any entree (including sandwiches and entree salads) by either reducing the standard portion size of entrees or offering smaller portion sizes in addition to standard portion sizes within local government facilities within a local jurisdiction.
Strategy 9	Communities should limit advertisements of less healthy foods and beverages.
Suggested measurement	A policy exists that limits advertising and promotion of less healthy foods and beverages within local government facilities in a local jurisdiction or on public school campuses during the school day within the largest school district in a local jurisdiction.
Strategy 10	Communities should discourage consumption of sugar-sweetened beverages.
Suggested measurement	Licensed child care facilities within the local jurisdiction are required to ban sugar-sweetened beverages, including flavored/sweetened milk and limit the portion size of 100% juice.

Strategy to encourage breastfeeding

Strategy 11	Communities should increase support for breastfeeding.
Suggested measurement	Local government has a policy requiring local government facilities to provide breastfeeding accommodations for employees that include both time and private space for breastfeeding during working hours.

Strategies to encourage physical activity or limit sedentary activity among children and youth

Strategy 12	Communities should require physical education in schools.
Suggested measurement	The largest school district located within the local jurisdiction has a policy that requires a minimum of 150 minutes per week of PE in public elementary schools and a minimum of 225 minutes per week of PE in public middle schools and high schools throughout the school year (as recommended by the National Association of Sports and Physical Education).
Strategy 13	Communities should increase the amount of physical activity in PE programs in schools.
Suggested measurement	The largest school district located within the local jurisdiction has a policy that requires K–12 students to be physically active for at least 50% of time spent in PE classes in public schools.
Strategy 14	Communities should increase opportunities for extracurricular physical activity.
Suggested measurement	The percentage of public schools within the largest school district in a local jurisdiction that allow the use of their athletic facilities by the public during non-school hours on a regular basis.
Strategy 15	Communities should reduce screen time in public service venues.
Suggested measurement	Licensed child care facilities within the local jurisdiction are required to limit screen viewing time to no more than 2 hours per day for children aged ≥2 years.

more vegetables, fruits, whole grains, fat-free and low-fat dairy products, and seafood, and to consume less sodium, saturated and trans fats, added sugars, and refined grains.

The 2010 dietary guidelines present 23 key recommendations for the general population and six additional recommendations for specific populations, such as pregnant women. The guidelines advise Americans to reduce:

TABLE 10.1

Community strategies and measurements to prevent obesity, 2009 [CONTINUED]

Strategies to create safe communities that support physical activity

Strategy 16	Communities should improve access to outdoor recreational facilities.
Suggested measurement	The percentage of residential parcels within a local jurisdiction that are located within a half-mile network distance of at least one outdoor public recreational facility.
Strategy 17	Communities should enhance infrastructure supporting bicycling.
Suggested measurement	Total miles of designated shared-use paths and bike lanes relative to the total street miles (excluding limited access highways) that are maintained by a local jurisdiction.
Strategy 18	Communities should enhance infrastructure supporting walking.
Suggested measurement	Total miles of paved sidewalks relative to the total street miles (excluding limited access highways) that are maintained by a local jurisdiction.
Strategy 19	Communities should support locating schools within easy walking distance of residential areas.
Suggested measurement	The largest school district in the local jurisdiction has a policy that supports locating new schools, and/or repairing or expanding existing schools, within easy walking or biking distance of residential areas.
Strategy 20	Communities should improve access to public transportation.
Suggested measurement	The percentage of residential and commercial parcels in a local jurisdiction that are located either within a quarter-mile network distance of at least one bus stop or within a half-mile network distance of at least one train stop (including commuter and passenger trains, light rail, subways, and street cars).
Strategy 21	Communities should zone for mixed use development.
Suggested measurement	Percentage of zoned land area (in acres) within a local jurisdiction that is zoned for mixed use that specifically combines residential land use with one or more commercial, institutional, or other public land uses.
Strategy 22	Communities should enhance personal safety in areas where persons are or could be physically active.
Suggested measurement	The number of vacant or abandoned buildings (residential and commercial) relative to the total number of buildings located within a local jurisdiction.
Strategy 23	Communities should enhance traffic safety in areas where persons are or could be physically active.
Suggested measurement	Local government has a policy for designing and operating streets with safe access for all users which includes at least one element suggested by the national complete streets coalition (http://www.completestreets.org)

Strategy to encourage communities to organize for change

Strategy 24	Communities should participate in community coalitions or partnerships to address obesity.
Suggested measurement	Local government is an active member of at least one coalition or partnership that aims to promote environmental and policy change to promote active living and/or healthy eating (excluding personal health programs such as health fairs).

SOURCE: Laura Kettel Khan et al., "Table. Summary of Recommended Community Strategies and Measurements to Prevent Obesity in the United States," in "Recommended Community Strategies and Measurements to Prevent Obesity in the United States," *MMWR Recommendations and Reports*, vol. 58, no. RR07, July 24, 2009, http://www.cdc.gov/mmwr/preview/mmwrhtml/rr5807a1.htm#box1 (accessed November 18, 2011)

- Consumption of sodium to less than 2,300 milligrams per day and cholesterol to less than 300 milligrams per day

- Saturated fats by replacing them with monounsaturated and polyunsaturated fats

- Consumption of trans fatty acids by sharply limiting the intake of partially hydrogenated oils and other solid fats (see Figure 10.2, which shows commonly used solid fats and oils and their composition in terms of saturated fat, monounsaturated fat, and polyunsaturated fat)

- Intake of refined grains and refined grain products with solid fats, added sugars, and sodium

- Alcohol consumption—one drink per day for women and two for men

The guidelines advise Americans to increase the consumption of:

- Nutrient-dense foods (e.g., fruits, lean meats and poultry, and eggs prepared without added solid fats, sugars, starches, and sodium) that provide the full range of essential nutrients and fiber, without excessive calories (see Figure 10.3, which compares the calorie content in some commonly consumed nutrient-dense foods with foods that are not nutrient dense)

- Vegetables (especially dark green, red, and orange vegetables), beans, peas, and fruits

- Whole grains and fat-free or low-fat dairy or fortified soy beverages

- Fish and other seafood

- A variety of foods high in protein, including eggs, beans, peas, soy products, and unsalted nuts and seeds

- Foods that are rich in potassium, dietary fiber, calcium, and vitamin D, including vegetables, fruits, whole grains, and dairy

The guidelines advise "appropriate calorie balance during each stage of life—childhood, adolescence, adulthood, pregnancy and breastfeeding, and older age." Women who may become pregnant are advised to choose foods that are rich in iron and folate and to take 400

FIGURE 10.2

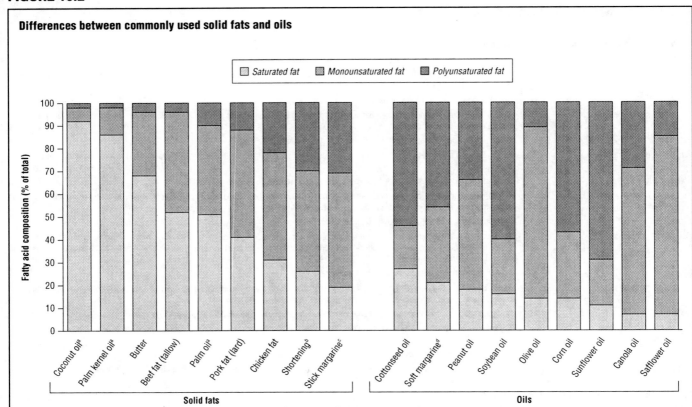

Differences between commonly used solid fats and oils

☐ Saturated fat   ▨ Monounsaturated fat   ▨ Polyunsaturated fat

[a]Coconut oil, palm kernel oil, and palm oil are called oils because they come from plants. However, they are semi-solid at room temperature due to their high content of short-chain saturated fatty acids. They are considered solid fats for nutritional purposes.
[b]Partially hydrogenated vegetable oil shortening, which contains transfats.
[c]Most stick margarines contain partially hydrogenated vegetable oil, a source of transfats.
[d]The primary ingredient in soft margarine with no transfats is liquid vegetable oil.

SOURCE: "Figure 3-3. Fatty Acid Profiles of Common Fats and Oils," in *Dietary Guidelines for Americans, 2010*, 7th ed., U.S. Department of Health and Human Services and U.S. Department of Agriculture, December 2010, http://health.gov/dietaryguidelines/dga2010/dietaryguidelines2010.pdf (accessed October 21, 2011)

micrograms of folic acid per day. Women who are pregnant are advised to take an iron supplement and those who are pregnant or breastfeeding are cautioned to limit their consumption of white tuna to just 6 ounces per week and to avoid eating tilefish, shark, swordfish, and mackerel, because these fish contain high mercury content. Adults aged 50 years and older are encouraged to choose foods that are fortified with vitamin B12, such as fortified cereals, or to take dietary supplements to ensure adequate B12 intake.

MyPlate Is Also for Children

In June 2011 MyPlate replaced MyPyramid for Kids, which, like the food pyramid for adults, provided guidance for children's diets. (See Figure 5.2 in Chapter 5.) The website ChooseMyPlate.gov replaces much of the information that was formerly available on MyPyramid.gov and, to engage children, includes a coloring sheet for children. It also has an interactive feature to help with meal planning. MyPlate is part of a larger communications initiative based on the 2010 dietary guidelines to help consumers of all ages make better food choices.

The dietary guidelines observe that healthy diets and adequate physical activity are vitally important for children in view of the fact that risk factors for adult chronic diseases are increasingly found in younger ages. The guidelines assert that "eating patterns established in childhood often track into later life, making early intervention on adopting healthy nutrition and physical activity behaviors a priority." The guidelines advise that young children consume between 1,000 and 2,000 calories per day and older children and adolescents between 1,400 and 3,200 calories per day. Table 10.2 shows the estimated calories needed of children, adolescents, and adults by sex and physical activity level. The proportion of recommended macronutrients (carbohydrate, fat, and protein) changes with advancing age. For example, children aged one to three years require less protein and more fat in their diet than do older children. (See Table 5.3 in Chapter 5.)

Children aged six years and older are encouraged to play hard and be more physically active to meet the government's recommended 60 minutes of exercise per day. Even though the guidelines do not offer specific

FIGURE 10.3

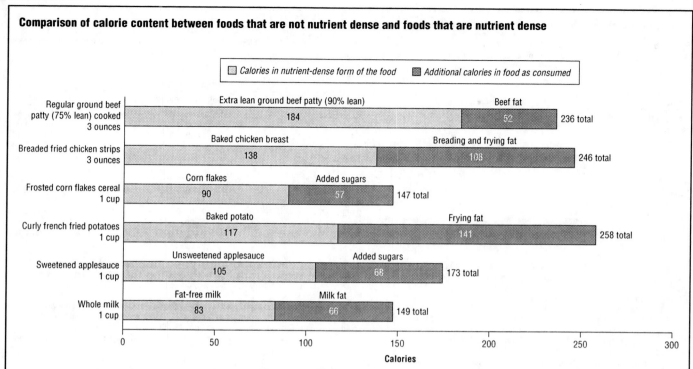

Comparison of calorie content between foods that are not nutrient dense and foods that are nutrient dense

☐ Calories in nutrient-dense form of the food   ▨ Additional calories in food as consumed

Regular ground beef patty (75% lean) cooked 3 ounces — Extra lean ground beef patty (90% lean) 184 | Beef fat 52 | 236 total

Breaded fried chicken strips 3 ounces — Baked chicken breast 138 | Breading and frying fat 108 | 246 total

Frosted corn flakes cereal 1 cup — Corn flakes 90 | Added sugars 57 | 147 total

Curly french fried potatoes 1 cup — Baked potato 117 | Frying fat 141 | 258 total

Sweetened applesauce 1 cup — Unsweetened applesauce 105 | Added sugars 68 | 173 total

Whole milk 1 cup — Fat-free milk 83 | Milk fat 66 | 149 total

Calories: 0 50 100 150 200 250 300

SOURCE: "Figure 5-2. Examples of the Calories in Food Choices That Are Not in Nutrient Dense Forms and the Calories in Nutrient Dense Forms of These Foods," in *Dietary Guidelines for Americans, 2010*, 7th ed., U.S. Department of Health and Human Services and U.S. Department of Agriculture, December 2010, http://health.gov/dietaryguidelines/dga2010/dietaryguidelines2010.pdf (accessed October 21, 2011)

recommendations about the duration of physical activity for children aged two to five years, they advise that young children should play actively several times each day. Because children and teens are often active in short bursts of time rather than for sustained periods of time, these short bursts accumulate to meet physical activity requirements.

Praise and Criticism for MyPlate

Like MyPyramid, MyPlate has garnered praise and criticism. In "Why It's Good That the Food Pyramid Became a Plate" (*Atlantic*, June 3, 2011), Marion Nestle of New York University praises the new icon, explaining that it is easy enough for a child to use. Nestle approves of the fact that vegetables are the largest sector on the plate, that vegetables and fruits together consume half the plate, and that dairy foods are off to the side so they may be considered discretionary. Nestle also likes the fact that unless one chooses a very large plate, there's no need to count servings or measure portion sizes. She has just one criticism of MyPlate: its categorization of protein as a food group. Nestle explains that "protein is a nutrient, not a food," and observes that "protein is not exactly lacking in American diets. The average American consumes twice the protein needed." Nestle is concerned that Americans may equate protein exclusively with meat rather than with a larger group of foods including beans,

nuts, poultry, fish, grains, and dairy (which have separate sectors on the plate) that are also sources of protein in American diets.

The Physicians Committee for Responsible Medicine (PCRM) concurs in "Breaking News! USDA Replaces Food Pyramid with MyPlate" (June 2011, http://www.pcrm.org/media/online/jun2011/breaking-news-usda-replaces-food-pyramid-with) with Nestle about the protein portion of the plate, observing that beans, whole grains, and vegetables contain protein. The PCRM objects to the inclusion of dairy, which is often a source of fat and cholesterol, and opines that there are more healthful sources of dietary calcium. The PCRM nutritionist Kathryn Strong asserts that "the USDA's new plate icon couldn't be more at odds with federal food subsidies. The plate icon advises Americans to limit high-fat products like meat and cheese, but the federal government is subsidizing these very products with billions of tax dollars and giving almost no support to fruits and vegetables." Nearly two-thirds (63%) of federal agricultural subsidies support meat and dairy production and less than 1% of subsidies support the cultivation of fruits and vegetables.

In "What's on Your Plate? MyPlate Replaces the Food Pyramid" (*Shape*, June 2011), Jennipher Walters laments that MyPlate fails to address Americans'

TABLE 10.2

Estimated calorie needs by age, sex, and physical activity

Estimated amounts of calories needed to maintain calorie balance for various gender and age groups at three different levels of physical activity. The estimates are rounded to the nearest 200 calories. An individual's calorie needs may be higher or lower than these average estimates.

Gender	Age (years)	Physical activity level[a]		
		Sedentary	Moderately active	Active
Child (female and male)	2–3	1,000–1,200[b]	1,000–1,400[b]	1,000–1,400[b]
Female[c]	4–8	1,200–1,400	1,400–1,600	1,400–1,800
	9–13	1,400–1,600	1,600–2,000	1,800–2,200
	14–18	1,800	2,000	2,400
	19–30	1,800–2,000	2,000–2,200	2,400
	31–50	1,800	2,000	2,200
	51+	1,600	1,800	2,000–2,200
Male	4–8	1,200–1,400	1,400–1,600	1,600–2,000
	9–13	1,600–2,000	1,800–2,200	2,000–2,600
	14–18	2,000–2,400	2,400–2,800	2,800–3,200
	19–30	2,400–2,600	2,600–2,800	3,000
	31–50	2,200–2,400	2,400–2,600	2,800–3,000
	51+	2,000–2,200	2,200–2,400	2,400–2,800

Notes: Based on Estimated Energy Requirements (EER) equations, using reference heights (average) and reference weights (healthy) for each age/gender group. For children and adolescents, reference height and weight vary. For adults, the reference man is 5 feet 10 inches tall and weighs 154 pounds. The reference woman is 5 feet 4 inches tall and weighs 126 pounds. EER equations are from the Institute of Medicine's *Dietary Reference Intakes for Energy, Carbohydrate, Fiber, Fat, Fatty Acids, Cholesterol, Protein, and Amino Acids.* Washington (DC): The National Academies Press; 2002.
[a]Sedentary means a lifestyle that includes only the light physical activity associated with typical day-to-day life. Moderately active means a lifestyle that includes physical activity equivalent to walking about 1.5 to 3 miles per day at 3 to 4 miles per hour, in addition to the light physical activity associated with typical day-to-day life. Active means a lifestyle that includes physical activity equivalent to walking more than 3 miles per day at 3 to 4 miles per hour, in addition to the light physical activity associated with typical day-to-day life.
[b]The calorie ranges shown are to accommodate needs of different ages within the group. For children and adolescents, more calories are needed at older ages. For adults, fewer calories are needed at older ages.
[c]Estimates for females do not include women who are pregnant or breastfeeding.

SOURCE: "Table 2-3. Estimated Calorie Needs per Day by Age, Gender, and Physical Activity Level," in *Dietary Guidelines for Americans, 2010*, 7th ed., U.S. Department of Health and Human Services and U.S. Department of Agriculture, December 2010, http://health.gov/dietaryguidelines/dga2010/dietaryguidelines2010.pdf (accessed October 21, 2011)

tendency to snack, does not suggest that fruits be eaten to increase fiber intake rather than consumed as juice, does not specify that grains should be whole grain, does not emphasize the importance of eating vegetables in a variety of colors, and does not indicate that protein may be derived from foods other than meat.

Walter Willett of the Harvard School of Public Health indicates in "The Nutrition Source: Out with the Pyramid, in with the Plate" (June 2011, http://www.hsph.harvard.edu/nutritionsource/what-should-you-eat/plate-replaces-pyramid/index.html) that the MyPlate icon is an improvement over previous nutrition icons and praises its effort to coax Americans to consume a diet that is more plant-based. Even though Willet believes the plate is better than the pyramid, he is also concerned about the information it lacks, asking, "What type of grain? What sources of proteins? What fats are used to prepare the vegetables and the grains?"

Fruits & Veggies: More Matters

Founded in 1991, the 5 a Day for Better Health Program was jointly sponsored by the National Cancer Institute and the Produce for Better Health Foundation, a nonprofit consumer-education foundation representing the fruit and vegetable industry. In 2005 the CDC became the lead authority for the program, and two years later the program was renamed the National Fruit and Vegetable Program. To reflect the changes and recommendations made in the new dietary guidelines that were released in 2010, the CDC revamped the program and gave it a new name: Fruits & Veggies: More Matters (http://www.fruitsandveggiesmatter.gov/).

The Fruits & Veggies: More Matters initiative (2012, http://www.fruitsandveggiesmatter.gov/health_professionals/about.html) aims to increase fruit and vegetable consumption. Its objectives are "increasing public awareness of the importance of eating a diet rich in fruits and vegetables every day for better health, providing consumers with specific information about how to include more servings of fruits and vegetables into their daily routines, and increasing the availability of fruits and vegetables at home, school, work, and other places where food is served." Studies indicate that the majority of American adults and adolescents are not eating the recommended two or more servings of fruit and three or more servings of vegetables per day. For example, in "Correlates of Fruit and Vegetable Intakes in US Children" (*Journal of the American Dietetic Association*, vol. 109, no. 3, March 2009), Barbara A. Lorson, Hugo R. Melgar-Quinonez, and Christopher A. Taylor find that fruit and vegetable consumption among children and teens varies by age, race, sex, ethnicity, and household income. The study of 6,513 children and adolescents aged two to 18 years finds that:

- Two- to five-year-olds consumed significantly more fruit and juice than six- to 11- and 12- to 18-year-olds.

- Total vegetable consumption was significantly higher among 12- to 18-year-olds than among younger children.

- A scant 8% of vegetables consumed by children of all groups were dark green or orange; fried potatoes accounted for nearly half (46%) of total vegetable consumption.

- Mexican-Americans consumed significantly more fruit than non-Hispanic white children and adolescents.

- African-American children and adolescents consumed significantly more dark-green vegetables and fewer deep-yellow vegetables than Mexican-American and non-Hispanic white children and adolescents.

- Children and teens who failed to meet the recommendations tended to be male, older, and living in households making between 130% and 350% of the federal poverty level.

- Male children and adolescents living in households below 350% of the poverty level were more likely to consume energy-dense fruits and vegetables, such as fruit juice and french fries, and were at greater risk for being overweight.

Along with reducing the risk for heart disease, high blood pressure, stroke, many cancers, and diabetes, diets rich in fruits and vegetables can help prevent overweight and obesity. Fruits and vegetables are naturally low in calories and fat, and their high water and fiber content produce feelings of satiety (the feeling of fullness or satisfaction after eating). Combined with an active lifestyle and a low-fat diet, eating greater amounts of fruits and vegetables and fewer high-calorie foods at meals can help control weight.

In "How Many Fruits & Vegetables Do You Need?" (2012, http://www.fruitsandveggiesmatter.gov/), the CDC offers information about the benefits of eating fruits and vegetables, recipes, interactive tools, and information about how to use fruits and vegetables to help consumers manage their weight. For example, Table 10.3 shows fruit and vegetable choices that total 100 calories or less. The CDC advocates in "How to Use Fruits and Vegetables to Help Manage Your Weight" (June 2009, http://www.cdc.gov/nccdphp/dnpa/nutrition/pdf/CDC_5-A-Day.pdf) lightening the calorie load of meals by substituting vegetables for some meat or cheese in meals and substituting a serving of fruits or vegetables for high-calorie snacks such as corn chips.

State and Community Funding for Prevention Efforts

The CDC Division of Nutrition, Physical Activity, and Obesity aims to help states prevent obesity and other

TABLE 10.3

Servings of fruit and vegetables with 100 calories or less

- a medium-size apple (72 calories)
- a medium-size banana (105 calories)
- 1 cup steamed green beans (44 calories)
- 1 cup blueberries (83 calories)
- 1 cup grapes (100 calories)
- 1 cup carrots (45 calories), broccoli (30 calories), or bell peppers (30 calories) with 2 tbsp. hummus (46 calories)

SOURCE: "About 100 Calories or Less," in *How to Use Fruits and Vegetables to Help Manage Your Weight*, Centers for Disease Control and Prevention, June 5, 2009, http://www.cdc.gov/nccdphp/dnpa/nutrition/pdf/CDC_5-A-Day.pdf (accessed November 19, 2011)

chronic diseases by focusing on poor nutrition and inadequate physical activity. The division assists states in developing and implementing nutrition and physical activity interventions, and sponsoring initiatives to help populations balance caloric intake and expenditure, increase physical activity, improve nutrition by increasing consumption of fruits and vegetables, reduce television time, and increase breastfeeding.

According to the HHS, in "American Recovery and Reinvestment Act Prevention and Wellness Initiative: Communities Putting Prevention to Work" (March 19, 2010, http://www.cdc.gov/chronicdisease/recovery/PDF/HHS_CPPW_CommunityFactSheet.pdf), 44 communities received funding for obesity prevention programs totaling $230 million in 2010. The dollar amount of the awards ranged from $16.1 million for the County of San Diego Health and Human Services Agency in California and $15.9 million each for the Cook County Department of Public Health/Public Health Institute of Metropolitan Chicago, Illinois, and the County of Los Angeles Department of Public Health in California, to $1 million for the Cherokee Nation Health Service Group in Oklahoma and $900,000 for the Pueblo of Jemez, New Mexico.

In "Communities Putting Prevention to Work" (November 29, 2011, http://www.cdc.gov/Communities PuttingPreventiontoWork/success_stories/index.htm), the CDC provides examples of obesity prevention community initiatives, such as San Diego, California, which used its funding to encourage farmers' markets to accept food stamps and the electronic benefits transfer card (a kind of debit card that is for food-stamp credits) to increase access to healthy, local produce.

IS NUTRITION EDUCATION WORKING TO IMPROVE AMERICANS' DIETS?

The Healthy Eating Index (HEI) is a measure developed in 1990 by the USDA to assess the overall health value of Americans' diets. It captures the type and quantity of foods people eat and the degree to which diets comply with specific recommendations in the USDA dietary guidelines. The HEI assigns points for eating consistently within USDA guidelines. It assesses 10 dietary components—grains, vegetables, fruits, milk, meat, total fat, total saturated fat, cholesterol, sodium, and a varied diet—on a scale of 0 to 10. Individuals who eat grains, vegetables, fruits, milk, meat (including chicken and fish), as well as a variety of foods at or above the USDA-recommended levels receive a maximum score of 10. A score of 0 is assigned when the recommended amount of those components is not eaten. For fat, saturated fat, cholesterol, and sodium, a score of 10 is awarded for eating the recommended amount or less. The highest possible score is 100; a score of 80 or above is considered a healthy diet, scores between 51 and 80 show a need for dietary improvement, and scores below 50 indicate poor diets.

Researchers use the HEI to evaluate Americans' diets. For example, Colin D. Rehm, Pablo Monsivais, and Adam Drewnowski of the University of Washington, Seattle, looked at the distribution of diet cost and diet quality and reported their findings in "The Quality and Monetary Value of Diets Consumed by Adults in the United States" (*American Journal of Clinical Nutrition*, vol. 94, no. 5, November 2011). The researchers find that higher diet costs are associated with higher HEI scores and that "higher diet cost was strongly associated with consuming more servings of fruit and vegetables and fewer calories from solid fat, alcoholic beverages, and added sugars."

The market research firm NPD Group reports in *26th Annual Eating Patterns in America* (2011, http://www.npdgroup.com/lps/epa/) that Americans have changed some, but not all, of their food purchasing and eating habits. Adults surveyed in 2011 said they were:

- Skipping fewer meals and eating dinner at least five times per week around the family table

- Drinking more bottled water and eating more pizza, fruit, salty snacks, and yogurt at home

- Purchasing more breakfast sandwiches, hot cereal, iced tea, and burritos from restaurants

- Taking more vitamins and supplements than ever before—54% reported daily dietary use of nutritional supplements

- Continuing to favor easy meal preparation methods and one-dish meals when eating at home

- Cooking on the stove top—90% of dinners were cooked on the stove top

- Less likely to use fresh products to prepare meals at home—60% reported cooking with fresh products in 2011, compared with 75% during the late 1980s

- Consuming less salt—the proportion of Americans consuming products labeled low or reduced salt/

sodium (34%) remained unchanged since 2007, but was lower than the 60% reported during the early 1990s

Even though restaurants saw some slight gains in 2010, the NPD Group reports that restaurant traffic stalled during the second quarter of 2011 in response to persistent "unemployment, rising gas and commodity prices and low consumer confidence." As a result, the number of restaurants in the United States declined. In total, U.S. restaurant unit counts declined by 9,450, or 2%. Of this total, 8,650 were independent restaurants as opposed to chain restaurants. Quick-service restaurants declined by 3,485 restaurants, or 1%.

Americans Skipping Breakfast

In the press release "31 Million U.S. Consumers Skip Breakfast Each Day, Reports NPD" (October 11, 2011, https://www.npd.com/wps/portal/npd/us/news/pressreleases/pr_111011b), the NPD Group indicates that one out of 10, or 31 million Americans, skipped breakfast in 2011. Twenty-eight percent of young men and 18% of young women skipped the morning meal, compared with 11% of men and 10% of women aged 55 years and older. The likelihood of children skipping breakfast increased with advancing age: 14% of teens aged 13 to 17 years did not eat breakfast. The most common reasons offered for skipping breakfast included "not feeling hungry/thirsty" and "didn't feel like eating or drinking." Other respondents, most often adult females, said they did not have time or were too busy, rushing, or running late to eat breakfast. Approximately one out of five adults consumed foods and beverages during the morning both at home and away from home on a typical day; and 14% of adults had breakfast outside the home.

Americans' Interest in Healthy Eating

The NPD Group reports in the press release "Portion Control of Growing Interest to U.S. Consumers, Reports NPD" (July 26, 2011, https://www.npd.com/press/releases/press_110726a.html) that of 30 healthy lifestyle strategies, Americans named regular exercise, well-balanced meals, eating all things in moderation, limiting or avoiding foods with saturated fat or cholesterol or trans fats, and drinking eight glasses of water per day as the top five ways to maintain a healthy lifestyle. Portion control, or eating smaller portions, ranked 11th in importance among people of all ages and seventh among those aged 21 to 34 years. Among people aged 46 to 54 years portion control dropped to 12th place. More women than men said portion control is important. Among restaurant goers interested in a healthful diet, portion control and smaller portions was named as the third most important characteristic. Among fast-food purchasers, it rose to second place.

Americans' Snack Food Choices

The NPD Group predicts in the press release "NPD Looks into the Future of Eating and Finds a Whole Lot of Snacking Going On" (August 31, 2009, http://www.npd.com/press/releases/press_090831.html) that snacking at home will outpace population growth during the second decade of the 21st century. Between 2008 and 2018 snacking at home is projected to increase by 19%. Snacking at home during the morning is projected to increase by 23%, afternoon snacking is expected to rise by 20%, and evening snacking is forecasted to increase by 15%. Besides predicting increasing reliance on convenience foods, the NPD Group believes that the use of frozen foods, canned ingredients, and completely home-cooked dinners will decline.

Snacking remains popular among U.S. consumers. In "Top 10 Food Trends" (*IFT*, vol. 65, no. 4, April 2011), A. Elizabeth Sloan reports that "among the 10 largest consumer packaged goods...food categories, chocolate candy, salty snacks, and bottled water made significant gains...in 2010." According to Sloan, baby boomers (people born between 1946 and 1964) want to snack on fruits and vegetables, nuts, cookies, crackers, chocolate candy, and diet soda. In contrast, generation Yers (people born between the mid-1970s and the early 1990s) prefer salty and savory snacks, sweet gourmet snacks, and ethnic and spicy foods. Abbie Westra reports in "Snackdown" (CSPnet.com, October 2011) that in 2011 the NPD Group found that afternoon snacking is growing, presumably because people are eating smaller lunches to save time and money and some substitute snacks for lunch in an effort to control portion size and calories consumed. The food choices for afternoon snacks have changed: 10% of afternoon snacks are burgers, 8% are french fries, and pizza and breaded chicken sandwiches account for 3% each.

Interventions to Promote Healthy Weight

In "Obesity Prevention and Control: Interventions in Community Settings" (January 26, 2011, http://www.thecommunityguide.org/obesity/communitysettings.html), the CDC's Community Preventive Services Task Force reviews the effectiveness of interventions that prevent obesity and promote healthy eating and physical activity. The task force considers the effectiveness of population-based interventions that promote healthy growth and development of children and adolescents and that support healthy weights among adults. It also focuses on school-based strategies, work-site programs, health care system interventions, and community-wide initiatives.

The task force recommends interventions that reduce the time children and teens spend watching television, playing video or computer games, and surfing the Internet. It endorses work-site programs that combine nutri-tion and physical activity as effective strategies to reduce and control overweight and obesity. It also indicates that more research is needed to determine the extent to which school-based programs help control overweight and obesity. Table 10.4 is an overview of the interventions and task force ratings.

PREVENTION PROGRAMS AT THE WORK SITE

Along with school-based nutrition programs and education initiatives aimed at the public at large, several notable obesity prevention efforts involve developing and implementing strategies to integrate physical activity and healthy food choices into routine work-site activities. Examples of such activities include incorporating planned activity breaks with music into long meetings; offering healthy food choices during meetings and breaks and in employee cafeterias: and hosting walking meetings.

Because more than 100 million Americans (over one out of every three people in the United States, as of the end of 2011) spend a large number of their waking hours at work, the work site presents another opportunity for prevention programs. In "Obesity Prevention and Control: Interventions in Community Settings," the Community Preventive Services Task Force advises moving beyond traditional workplace health education programs. It recommends more intensive and comprehensive efforts such as modifying physical and social environments, instituting policies consistent with the objective of preventing overweight and obesity, and extending work-site prevention efforts not only to employees but also to the families of employees and their communities.

Examples of work-site obesity prevention and weight-control strategies include:

- Educating workers using lectures, written materials provided in print or online, and educational software

- Ensuring that healthy food options are available in cafeterias and vending machines

- Establishing work-site exercise facilities or creating incentives for employees to join local fitness centers

- Developing incentives, rewards, and reinforcements for workers to achieve and maintain a healthy body weight

- Encouraging employers to require weight management and physical activity counseling as covered benefits in health insurance contracts

- Providing individual or group behavioral counseling

Research suggests that obesity may begin at the office. W. Kerry Mummery et al. examine in the landmark study "Occupational Sitting Time and Overweight and Obesity in Australian Workers" (*American Journal of Preventive Medicine*, vol. 29, no. 2, August 2005) the

TABLE 10.4

Obesity prevention interventions and task force ratings, 2011

	Ratings
Interventions to reduce screen time (e.g., time in front of a TV, computer monitor)	
Behavioral interventions to reduce screen time	Recommended
These interventions may include:	
• Skills building, tips, goal setting, and reinforcement techniques	
• Parent or family support through provision of information on environmental strategies to reduce access to television, video games, and computers	
• A "TV turnoff challenge" in which participants are encouraged not to watch TV for a specified number of days	
Mass media interventions to reduce screen time	Insufficient evidence
In these campaigns, one or more components is designed to:	
• Increase knowledge about screen time	
• Influence attitudes	
• Change behavior by transmitting messages through newspapers, radio, television, and billboards	
Technology-supported interventions (e.g., computer or web applications)	
Technology-supported components may include use of the following:	
• Computers (e.g., internet, CD-ROM, e-mail, kiosk, computer program)	
• Video conferencing	
• Personal digital assistants	
• Pagers	
• Pedometers with computer interaction	
• Computerized telephone system interventions that target physical activity, nutrition, or weight.	
Non-technological components may include use of the following:	
• In-person counseling	
• Manual tracking	
• Printed lessons	
• Written feedback	
Multicomponent coaching or counseling interventions:	
• To reduce weight	Recommended
• To maintain weight loss	Recommended
Interventions in specific settings	
Worksite programs	Recommended
• Informational and educational strategies aim to increase knowledge about a healthy diet and physical activity. Examples include:	
Lectures	
Written materials (provided in print or online)	
Educational software	
• Behavioral and social strategies target the thoughts (e.g. awareness, self-efficacy) and social factors that effect behavior changes. Examples include:	
Individual or group behavioral counseling	
Skill-building activities such as cue control	
Rewards or reinforcement	
Inclusion of co-workers or family members to build support systems	
• Policy and environmental approaches aim to make healthy choices easier and target the entire workforce by changing physical or organizational structures. Examples of this include:	
Improving access to healthy foods (e.g. changing cafeteria options, vending machine content)	
Providing more opportunities to be physically active (e.g. providing on-site facilities for exercise)	
• Policy strategies may also change rules and procedures for employees such as health insurance benefits or costs or money for health club membership.	
• Worksite weight control strategies may occur separately or as part of a comprehensive worksite wellness program that addresses several health issues (e.g., smoking cessation, stress management, cholesterol reduction).	
School-based programs	Insufficient evidence
These interventions are conducted in the classroom and may seek to increase physical activity and/or improve nutrition, both in school and at home. Classroom and physical education teachers may receive special training to carry out the programs.	

SOURCE: Adapted from "Summary of Task Force Recommendations," in *The Guide to Community Preventive Services: Obesity Prevention and Control: Interventions in Community Settings*, Centers for Disease Control and Prevention, Office of Surveillance, Epidemiology, and Laboratory Services (OSELS), January 26, 2011, www.thecommunityguide.org/obesity/communitysettings.html (accessed November 19, 2011)

role of the workplace in the problem of overweight and obesity by studying the association between occupational sitting time and overweight and obesity in a sample of adults employed full time. The researchers find that the more time workers sat at their desk, the more likely they were to be overweight. Higher total daily sitting time was associated with a 68% increased risk of being overweight or obese.

Overall, men sat an average of 209 minutes while at work, 20 minutes more than the average for women. Mummery et al. suggest that the extra 20 minutes might make a difference because they find a significant association between sitting time and overweight and obesity in male workers, but not in female workers.

Mummery et al. assert that encouraging workers to exercise may favorably influence a company's bottom line. They conclude, "Time and productivity lost due to chronic diseases associated with overweight and obesity may make it financially worthwhile for employers to be more proactive in the health of their employees by promoting physical activity at work."

In "Poverty and Obesity in the U.S." (*Diabetes*, vol. 60, no. 11, November 2011), James A. Levine of the

Mayo Clinic in Rochester, Minnesota, observes that there is evidence of a link between a sedentary lifestyle, obesity, diabetes, other metabolic diseases, and premature death. People who are sedentary, like many office workers, move an average of two hours less per day than active people and as a result expend less energy, increasing their risk for obesity, chronic metabolic disease, and cardiovascular death. Levine notes that "more than half of county-to-county variance in obesity can be accounted for by variance in sedentariness."

Offices of the Future May Improve, Rather Than Imperil, Health and Fitness

Steve Karnowski notes in "Researcher Sees Future Where People Walk at Work" (Associated Press, June 7, 2005) that Levine, who studies nonexercise activity thermogenesis (NEAT; the calories people burn during everyday activities such as standing, walking, or even fidgeting), redesigned his office in 2005 to encourage physical activity to burn calories. Levine explains that because it is metabolically more effective and probably easier for most people to put more NEAT into their lives to achieve and maintain a healthy body weight than to seek organized exercise, the physically active office would be a natural outgrowth of NEAT research.

Levine's office of the future holds meetings while walking laps on a track rather than sitting around a conference table eating donuts. Workers at computers walk on a treadmill rather than sit, and presentations are made standing at magnetic marker boards rather than sitting at desks or conference tables.

Levine's retrofitted office even appeals to his colleagues who already exercise regularly because they assert that standing and moving keeps them alert and focused throughout the day. Levine admits that there is pressure in his office to work while standing and to keep moving throughout the day, but he contends that this positive peer pressure is preferable to the pressure to bring unhealthy snack foods to the work site.

James A. Levine and Selene Yeager explain in *Move a Little, Lose a Lot: New NEAT Science Reveals How to Be Thinner, Happier, and Smarter* (2009) that Americans' reliance on electronics and especially the Internet has deprived them of the opportunity to be physically active and burn calories. They assert that changing office workers' routines to include more standing, turning, and bending throughout the course of the workday can burn 2,100 calories per week, boost metabolism, reduce blood pressure, and increase mental clarity.

In "Effects of a Worksite Physical Activity Intervention for Hospital Nurses Who Are Working Mothers" (*AAOHN Journal*, vol. 59, no. 9, September 2011), Sharon J. Tucker et al. report the results of a study that tested an innovative 10-week work-site physical activity intervention that was incorporated into the work flow of hospital-based nurses. The intervention involved redesigning and changing the physical environment and providing social reinforcements and strategies for engaging in physical activities while at work and away from work. The nurses were given an intervention toolkit that contained a water bottle, tote bag, research-grade pedometer, resistance band, relaxation ball, relaxation CD, exercise DVD, nutrition and physical activity tips brochure, nutritious snack, walking meeting tag, and wellness journal. After a 30- to 60-minute introductory session, the nurses were asked to increase their overall physical activity for 10 weeks by one hour each workday, 30 minutes of which were to be through walking. The study met its objective: increasing overall daily hours of physical activity by one hour per day over the study period. Tucker et al. conclude that "it is feasible to target the worksite of hospital-based registered nurses to improve body composition and physical activity."

INTENSIFYING THE PREVENTION AGENDA IN THE HEALTH CARE SYSTEM

Interactions with health care professionals are important opportunities to deliver powerful prevention messages. Physicians' and other health professionals' prescriptions and recurring advice to maintain a healthy weight to prevent disease or reduce symptoms of existing disease are often powerful inducements for behavioral change. Most Americans have at least annual contact with a health care professional, and if this contact includes information about the importance of weight management, then it may reinforce prevention messages received in other settings such as schools and work sites. Furthermore, health care professionals are instrumental in shaping public policy and can leverage their expertise and credibility to present accurate messages in the media and catalyze sweeping changes in the community at large.

Examples of strategies to expand on prevention efforts in the health care delivery system include:

- Training health care providers and health profession students to use effective techniques to prevent and treat overweight and obesity

- Cultivating partnerships between health care providers, schools, faith-based groups, and other community organizations to target social and environmental causes of overweight and obesity

- Classifying obesity as a disease to enable reimbursement for prevention efforts

- Partially or fully covering weight-management services including nutrition education and physical activity programs as health plan benefits

The Patient Protection and Affordable Care Act (PPACA), a 10-year, $1.1 trillion bill to provide near-universal health care coverage, was signed into law in March 2010. The bill effectively eliminates insurers' ability to deny or cancel coverage because of preexisting medical conditions. It also emphasizes community prevention as an important strategy for improving the nation's health and curbing the huge costs that are associated with untreated chronic disease.

In "Promoting Prevention through the Affordable Care Act" (*New England Journal of Medicine*, vol. 363, no. 14, September 30, 2010), Howard Koh (1952–), the assistant secretary for health, and Kathleen Sebelius (1948–), the secretary of the HHS, opine that the PPACA will "reinvigorate public health on behalf of individuals, worksites, communities, and the nation at large—and will usher in a revitalized era for prevention at every level of society." The act requires health plans to offer obesity screening and counseling for adults and children, appropriates funds for fiscal years 2010 through 2014 for demonstration projects to develop model programs for reducing childhood obesity, and requires the disclosure of specified nutrient information for food sold in many chain restaurants and vending machines.

USING THE MEDIA TO COMMUNICATE THE PREVENTION MESSAGE

The media play a pivotal role in prevention efforts. The media can communicate and educate the public about healthy behaviors and health risks that are associated with overweight and obesity, introduce and reinforce prevention messages from health care professionals, and assist to alter attitudes and perceptions by celebrating healthy eating and physical activity.

The International Food Information Council (IFIC) has tracked media coverage of diet, nutrition, and food safety since 1995. In its first report, *Food for Thought* (1995), the IFIC noted that the leading nutrition and food issues receiving newspaper, television, and other media coverage during the previous 12 months were reducing fat intake; the impact of diet on disease risks; and discussions of foodborne illnesses, vitamin and mineral intake, disease causation, caloric intake, antioxidants, cholesterol intake, sugar intake, and fiber intake. As obesity became a more prominent issue during the late 1990s, the IFIC reports in "Executive Summary" (*Food for Thought VI* [December 2005, http://www.foodinsight .org/Content/3651/ExecSummaryFFTVI.pdf]) that the number of stories about diet, weight loss, nutrition, and obesity increased from 1,270 in 1995 to 2,412 in 2005. This increase reflected both a rising volume of coverage and an escalation in the number of media outlets reporting about diet, overweight, and obesity. In *Food for Thought VI*, the IFIC reports that obesity was the leading topic in food and nutrition media stories during 2004, followed by disease prevention, physical activity, weight

management, disease causation, vitamin and mineral intake, fat intake, functional foods, mad cow disease, calorie intake, and biotechnology.

Six years later, the IFIC published *2011 Food and Health Survey* (May 5, 2011, http://www.foodinsight.org/Content/3840/2011%20IFIC%20FDTN%20Food%20and%20Health%20Survey.pdf), which looks at trends in consumer attitudes toward food safety, nutrition, and health. The IFIC notes that even though more than two-thirds (68%) of Americans look to the media for information about food and nutrition, just 4% cite the popular media as a motivator to take action to manage their weight.

The media have responded with advertising and public service campaigns intended to heighten awareness of the risks that are associated with obesity and help Americans make healthier choices. However, by early 2012 it was not yet known if these antiobesity advertising campaigns were effective. For example, in "Georgia's Campaign to Address Childhood Obesity: The Controversy Continues" (*Sizable Issues*, January 4, 2012), Rebecca M. Puhl of Yale University comments on an antiobesity campaign that was launched in Georgia in 2011. The campaign features overweight children who describe their experiences of overeating or being bullied and advertises these children in web clips and on billboards. The striking black-and-white ads feature the slogans "Stocky, Chubby, and Chunky Are Still Fat" and "Big Bones Didn't Make Me This Way, Big Meals Did." Puhl observes that even though the campaign is intended to shock Georgia residents and issue a "wake up call" about the problem of childhood obesity, the campaign "stigmatizes and shames children and their families." Puhl characterizes the campaign as misguided and opines that it "has the potential to harm those most in need of help. The messages are not constructive, they are unlikely to be effective, and they offer no support or solutions for families struggling with obesity."

TARGETING CHILDHOOD OBESITY

I applaud the Alliance for a Healthier Generation for their advocacy on behalf of our kids and their efforts to make healthier school meals more affordable and accessible. Everyone has a role to play to help address the epidemic of childhood obesity—from the companies that supply our food to the parents who deserve to know what their kids are being served at school.

—First Lady Michelle Obama (January 21, 2011)

In 2005 the American Heart Association and the William J. Clinton Foundation launched a new initiative, the Alliance for a Healthier Generation (2011, http://www.healthiergeneration.org/about.aspx), to combat childhood obesity. The alliance's mission is to "reduce the nationwide prevalence of childhood obesity by 2015 and to empower kids nationwide to make healthy lifestyle choices." Working with companies that influence children's lives—food, beverage, fitness, gaming, and technology—the alliance seeks to improve children's health and nutrition at home, in school, in physicians' offices, and in the community at large.

The alliance's Healthy Schools Program supports administrators, teachers, parents, and students to institute policies and programs that enable students to eat better and move more. It involves insurers, employers, and health care provider associations to encourage reimbursement to physicians and registered dietitians for obesity prevention-related services. The alliance has helped forge voluntary agreements with the beverage, snack food, and dairy industries to significantly reduce the amount of high-calorie foods that are available to students in schools. It also champions the empowerME campaign (http://www.healthiergeneration.org/teens.aspx?id=3377) to inspire and motivate children "to eat healthier and move more."

CHAPTER 11
PUBLIC OPINION AND ACTION ABOUT DIET, WEIGHT, NUTRITION, AND PHYSICAL ACTIVITY

Overweight and obesity are among the most urgent health challenges facing our country today. Excess weight contributes to many of the leading causes of death in the United States, including heart disease, stroke, diabetes, and some types of cancer. More than a third of adults in the U.S.—over 72 million people—and 17% of children in the U.S. are obese.

—Thomas R. Frieden, Director of the Centers for Disease Control and Prevention (January 14, 2011)

Americans are growing heavier each year. Elizabeth Mendes of the Gallup Organization notes in *In U.S., Self-Reported Weight up Nearly 20 Pounds since 1990* (November 23, 2011, http://www.gallup.com/poll/150947/Self-Reported-Weight-Nearly-Pounds-1990.aspx) that a November 2011 Gallup poll finds American men and women the heaviest since the Gallup Organization began measuring body weight. The poll indicates that men's and women's self-reported weight had increased by about 20 pounds (9.1 kg) between 1990 and 2011. Interestingly, as their self-reported weight has increased, men and women have increased the weight they deem "ideal." In 2011 American men said they weigh on average 196 pounds (88.9 kg), about 15 pounds (6.8 kg) more than the 181 pounds (82.1 kg) they consider an ideal weight. Figure 11.1 shows American men's increasing self-reported weight, which along with their ideal weight has increased over the past two decades. In 1990 men weighed about 9 pounds (4.1 kg) more than their ideal weight, by 2011 men were an average of 15 pounds heavier than their ideal weight.

Women's weight also increased from an average of 142 pounds (64.4 kg) in 1990 to 160 pounds (72.6 kg) in 2011. (See Figure 11.2.) Their ideal average weight rose from 129 pounds (58.5 kg) to 138 pounds (62.6 kg). On average, American women are about 22 pounds (10 kg) heavier than their ideal weight, compared with 13 pounds (5.9 kg) heavier in 1990.

Based on Americans' self-reported and ideal weights in 2011, 67% of men and women were heavier than their ideal weight—up 5% from one year earlier. (See Table 11.1.) More than two-thirds of men (64%) and women (68%) were above their ideal weight. Despite the gap between their ideal and actual weight, when asked if they were overweight, just 39% of adults said they are somewhat or very overweight—more women (42%) than men (35%) described themselves as overweight. (See Table 11.2.) More than half (56%) of Americans considered themselves "about right"—60% of men and 52% of women. Interestingly, in 2011 more Americans saw themselves as "about right" in terms of weight than they did in 1991 and fewer viewed themselves as overweight. (See Figure 11.3.) Mendes observes that "the percentage of Americans who describe themselves as overweight has remained essentially unchanged over the past 20 years. While Americans are getting heavier, many may not recognize it or acknowledge it."

Even though the majority of Americans are overweight or obese, during the third quarter of 2011 the percentage of overweight and obese declined slightly and the percentage of people of normal weight increased. In *More Americans Now Normal Weight Than Overweight* (October 7, 2011, http://www.gallup.com/poll/149975/Americans-Normal-Weight-Overweight.aspx), Mendes points out that "for the first time in more than three years, more Americans are a normal weight (36.6%) than are overweight (35.8%)." (See Figure 11.4.) It is too early to tell whether this decline will continue, but it is a promising sign and a sharp contrast to previous years, during which rates of overweight and obesity increased.

According to Mendes, even though obesity rates slightly declined across all demographic groups, African-Americans, people aged 45 to 64 years, and those with low incomes were the most likely to be obese. (See Table 11.3.) Mendes posits that economic constraints may be a factor in the modest declines observed—people may be eating out less and choosing healthier foods to prepare at home. It is

FIGURE 11.1

Male poll respondents' average self-reported and ideal weight, 1991–2011

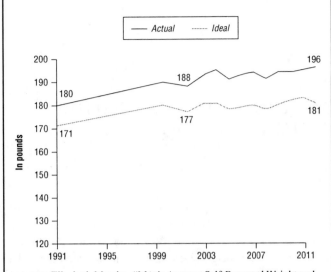

SOURCE: Elizabeth Mendes, "Men's Average Self-Reported Weight and Average Ideal Weight," in *In U.S., Self-Reported Weight up Nearly 20 Pounds since 1990*, The Gallup Organization, November 23, 2011, http://www.gallup.com/poll/150947/Self-Reported-Weight-Nearly-Pounds-1990.aspx (accessed November 28, 2011). Copyright © 2011 by The Gallup Organization. Reproduced by permission of The Gallup Organization.

FIGURE 11.2

Female poll respondents' average self-reported and ideal weight, 1991–2011

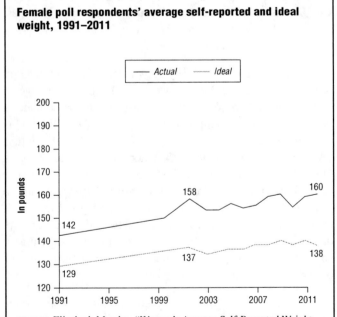

SOURCE: Elizabeth Mendes, "Women's Average Self-Reported Weight and Average Ideal Weight," in *In U.S., Self-Reported Weight up Nearly 20 Pounds since 1990*, The Gallup Organization, November 23, 2011, http://www.gallup.com/poll/150947/Self-Reported-Weight-Nearly-Pounds-1990.aspx (accessed November 28, 2011). Copyright © 2011 by The Gallup Organization. Reproduced by permission of The Gallup Organization.

TABLE 11.1

Poll respondents who are below, at, or above their ideal weight, November 2011

Based on Americans' average ideal weight minus their average self-reported actual weight

	Under ideal weight	At ideal weight	Over ideal weight
National adults	9%	18%	67%
Men	12%	20%	64%
Women	5%	17%	68%

SOURCE: Elizabeth Mendes, "Percentage of Americans Who Are under, at, and over Their Ideal Weight," in *In U.S., Self-Reported Weight up Nearly 20 Pounds since 1990* The Gallup Organization, November 23, 2011, http://www.gallup.com/poll/150947/Self-Reported-Weight-Nearly-Pounds-1990.aspx (accessed November 28, 2011). Copyright © 2011 by The Gallup Organization. Reproduced by permission of The Gallup Organization.

TABLE 11.2

Poll respondents who say they are overweight, about right, or underweight, November 2011

HOW WOULD YOU DESCRIBE YOUR OWN PERSONAL WEIGHT SITUATION RIGHT NOW?

	Very/somewhat overweight	About right	Very/somewhat underweight
National adults	39%	56%	5%
Men	35%	60%	5%
Women	42%	52%	5%

SOURCE: Elizabeth Mendes, "How Would You Describe Your Own Personal Weight Situation Right Now?" in *In U.S., Self-Reported Weight up Nearly 20 Pounds since 1990*, The Gallup Organization, November 23, 2011, http://www.gallup.com/poll/150947/Self-Reported-Weight-Nearly-Pounds-1990.aspx (accessed November 28, 2011). Copyright © 2011 by The Gallup Organization. Reproduced by permission of The Gallup Organization.

also possible that some of the nutrition education and health promotion initiatives instituted in recent years, such as First Lady Michelle Obama's (1964–) Let's Move! campaign, have contributed to the decline in obesity.

AMERICANS' DIETS HAVE NOT IMPROVED

There is considerable room for improvement in Americans' eating habits. The Gallup-Healthways Well-Being Index, which tracks health behaviors, finds that fewer Americans consumed a healthy diet in 2011 than they did in 2010. Specifically, fruit and vegetable consumption declined by about 2%, with the biggest decreases among women, young adults, older adults, and Hispanics. Dan Witter of the Gallup Organization speculates in *Americans' Eating Habits Worse This Year Compared with Last* (June 9, 2011, http://www.gallup.com/poll/147989/Americans-Eating-Habits-Worse-Year-Compared-Last.aspx) that higher gas prices may have prompted many Americans to forgo fresh produce in favor of less expensive food choices.

FIGURE 11.3

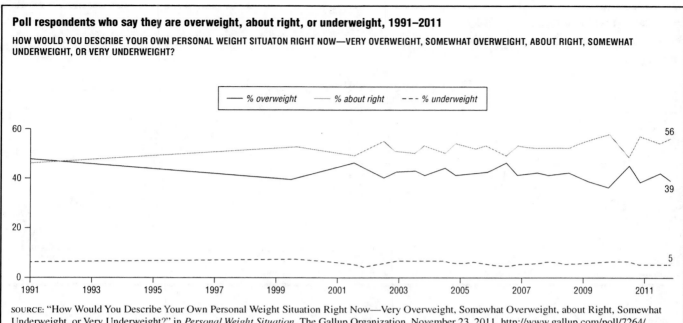

Poll respondents who say they are overweight, about right, or underweight, 1991–2011

HOW WOULD YOU DESCRIBE YOUR OWN PERSONAL WEIGHT SITUATON RIGHT NOW—VERY OVERWEIGHT, SOMEWHAT OVERWEIGHT, ABOUT RIGHT, SOMEWHAT UNDERWEIGHT, OR VERY UNDERWEIGHT?

SOURCE: "How Would You Describe Your Own Personal Weight Situation Right Now—Very Overweight, Somewhat Overweight, about Right, Somewhat Underweight, or Very Underweight?" in *Personal Weight Situation*, The Gallup Organization, November 23, 2011, http://www.gallup.com/poll/7264/Personal-Weight-Situation.aspx (accessed November 28, 2011). Copyright © 2011 by The Gallup Organization. Reproduced by permission of The Gallup Organization.

FIGURE 11.4

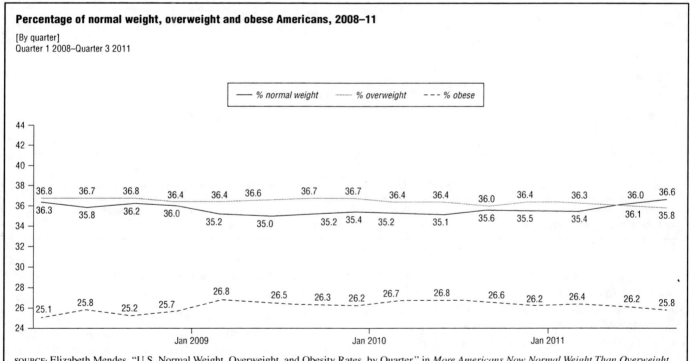

Percentage of normal weight, overweight and obese Americans, 2008–11

[By quarter]
Quarter 1 2008–Quarter 3 2011

SOURCE: Elizabeth Mendes, "U.S. Normal Weight, Overweight, and Obesity Rates, by Quarter," in *More Americans Now Normal Weight Than Overweight*, The Gallup Organization, October 7, 2011, http://www.gallup.com/poll/149975/Americans-Normal-Weight-Overweight.aspx (accessed November 28, 2011). Copyright © 2011 by The Gallup Organization. Reproduced by permission of The Gallup Organization.

Furthermore, in late 2011 the percentage of Americans who said they had enough money to purchase food for themselves and their family declined, approaching the record low that was reported in 2008 during the economic recession (which lasted from late 2007 to mid-2009). In *Americans' Ability to Afford Food Nears Three-Year Low* (November 10,

TABLE 11.3

Percentage obese by demographics, 2008–11

[Sorted by most to least obese in 2011. Among adults aged 18 and older.]

	2008	2009	2010	2011 Jan–Sep	Change, 2011 vs. 2010
Blacks	35.1	36.2	36.0	35.4	−0.6
Aged 45–64	29.5	30.6	30.9	30.7	−0.2
Annual income less than $36,000	30.0	30.9	31.1	30.3	−0.8
Aged 30–44	27.0	27.7	28.1	27.9	−0.2
Men	27.0	27.8	28.1	27.7	−0.4
Hispanics	27.4	28.3	28.2	27.4	−0.8
Annual income $36,0 00–$89,999	25.8	26.9	26.8	25.8	−1.0
Whites	24.2	25.2	25.4	24.8	−0.6
Aged 65+	23.4	24.2	24.6	24.6	0.0
Women	23.9	25.2	25.1	24.6	−0.5
Annual income $90,000+	21.1	21.4	21.6	21.0	−0.6
Aged 18–29	17.4	18.3	18.0	17.5	−0.5
Asians	8.6	9.6	8.2	11.5	+3.3

SOURCE: Elizabeth Mendes, "Percentage Obese in U.S. among Various Demographic Groups," in *More Americans Now Normal Weight Than Overweight*, The Gallup Organization, October 7, 2011, http://www.gallup.com/poll/149975/Americans-Normal-Weight-Overweight.aspx (accessed November 28, 2011). Copyright © 2011 by The Gallup Organization. Reproduced by permission of The Gallup Organization.

FIGURE 11.5

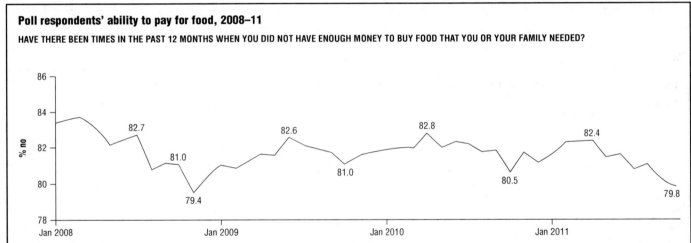

Poll respondents' ability to pay for food, 2008–11

HAVE THERE BEEN TIMES IN THE PAST 12 MONTHS WHEN YOU DID NOT HAVE ENOUGH MONEY TO BUY FOOD THAT YOU OR YOUR FAMILY NEEDED?

SOURCE: Lymari Morales, "Have There Been Times in the Past 12 Months When You Did Not Have Enough Money to Buy Food That You or Your Family Needed?" in *Americans' Ability to Afford Food Nears Three-Year Low*, The Gallup Organization, November 10, 2011, http://www.gallup.com/poll/150689/Americans-Ability-Afford-Food-Nears-Three-Year-Low.aspx (accessed November 28, 2011). Copyright © 2011 by The Gallup Organization. Reproduced by permission of The Gallup Organization.

2011, http://www.gallup.com/poll/150689/Americans-Ability-Afford-Food-Nears-Three-Year-Low.aspx), Lymari Morales of the Gallup Organization reports that during the third quarter of 2011, 20.2% of those surveyed said they did not have sufficient money for food. (See Figure 11.5.)

HOW AMERICANS ATTEMPT TO LOSE WEIGHT

A November 2011 Gallup poll asked Americans who claim to have successfully lost weight which strategies they used. The most popular responses were exercise (31%) and simply eating less (23%). (See Table 11.4.) Twelve percent said they had counted calories and/or used portion control and 10% said they "ate more natural foods" to achieve weight loss.

The poll also indicates that even though two-thirds of Americans described themselves as being heavier than their ideal weight, only 29% were actively trying to lose weight in 2011. (See Figure 11.6.) This percentage has remained relatively constant since 2004.

The Gallup Organization also confirms the finding that the majority of Americans have made at least one serious attempt to lose weight at some point during their life: one-quarter report one or two attempts, 30% have tried between three and 10 times, and 8% have made

TABLE 11.4

Strategies used by poll respondents who succeeded in losing weight, 2011

MOST EFFECTIVE STRATEGIES OR METHODS OF LOSING WEIGHT NAMES BY AMERICANS WHO HAVE EVER SUCCEEDED IN LOSING WEIGHT

	Nov. 3–6, 2011 %
Dietary changes	
Ate less/dieted (non-specific)	23
Counted calories/portion control	12
Ate more natural foods	10
Avoided sugar, sweets, soda	6
Did Weight Watchers program	5
Did Atkins Diet/low carb/high protein	4
Ate more fruits, vegetables/salads	3
Ate low fat diet	2
Exercise	
Worked out/exercises (non-specific)	31
Walked	5
Ran/jogged	3
Other	
Diet and exercise (non-specific)	8
Took diet pills/drugs	4
Pregnancy/birth-related weight loss	2
Attitude/discipline	1
Had gastric bypass surgery	1
Other	8

The base is 52% of Americans who have ever succeeded in losing weight. Percentages total more than 100% as a result of multiple responses.

SOURCE: Lydia Saad, "Most Effective Strategies or Methods of Losing Weight Named by Americans Who Have Ever Succeeded in Losing Weight," in *To Lose Weight, Americans Rely More on Dieting Than Exercise*, The Gallup Organization, November 28, 2011, http://www.gallup.com/poll/150986/Lose-Weight-Americans-Rely-Dieting-Exercise.aspx (accessed November 28, 2011). Copyright © 2011 by The Gallup Organization. Reproduced by permission of The Gallup Organization.

more than 10 attempts to shed pounds. (See Table 11.5.) More women (73%) than men (55%) said they have ever tried to lose weight. Women have also tried more often—on average making seven attempts, compared with men, who have made an average of fewer than four attempts.

CONSUMER ATTITUDES AND BEHAVIORS TOWARD DIET AND HEALTH

In *Nutrition and You: Trends 2011* (May 2011, http://www.eatright.org/media/content.aspx?id=7639), the Academy of Nutrition and Dietetics (formerly the American Dietetic Association) reports the findings from eight surveys conducted since 1991 that considered consumer attitudes and behaviors toward diet and health. The most recent survey of more than 750 adults aged 25 years and older was conducted by Mintel International Group Ltd. in May 2011. The academy observes that "Americans' desire to eat better and efforts to do so have not changed much since 2008."

Since 1991 the Academy of Nutrition and Dietetics has categorized respondents into three distinct groups—"I'm already doing it," "I know I should...," and "Don't bother me"—that describe their attitudes about maintaining a healthy diet and getting regular exercise. The 2011 survey finds that 42% of respondents were in the first group—"I'm already doing it." This group tends to have more females, is likely to have someone in the home who is on a diet for health reasons, and is likely to seek nutrition information from magazines. About two-thirds (62%) of this group said nutrition is very important.

The second group—"I know I should..."—consists of people aged 35 to 54 years and those who live in a four-person household. Nearly four out of 10 (38%) survey

FIGURE 11.6

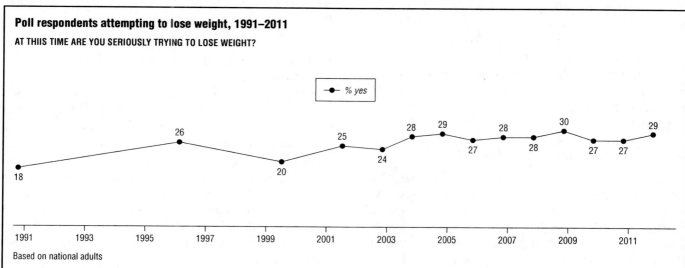

Poll respondents attempting to lose weight, 1991–2011

AT THIIS TIME ARE YOU SERIOUSLY TRYING TO LOSE WEIGHT?

Based on national adults

SOURCE: Lydia Saad, "At This Time Are You Seriously Trying to Lose Weight?" in *To Lose Weight, Americans Rely More on Dieting Than Exercise*, The Gallup Organization, November 28, 2011, http://www.gallup.com/poll/150986/Lose-Weight-Americans-Rely-Dieting-Exercise.aspx (accessed November 28, 2011). Copyright © 2011 by The Gallup Organization. Reproduced by permission of The Gallup Organization.

TABLE 11.5

Poll respondents' number of serious weight loss attempts, 2011

HOW MANY DIFFERENT TIMES, IF ANY, HAVE YOU SERIOUSLY TRIED TO LOSE WEIGHT IN YOUR LIFE?

Based on national adults

	Once or twice	3–10 times	Move than 10 times	Never	No opinion	Mean
	%	%	%	%	%	
National adults	25	30	8	33	4	5.3
Men	25	23	7	44	1	3.6
Women	26	37	10	22	6	7.0

SOURCE: Lydia Saad, "How Many Different Times, If Any, Have You Seriously Tried to Lose Weight in Your Life?" in *To Lose Weight, Americans Rely More on Dieting Than Exercise*, The Gallup Organization, November 28, 2011, http://www.gallup.com/poll/150986/Lose-Weight-Americans-Rely-Dieting-Exercise.aspx (accessed November 28, 2011). Copyright © 2011 by The Gallup Organization. Reproduced by permission of The Gallup Organization.

respondents were in this group. Forty-one percent said nutrition is very important but would like practical tips about how to improve their diet. People in this group were the most likely to appreciate the benefits of organic food and more likely to use magazines and the Internet to obtain nutrition information.

The third group—"Don't bother me"—consists largely of young men aged 18 to 24 years with less than a college education. One-fifth of respondents were in this group. People in this group were the least likely to be married or living with a partner.

The 2011 survey finds that about half (49%) of Americans said they are doing all they can to achieve balanced nutrition and a healthy diet. This represents an increase of five percentage points from 1991, when just 44% made this claim. Adults aged 65 years and older (66%) were the most likely to make this claim; people aged 45 to 54 years were the least likely (40%). Households with children were significantly less likely to report that they are "doing all they can."

The most frequently named reason for not eating healthier was "I don't want to give up the foods I like" (82%), followed by "I am satisfied with the way I currently eat" (75%) and "It takes too much time to keep track of my diet" (62%). In contrast, almost half (46%) said they are actively seeking information about nutrition and healthful eating and about the same proportion (41%) said they feel weight is an indicator of a healthy diet and that taking vitamins is necessary to ensure good health (42%). About one-third (35%) said "It seems like I'm always hearing information about what not to eat, rather than what I should eat."

Among the most promising findings were that 43% of respondents said they had increased consumption of low-fat foods during the past five years as well as low-sugar foods (34%), low-sodium foods (31%), and low-carbohydrate foods (28%). Nearly half said they had increased consumption of vegetables (49%), whole-grain foods (48%), fish (46%), chicken (44%), and fruits (41%).

Television remained the leading source of nutrition information (67% of respondents), followed by magazines

(41%) and the Internet (40%). Just 1% of respondents said they obtain nutrition information from nurses, health clubs, registered dieticians, or personal trainers and 2% named nutritionists as their source of information about diet and healthful eating.

Are Americans Getting Enough Exercise to Help Them Manage Their Weight?

In *Americans Still Exercising Less Than before Financial Crisis* (July 13, 2011, http://www.gallup.com/poll/148466/Americans-Exercising-Less-Financial-Crisis.aspx), Mendes reports that about half (53.4%) of Americans were exercising at least 30 minutes on three or more days per week in 2011. (See Figure 11.7.) According to Mendes, the overall rates of exercise have declined since 2008, with the exception of young adults aged 18 to 29 years, where there was a slight uptick in the percentage reporting regular exercise. (See Table 11.6.) There was also a slight increase in the percentage of African-Americans reporting participation in regular exercise, but this group along with people with less than a high school education, those earning less than $36,000 per year, women, and older adults remain the least likely to engage in frequent exercise.

OBESITY COMPROMISES EMOTIONAL WELL-BEING

The 2010 Gallup-Healthways Well-Being Index indicates that Americans who are obese are more likely to report being diagnosed with depression and to suffer from stress, worry, anger, and sadness than overweight or normal-weight adults. Nearly one-quarter (23.2%) of people who are obese said they have been diagnosed with depression, compared with 14.3% of people who are normal weight, 14.9% of people who are overweight, and 19.1% of people who are underweight. (See Table 11.7.) Interestingly, people who are overweight and those who are underweight suffer from comparable rates of stress, worry, anger, and sadness.

In view of these findings, it is not unexpected that people who are obese and those who are underweight report less happiness and enjoyment in life than their overweight

FIGURE 11.7

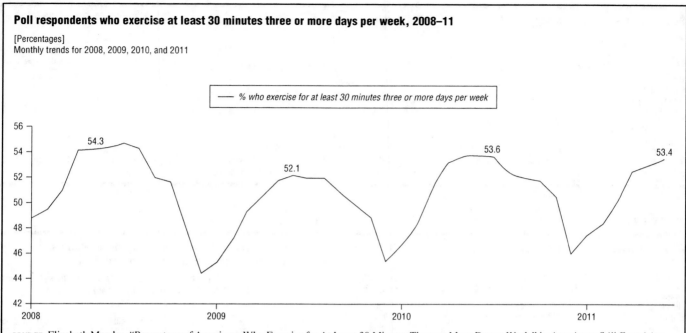

Poll respondents who exercise at least 30 minutes three or more days per week, 2008–11

[Percentages]
Monthly trends for 2008, 2009, 2010, and 2011

—— % who exercise for at least 30 minutes three or more days per week

SOURCE: Elizabeth Mendes, "Percentage of Americans Who Exercise for At Least 30 Minutes Three or More Days a Week," in *Americans Still Exercising Less Than before Financial Crisis*, The Gallup Organization, July 13, 2011, http://www.gallup.com/poll/148466/Americans-Exercising-Less-Financial-Crisis.aspx (accessed November 28, 2011). Copyright © 2011 by The Gallup Organization. Reproduced by permission of The Gallup Organization.

TABLE 11.6

Poll respondents who exercise at least 30 minutes three or more days per week, by demographics, 2008–11

[Percentages]

In order by percent change

	2008	2009	2010	2011 (January–June)	Change (in pct. pts.) 2011 vs. 2008
Aged 65 years old and older	50.9	48.8	49.0	48.4	−2.5
45- to 64-year-olds	51.0	48.9	50.2	49.6	−1.4
Hispanic	52.9	50.4	51.6	51.5	−1.4
East	50.8	49.2	50.3	49.6	−1.2
High school or less	49.0	46.7	48.1	48.0	−1.0
White	51.8	49.9	51.2	50.9	−0.9
Women	50.0	48.4	49.8	49.3	−0.7
West	55.4	53.8	55.2	54.7	−0.7
Postgraduate	57.1	55.8	57.6	56.4	−0.7
South	51.0	48.7	50.2	50.3	−0.7
Men	53.7	51.5	53.1	53.1	−0.6
$36,000 to $89,999 per year	51.9	50.0	51.5	51.3	−0.6
Less than $36,000 per year	48.9	46.9	48.4	48.3	−0.6
Technical/vocational some college	52.0	50.1	51.6	51.4	−0.6
College graduate	54.2	52.5	53.8	53.8	−0.4
Midwest	50.2	48.2	50.1	50.1	−0.1
30- to 44-year-olds	50.7	49.1	51.0	50.7	0.0
$90,000 or more per year	55.2	54.4	55.7	55.4	+0.2
Black	48.7	47.8	49.6	49.9	+1.2
18- to 29-year-olds	55.3	54.1	56.5	56.7	+1.4

SOURCE: Elizabeth Mendes, "Percentage of Americans Who Report Exercising At Least 30 Minutes Three or More Days a Week by Demographic Group," in *Americans Still Exercising Less Than Before Financial Crisis*, The Gallup Organization, July 13, 2011, http://www.gallup.com/poll/148466/Americans-Exercising-Less-Financial-Crisis.aspx (accessed November 28, 2011). Copyright © 2011 by The Gallup Organization. Reproduced by permission of The Gallup Organization.

and normal-weight peers. (See Table 11.8.) In *Obesity Linked to Lower Emotional Wellbeing* (September 17, 2010, http://www.gallup.com/poll/143045/Obesity-Linked-Lower-Emotional-Wellbeing.aspx), Mendes explains that even though it remains unclear whether people who are stressed, worried, or depressed are more likely to become

TABLE 11.7

Poll respondents experiencing negative emotions by BMI, 2010

	% stress	% worry	% anger	% sadness	% diagnosed with depression
Obese	41.6	34.5	15.7	19.9	23.2
Overweight	37.4	29.5	13.1	15.8	14.9
Normal weight	39.4	30.6	12.6	16.3	14.3
Underweight	42.0	35.9	16.0	21.3	19.1

BMI = Body mass index.

SOURCE: Elizabeth Mendes, "Percentage of Americans Experiencing Negative Emotions, by BMI Category," in *Obesity Linked to Lower Emotional Wellbeing*, The Gallup Organization, September 17, 2010, http://www.gallup.com/poll/143045/Obesity-Linked-Lower-Emotional-Wellbeing.aspx (accessed November 28, 2011). Copyright © 2011 by The Gallup Organization. Reproduced by permission of The Gallup Organization.

TABLE 11.8

Poll respondents experiencing positive emotions by BMI, 2010

	% enjoyment	% happiness
Obese	82.1	85.9
Overweight	85.3	88.4
Normal weight	86.3	89.5
Underweight	82.0	87.2

BMI = Body mass index.

SOURCE: Elizabeth Mendes, "Percentage of Americans Experiencing Positive Emotions, by BMI Category," in *Obesity Linked to Lower Emotional Wellbeing*, The Gallup Organization, September 17, 2010, http://www.gallup.com/poll/143045/Obesity-Linked-Lower-Emotional-Wellbeing.aspx (accessed November 28, 2011). Copyright © 2011 by The Gallup Organization. Reproduced by permission of The Gallup Organization.

TABLE 11.9

Poll respondents who feel companies should be allowed to refuse to hire workers who are significantly overweight, 2011

DO YOU THINK COMPANIES SHOULD BE ALLOWED TO REFUSE TO HIRE PEOPLE JUST BECAUSE THEY ARE SIGNIFCANTLY OVERWEIGHT/THEY SMOKE, OR NOT?

	Yes, should	No, should not
They are significantly overweight	14%	84%
They smoke	14%	85%

SOURCE: Elizabeth Mendes, "Do You Think Companies Should Be Allowed to Refuse to Hire People Just Because They Are Significantly Overweight/They Smoke or Not?" in *Americans Don't Want Biases in Hiring Smokers, the Overweight*, The Gallup Organization, July 22, 2011, http://www.gallup.com/poll/148619/Americans-Don-Biases-Hiring-Smokers-Overweight.aspx (accessed November 28, 2011). Copyright © 2011 by The Gallup Organization. Reproduced by permission of The Gallup Organization.

obese or these emotional states are a consequence of obesity, elevated levels of "stress, worry, anger, sadness, and depression in particular decrease a person's quality of life" and can compromise the affected individual's engagement in society and work.

How Do Americans Feel about People Who Are Overweight?

In view of instances of discrimination against people who are overweight or obese and the stigma that is associated with being overweight, Mendes indicates in *Americans Don't Want Biases in Hiring Smokers, the Overweight* (July 22, 2011, http://www.gallup.com/poll/148619/Americans-Don-Biases-Hiring-Smokers-Overweight.aspx) that an overwhelming majority (84%) of Americans claimed in a July 2011 Gallup poll that companies should not be allowed to refuse to hire people who are significantly overweight. (See Table 11.9.)

Even though Americans clearly do not want to see employers discriminate against people who are significantly overweight, they are divided about charging people who are significantly overweight higher health insurance premiums. Over four out of 10 (42%) of those polled in July 2011 said higher health insurance rates are justified, whereas 57% felt higher rates are unjustified. (See Table 11.10.) Mendes

observes that Americans with higher incomes and levels of educational attainment are more inclined to favor higher health insurance rates for people who are overweight than people with lower incomes and educational attainment. More men (50%) than women (35%) felt higher rates are justified for people who are overweight. (See Table 11.11.) Similarly, nearly twice as many men (19%) as women (10%) said employers should be permitted to discriminate against job applicants who are significantly overweight.

How Do People Who Are Obese View Obesity?

Rebecca M. Puhl et al. of Yale University looked at how people who are obese view obesity and reported their results in "Attitudes toward Obesity in Obese Persons: A Matched Comparison of Obese Women with and without Binge Eating" (*Eating and Weight Disorders*, vol. 15, no. 3, September 2010). The researchers also sought to compare weight bias in two distinct groups: women who are obese and women who are obese and suffer from binge eating disorder. Both groups of women were screened for symptoms of depression, completed two measures of attitudes about obesity that asked respondents to express agreement or disagreement with certain statements about obese people, and completed a questionnaire to assess their self-esteem.

TABLE 11.10

Public opinion about whether persons who are significantly overweight should pay higher insurance rates, July 2011

DO YOU THINK IT WOULD BE JUSTIFIED OR UNJUSTIFIED TO SET HIGHER HEALTH INSURANCE RATES FOR PEOPLE WHO ARE SIGNIFCANTLY OVERWEIGHT/SMOKE?

	Justified	Unjustified
Are significantly overweight	42%	57%
Smoke	60%	38%

SOURCE: Elizabeth Mendes, "Do You Think It Would Be Justified or Unjustified to Set Higher Health Insurance Rates for People Who Are Significantly Overweight/They Smoke?" in *Americans Don't Want Biases in Hiring Smokers, the Overweight*, The Gallup Organization, July 22, 2011, http://www.gallup.com/poll/148619/Americans-Don-Biases-Hiring-Smokers-Overweight.aspx (accessed November 28, 2011). Copyright © 2011 by The Gallup Organization. Reproduced by permission of The Gallup Organization.

TABLE 11.11

Public opinion about whether persons who are significantly overweight should pay higher insurance rates or be discriminated against in hiring, by sex, 2011

Gender views toward significantly overweight people

	Men	Women
It is justified to set higher health insurance rates for them	50%	35%
Companies should be allowed to refuse to hire them	19%	10%

SOURCE: Elizabeth Mendes, "Gender Views toward Significantly Overweight People," in *Americans Don't Want Biases in Hiring Smokers, the Overweight*, The Gallup Organization, July 22, 2011, http://www.gallup.com/poll/148619/Americans-Don-Biases-Hiring-Smokers-Overweight.aspx (accessed November 28, 2011). Copyright © 2011 by The Gallup Organization. Reproduced by permission of The Gallup Organization.

Puhl et al. find no differences in attitudes toward obese people between the two groups of women, but they note that both groups endorsed many anti-fat attitudes and negative weight-based stereotypes. The most prominent difference between the groups was that women with binge eating disorder who reported more favorable attitudes toward obese people had higher self-esteem and lower levels of depression. Puhl et al. conclude, "The presence of weight bias among obese persons suggests the need for stigma-reduction interventions to target all individuals, including obese persons. Interventions may need to be tailored in ways that address potential internalization of weight bias among obese individuals."

Many People Who Are Overweight and Obese Do Not Feel Their Weight Increases Health Risks

The results of a study presented at the American College of Emergency Physicians meeting in San Francisco, California, in October 2011 suggest that many people who are overweight or obese do not believe their weight poses a health risk. Jenifer Goodwin reports in "Many Don't Believe Their Obesity Poses Health Risks: Study" (HealthDay, October 15, 2011) that researchers at the University of Florida, Gainesville, asked 450 patients visiting the emergency department at a Florida hospital whether they believed their weight endangered their health and whether a physician or other health professional ever told them that they are overweight. More than half (53%) of the overweight and obese men and far fewer women (38%) surveyed felt their weight was not a problem. Among the obese people who were surveyed, a higher proportion (70%) said their weight posed a health risk.

Slightly more than one-third of men and half of the women said their physicians had discussed their weight with them. Of those who perceived their weight as a health problem, just 19% reported talking about it with a health professional.

Americans Are Concerned about Childhood Obesity

According to the report "Drug Abuse Now Equals Childhood Obesity as Top Health Concern for Kids" (August 15, 2011, http://www.med.umich.edu/mott/npch/pdf/081511top tenreport.pdf), childhood obesity is number one on the list of the top-10 health concerns for children named by the C.S. Mott Children's Hospital (University of Michigan Health System) National Poll on Children's Health issues. In May 2011 adults were asked to rate 23 health concerns affecting children. The list included some relatively recent threats such as Internet safety and children's use of technology, but obesity was named by 33% of respondents, followed by drug abuse (33%) and smoking and tobacco use (25%).

Are Parents to Blame for Children's Obesity?

There is no question that parents play a pivotal role in terms of preventing childhood obesity by shaping their children's early eating and physical activity habits. However, should overweight children be taken away from their parents? Gaëlle Faure reports in "Should Parents of Overweight Kids Lose Custody?" (*Time*, October 16, 2009) that in recent years there have been several cases in which a child's obesity resulted in parents losing custody of the child. Removing children from their home is a controversial move, but some health professionals believe there are instances in which it can literally save a child's life or at least prevent the development of serious health problems such as type 2 diabetes, hypertension, sleep apnea, and high cholesterol. For example, in South Carolina a 14-year-old boy who weighed 555 pounds (252 kg) was removed from his mother's custody in May 2009, and child-neglect charges were leveled against the mother.

According to Faure, health professionals who do not support the practice of removing obese children from their home observe that multiple factors affect a child's weight and that parents are but one of these influences. They point to genetic predisposition, socioeconomic status, and environmental factors as contributing to children's excess weight. They also note that children of all ages have been found to undermine their parents' best intentions by "sneaking extra food behind their parents' backs."

Faure indicates that many parents deny that their obese children have a weight problem. The parents of obese children, who often are overweight or obese themselves, may be reluctant to address the many challenges inherent in modifying their diet and increasing physical activity. Parents may also be hampered in their efforts by a lack of community resources. In some communities there are no weight-loss programs for children and teens with clinically severe obesity. For example, in the case of the South Carolina teen, all the services for obese children considered him beyond the maximum weight their programs could accommodate.

Todd Varness et al. of the University of Wisconsin School of Medicine and Public Health suggest in "Childhood Obesity and Medical Neglect" (*Pediatrics*, vol. 123, no. 1, January 1, 2009) that removal of a child from the home is only justified when three of the following conditions are met:

1. A high likelihood that serious imminent harm will occur;

2. A reasonable likelihood that coercive state intervention will result in effective treatment; and

3. The absence of alternative options for addressing the problem.

The researchers indicate that even though all three criteria are met quite infrequently, when they are, "a trial of enforced treatment outside the home may be indicated, to protect the child from irreversible harm."

In "State Intervention in Life-Threatening Childhood Obesity" (*Journal of the American Medical Association*, vol. 306, no. 2, July 13, 2011), Lindsey Murtagh and David S. Ludwig support the use of state intervention in cases of life-threatening obesity. They observe, "Improper feeding practices, causing undernourishment and failure to thrive, have long been addressed through the child abuse and neglect framework." Murtagh and Ludwig assert that physicians are, or should be obligated, to inform child protective services in "cases of children for whom chronic parental neglect has resulted in severe weight-related health complications." In contrast, Susan Z. Yanovski, Jack A. Yanovski, and Mary Horlick point out in "Life-Threatening Childhood Obesity and Legal Intervention" (*Journal of the American Medical Association*, vol. 306, no. 16, October 26, 2011) that obesity is highly heritable and that genetic factors play a key role in risk for obesity.

The article "200 Pound Child Removed from Home Because of Weight" (UPI.com, November 28, 2011) reports that in November 2011 an eight-year-old boy who weighed more than 200 pounds (91 kg) was removed from his home in Ohio and placed in foster care. This was the first recorded instance of a government agency intervening to remove a child from his or her home because of concern about the child's physical health. According to a spokesperson for the Cuyahoga County Department of Children and Family Services, the third grader was removed because his mother had not done enough to help him lose weight and failed to comply with his physician's orders. As a result, "case workers considered his mother's failure to reduce his weight a

form of medical neglect." A lawyer representing the boy's mother argued that the boy's weight does not pose an imminent danger to his health and that removing him from his family, school, and friends could result in emotional distress.

According to Tara Dodrill, in "Ohio Boy Removed from Home Because of Obesity Concerns" (Yahoo News, November 28, 2011), the case created a firestorm of commentary in the blogosphere via e-mail, Twitter, and other social media. Many people spoke out in favor of protecting the boy's health and preventing increasingly dire consequences of obesity, whereas others decried removing the child from his home because they fear the trauma will only serve to compound his problems. Still others called for support services and counseling to help parents and children who are overweight or obese.

Parents Misjudge Children's Weight

Several studies find that parents often misperceive their children's weight and underestimate their risk for obesity in adulthood. For example, Jessica Doolen, Patricia T. Alpert, and Sally K. Miller of the University of Nevada, Las Vegas, find in "Parental Disconnect between Perceived and Actual Weight Status of Children: A Metasynthesis of the Current Research" (*Journal of the American Academy of Nurse Practitioners*, vol. 21, no, 3, March 2009) that parents were less able to recognize their child's risk for obesity if they themselves were overweight. The researchers also note that cultural influences had an impact on parents' perceptions of children's weight, in that African-American mothers were more satisfied with their larger children than were white mothers. Doolen, Alpert, and Miller conclude, "If parents do not recognize their child as at risk for overweight or overweight, they cannot intervene to diminish the risk factors for pediatric obesity and its related complications. More research is needed to identify why this phenomenon occurs. Only then can effective interventions be initiated."

Another study examined the relationship between parents' underestimation of their child's weight and concerns about their child's weight and health. Jillian M. Tschamler et al. interviewed parents in a pediatric clinic, measured the height and weight of the children, and reported their findings in "Underestimation of Children's Weight Status: Views of Parents in an Urban Community" (*Clinical Pediatrics*, vol. 49, no. 5, May 2010). The researchers find that many parents—nearly half of the parents of overweight children and about one-quarter of the parents of normal-weight children—underestimated their child's weight. Parents of normal-weight children who underestimated their child's weight were more likely to be concerned about their child's weight than those who did not underestimate. Parents of overweight children who underestimated were less likely to be concerned about their child's weight than those who recognized their children as being overweight. Tschamler et al. conclude that parents who underestimate their children's weight status are not likely to be receptive to initiatives that are aimed at preventing childhood obesity.

IMPORTANT NAMES
AND ADDRESSES

Academy for Eating Disorders
111 Deer Lake Rd., Ste. 100
Deerfield, IL 60015
(847) 498-4274
FAX: (847) 480-9282
E-mail: info@aedweb.org
URL: http://www.aedweb.org/

Academy of Nutrition and Dietetics
120 S. Riverside Plaza, Ste. 2000
Chicago, IL 60606-6995
(312) 899-0040
1-800-877-1600
URL: http://www.eatright.org/

American Academy of Sleep Medicine
2510 N. Frontage Rd.
Darien, IL 60561
(603) 737-9700
FAX: (603) 737-9790
URL: http://www.aasmnet.org/

American Cancer Society
250 Williams St. NW
Atlanta, GA 30303
1-800-227-2345
URL: http://www.cancer.org/

American Diabetes Association
1701 N. Beauregard St.
Alexandria, VA 22311
1-800-342-2383
E-mail: AskADA@diabetes.org
URL: http://www.diabetes.org/

American Heart Association
7272 Greenville Ave.
Dallas, TX 75231
(214) 570-5978
1-800-242-8721
URL: http://www.americanheart.org/

American Society of Bariatric Physicians
2821 S. Parker Rd., Ste. 625
Aurora, CO 80014
(303) 770-2526

FAX: (303) 779-4834
URL: http://www.asbp.org/

**American Society for Metabolic
and Bariatric Surgery**
100 SW. 75th St., Ste. 201
Gainesville, FL 32607
(352) 331-4900
FAX: (352) 331-4975
E-mail: info@asbs.org
URL: http://www.asmbs.org/

Arthritis Foundation
PO Box 7669
Atlanta, GA 30357-0669
1-800-283-7800
URL: http://www.arthritis.org/

Atkins Nutritionals Inc.
1050 17th St., Ste. 1000
Denver, CO 80265
1-800-628-5467
URL: http://www.atkins.com/

Center for Science in the Public Interest
1220 L St. NW
Washington, DC 20005
(202) 332-9110
FAX: (202) 265-4954
E-mail: cspi@cspinet.org
URL: http://www.cspinet.org/

**Centers for Disease Control and
Prevention**
1600 Clifton Rd.
Atlanta, GA 30333
1-800-232-4636
URL: http://www.cdc.gov/

**Council on Size and Weight
Discrimination**
PO Box 305
Mt. Marion, NY 12456
(845) 679-1209
FAX: (845) 679-1206

E-mail: info@cswd.org
URL: http://www.cswd.org/

Eating Disorders Coalition
720 Seventh St. NW, Ste. 300
Washington, DC 20001
(202) 543-9570
URL: http://www.eatingdisorderscoalition.org/

Federal Trade Commission
600 Pennsylvania Ave. NW
Washington, DC 20580
1-877-382-4357
URL: http://www.ftc.gov/

International Food Information Council
1100 Connecticut Ave. NW, Ste. 430
Washington, DC 20036
(202) 296-6540
E-mail: info@foodinsight.org
URL: http://www.foodinsight.org/

**National Association to Advance Fat
Acceptance**
PO Box 4662
Foster City, CA 94404-0662
(916) 558-6880
URL: http://www.naafa.org/

**National Association of Anorexia Nervosa
and Associated Disorders**
PO Box 640
Naperville, IL 60566
(630) 577-1333
E-mail: anadhelp@anad.org
URL: http://www.anad.org/

**National Association of Cognitive-
Behavioral Therapists**
203 Three Springs Dr., Ste. 4
Weirton, WV 26062
(304) 723-3982
1-800-853-1135
E-mail: nacbt@nacbt.org
URL: http://www.nacbt.org/

National Center for Health Statistics
3311 Toledo Rd.
Hyattsville, MD 20782
1-800-232-4636
URL: http://www.cdc.gov/nchs/

National Center on Sleep Disorders Research
National Heart, Lung, and Blood Institute
6701 Rockledge Dr.
Bethesda, MD 20892
(301) 435-0199
FAX: (301) 480-3451
E-mail: nhlbiinfo@nhlbi.nih.gov
URL: http://www.nhlbi.nih.gov/about/ncsdr/

National Diabetes Information Clearinghouse
One Information Way
Bethesda, MD 20892-3560
1-800-860-8747
FAX: (703) 738-4929
E-mail: ndic@info.niddk.nih.gov
URL: http://diabetes.niddk.nih.gov/

National Digestive Diseases Information Clearinghouse
Two Information Way
Bethesda, MD 20892-3570
1-800-891-5389
FAX: (703) 738-4929
E-mail: nddic@info.niddk.nih.gov
URL: http://digestive.niddk.nih.gov/

National Eating Disorders Association
165 West 46th St.
New York, NY 10036

(212) 575-6200
1-800-931-2237
FAX: (212) 575-1650
E-mail: info@NationalEatingDisorders.org
URL: http://www.nationaleatingdisorders.org/

National Heart, Lung, and Blood Institute
PO Box 30105
Bethesda, MD 20824-0105
(301) 592-8573
FAX: (240) 629-3246
E-mail: nhlbiinfo@nhlbi.nih.gov
URL: http://www.nhlbi.nih.gov/

National Institute of Diabetes and Digestive and Kidney Diseases
Bldg. 31, Rm. 9A06
31 Center Dr., MSC 2560
Bethesda, MD 20892-2560
(301) 496-3583
URL: http://www.niddk.nih.gov/

National Mental Health Association
2000 N. Beauregard St., Sixth Floor
Alexandria, VA 22311
(703) 684-7722
1-800-969-6642
FAX: (703) 684-5968
URL: http://www.nmha.org/

National Women's Health Information Center
8270 Willow Oaks Corporate Dr.
Fairfax, VA 22031
1-800-994-9662
URL: http://www.womenshealth.gov/

Obesity Society
8757 Georgia Ave., Ste. 1320
Silver Spring, MD 20910
(301) 563-6526
FAX: (301) 563-6595
URL: http://www.obesity.org/

Rudd Center for Food Policy and Obesity
Yale University
309 Edwards St.
New Haven, CT 06511
(203) 432-6700
FAX: (203) 432-9674
URL: http://www.yaleruddcenter.org/

TOPS Club Inc.
4575 S. Fifth St.
Milwaukee, WI 53207
(414) 482-4620
URL: http://www.tops.org/

Weight-Control Information Network
One WIN Way
Bethesda, MD 20892-3665
1-877-946-4627
FAX: (202) 828-1028
E-mail: win@info.niddk.nih.gov
URL: http://win.niddk.nih.gov/index.htm

Weight Watchers International Inc.
175 Crossways Park West
Woodbury, NY 11797
(516) 390-1400
URL: http://www.weightwatchers.com/

RESOURCES

The Centers for Disease Control and Prevention (CDC) tracks nationwide health trends, including overweight and obesity, and reports its findings in several periodicals, especially its *Health, United States* and *Morbidity and Mortality Weekly Reports*. The *National Vital Statistics Reports*, which is issued by the CDC's National Center for Health Statistics (NCHS), gives detailed information on U.S. births, birth weights, and death data and trends. The NCHS also compiles and analyzes demographic data—the heights and weights of a representative sample of the U.S. population—to develop standards for desirable weights. The National Health Interview Surveys, the National Health Examination Surveys, the National Health and Nutrition Examination Surveys, and the Behavioral Risk Factor Surveillance System offer ongoing information about the lifestyles, health behaviors, and health risks of Americans. Working with other agencies and professional organizations, the CDC produced *Healthy People 2020*, which serves as a blueprint for improving the health status of Americans.

The U.S. Department of Agriculture provides nutrition guidelines for Americans, and the Federal Trade Commission (FTC) has launched initiatives to educate consumers and the media about false and deceptive weight-loss advertising. The FTC is one of about 50 members of the Partnership for Healthy Weight Management, a coalition of scientific, academic, health care, government, commercial, and public-interest representatives, that aims to increase public awareness of the obesity epidemic and to promote responsible marketing of weight-loss products and programs.

The relationship between birth weight and future health risks has been examined by many researchers, and the studies cited in this text were reported in *American Journal of Epidemiology, American Journal of Obstetrics and Gynecology, Circulation, International Journal of Cancer, Journal of Clinical Endocrinology and Metabolism, Journal of Women's Health, Obesity,* and *Pediatrics*. Data from the CDC Pregnancy Nutrition Surveillance System show that very overweight women benefit from reduced weight gain during pregnancy to help reduce the risk for high-birth-weight infants.

The World Health Organization and the National Institutes of Health provide definitions, epidemiological data, and research findings about a comprehensive range of public health issues, including diet, nutrition, overweight, and obesity. The Central Intelligence Agency's *World Factbook* provides longevity estimates. The National Heart, Lung, and Blood Institute conducts research about obesity and overweight. Weight-control information and updated weight-for-height tables that incorporate height, weight, and body mass index are published by the National Institute of Diabetes and Digestive and Kidney Diseases (the part of the National Institutes of Health that is primarily responsible for obesity- and nutrition-related research). The National Institute of Mental Health offers information about eating disorders as well as the mental health issues that are related to obesity.

The origins, causes, and consequences of the obesity epidemic have been described in numerous professional and consumer publications, including *AAOHN Journal, Adolescent Medicine State of the Art Review, Advances in Clinical Chemistry, American Family Physician, American Journal of Clinical Nutrition, American Journal of Epidemiology, American Journal of Managed Care, American Journal of Obstetrics and Gynecology, American Journal of Preventive Medicine, American Journal of Psychiatry, American Journal of Public Health, Annals of Behavioral Medicine, Annals of Internal Medicine, Archives of General Psychiatry, Archives of Internal Medicine, Archives of Pediatrics and Adolescent Medicine, Archives of Physiology and Biochemistry, Archives of Surgery, Bariatric Nursing and Surgical Patient Care, Behaviour Research and Therapy, Biological Psychiatry, BMC Public Health, Bulletin of the American College of Surgeons, Canadian Medical Association Journal, Cancer Causes and Control, Cancer Epidemiology, Child* and Adolescent Psychiatry and Mental Health, Circulation, Clinical Gastroenterology and Hepatology, Complementary Therapies in Medicine, Critical Care Clinics, Current Oncology Reports, Current Opinions in Obstetrics and Gynecology, Demography, Diabetes, Diabetes Care, Diabetes, Metabolic Syndrome, and Obesity, Diabetes, Obesity, and Metabolism, Diabetologia, Drugs Today, Eating Behaviors, Endocrinology and Metabolism Clinics, Endocrinology Nutrition, European Eating Disorders Review, European Heart Journal, European Journal of Clinical Investigation, European Journal of Epidemiology, Expert Review of Anticancer Therapy, Fertility and Sterility, Genomics and Health, Global Health, Health Affairs, Health Technology Assessment, Human Reproduction, International Journal of Behavioral Nutrition and Physical Activity, International Journal of Cancer, International Journal of Eating Disorders, International Journal of Eating Disorders Review, International Journal of Obesity, International Journal of Women's Health, Journal of Abnormal Psychology, Journal of Alzheimer's Disease, Journal of the American Dietetic Association, Journal of the American Medical Association, Journal of Clinical Endocrinology and Metabolism, Journal of Clinical Nursing, Journal of Digestive Diseases, Journal of General Internal Medicine, Journal of Maternal-Fetal and Neonatal Medicine, Journal of Medicinal Food, Journal of Nutrition, Journal of Obesity, Journal of Occupational and Environmental Medicine, Journal of Paediatrics and Child Health, Journal of Pediatric Gastroenterology and Nutrition, Journal of Pediatric Surgery, Journal of the Pancreas, Journal of Women's Health, Lancet, Mediators of Inflammation, Medical Care, Medical Clinics of North America, Medical Hypotheses, Medical News Today, Medicine and Science in Sports and Exercise, Medscape Medical News, Nature, New England Journal of Medicine, Neuropsychopharmacology, Nutrition Action, Nutrition Journal, Nutrition, Metabolism, and Cardiovascular Diseases, Obesity, Obesity Reviews, Orthopedic Clinics of North America, Pediatrics, Pediatric Blood Cancers, Pediatric Clinics of North America, Physiology and Behavior, PLoS Medicine, PLoS One, Psychiatric Clinics of North America, Public Health Reports, Scandinavian Journal of Public Health, Seminars in Reproductive Medicine, Social Science Quarterly, Surgical Endoscopy, and Therapeutic Advances in Cardiovascular Disease.

Several excellent books and publications provided valuable insight into the obesity epidemic. Peter N. Stearns, in *Fat History: Bodies and Beauty in the Modern West* (1997), and Laura Fraser, in *Losing It: False Hopes and Fat Profits in the Diet Industry* (1998), offer detailed histories of magical cures and weight-loss fads. In *Diabesity: The Obesity-Diabetes Epidemic That Threatens America—And What We Must Do to Stop It* (2005), Francine Ratner Kaufman, the former president of the American Diabetes Association, contends that the diabesity epidemic "imperils human existence as we now know it." David A. Kessler, the former commissioner of the U.S. Food and Drug Administration, explains in *The End of Overeating: Taking Control of the Insatiable American Appetite* (2009) how the desire to eat and overeat originates in the brain and is triggered by a variety of combinations of salt, fat, and sugar in the American diet.

Medical and public health societies, along with advocacy organizations, professional associations, and foundations, offer a wealth of information about the relationship between weight, health, and disease. Sources cited in this edition include the Academy of Nutrition and Dietetics, the American Heart Association, the American Medical Association, the American Obesity Association, the Center for Consumer Freedom, the Center for Science in the Public Interest, the International Size Acceptance Association, the National Academy of Sciences, the National Association to Advance Fat Acceptance, the National Eating Disorders Association, the Pharmacy Benefit Management Institute, the Public Health Advocacy Institute, and the Trust for America's Health.

The Gallup Organization makes available valuable poll and survey data about Americans' attitudes about overweight, obesity, physical activity, diet, and nutrition. Finally, many professional associations, voluntary medical organizations, and foundations dedicated to research, education, and advocacy about eating disorders, overweight, and obesity provided up-to-date information that was included in this edition.

INDEX

Page references in italics refer to photographs. References with the letter t following them indicate the presence of a table. The letter f indicates a figure. If more than one table or figure appears on a particular page, the exact item number for the table or figure being referenced is provided.

Q

"The Quality and Monetary Value of Diets Consumed by Adults in the United States" (Rehm, Monsivais, & Drewnowski), 168

"Quest for a Long Life Gains Scientific Respect" (Wade), 158

R

Race/ethnicity
eating disorders and, 150–151
inactivity by, 104
low birthweights/very low birthweights by, 6*t*
obese adults and, 3–4
obese adults in selected communities by, 3*t*–4*t*
obesity and, 14
physical activity, percentage of adults age 18 and older who engaged in regular, by, 108*f*

Racine, Sarah E., 51

Ramlau-Hansen, Cecilia Høst, 45

Randell, Rebecca, 115

"A Randomized Trial Comparing Human E-Mail Counseling, Computer-Automated Tailored Counseling, and No Counseling in an Internet Weight Loss Program" (Tate, Jackvony, & Wing), 114

"A Randomized Trial of a Low-Carbohydrate Diet vs. Orlistat Plus a Low-Fat Diet for Weight Loss" (Yancy et al.), 150

Rankin, Judith, 45

Rankinen, Tuomo, 34

"Rapid Postnatal Weight Gain and Visceral Adiposity in Adulthood: The Fels Longitudinal Study" (Demerath), 7–8

Rasu, Rafia S., 127

"Recent Improvements in Bariatric Surgery Outcomes" (Encinosa et al.), 127

Recommendations for Preventive Pediatric Health Care by the American Academy of Pediatrics, 80

"Recommended Community Strategies and Measurements to Prevent Obesity in the United States" (Khan et al.), 161

Red Flag Campaign, 156–157

Reduced calorie menus
Asian-American cuisine, 98(*t*5.9)
lacto-ovo vegetarian cuisine, 99(*t*5.11)
Mexican-American cuisine, 99(*t*5.10)
southern cuisine, 98(*t*5.8)
traditional American cuisine—1,200 calories, 96*f*
traditional American cuisine—1,600 calories, 97*f*

Reed, Mary Jane, 42–43

Rehm, Colin D., 168

"Relationship between Body Mass Index and Perceived Insufficient Sleep among U.S. Adults: An Analysis of 2008 BRFSS Data" (Wheaton), 44

"Remarks by the President and First Lady at the Signing of the Healthy, Hunger-Free Kids Act" (White House press release), 137

Renn, Crystal, 59

"Reproductive Health of Women Electing Bariatric Surgery" (Gosman), 45

Research
funding for various research, conditions, disease categories, estimates of, 122*t*–126*t*
funding obesity research, 121

"Researcher Sees Future Where People Walk at Work" (Kamowski), 171

"Response of the Food and Beverage Industry to the Obesity Threat" (Koplan & Brownell), 139–140

Restaurants
decline in numbers, 168
eating out, 18–21
PPACA requirements for, 138
See also Fast food

Restrictive techniques, 111–112

"Retailers, NGOs, and Food and Beverage Industry Launch National Initiative to Help Reduce Obesity" (HWCF), 140

Reuser, Mieke, 121, 123

"A Review and Primer of Molecular Genetic Studies of Anorexia Nervosa" (Klump & Gobrogge), 57

Rhode Island, 118

The Rice Diet Cookbook (Rosati), 89

Ridgway, Charlotte L., 6–7

Rimonabant, 110

Rimonabant Briefing Document (FDA), 110

Ringdahl, Erika, 42

Risks. *See* Health risks

"Risks and Management of Obesity in Pregnancy: Current Controversies" (Wax), 46

Robinson, Malcolm K., 113

Rochman, Bonnie, 74–75

Rogers, Lois, 138

"The Role and Challenges of the Food Industry in Addressing Chronic Disease" (Yach), 140

"Role of Dietary Factors and Food Habits in the Development of Childhood Obesity: A Commentary by the ESPGHAN Committee on Nutrition" (Agostini et al.), 71

Rombauer, Irma S., 21

Root, Tammy L., 50

Rosati, Kitty Gurkin, 89

Rose, David P., 44

Rose, Michael R., 158

Roux-en-Y gastric bypass
description of, 111
diagram of, 111*f*
risks, side effects of, 112

Rubinstein, Tamar B., 54

Russell, George V., 117

S

Saccharin, 87

San Francisco, weight-based discrimination ban of, 143

San Francisco Human Rights Commission, 143

Santini, Ferruccio, 33

Saturated fats, 163

Schneider, Patrick L., 103

School Health Profiles 2010: Characteristics of Health Programs among Secondary Schools in Selected U.S. Sites (Brenner et al.), 73

"School Lunch Proposals Set off a Dispute" (Nixon), 137

School Meals: Building Blocks for Healthy Children (IOM), 137

Schools
children's diets, role of in, 73
overweight/obesity prevention in, 160–167
with physical education course in each grade, 76*f*
physical education programs of, 75–76
prevention efforts in, 160
promotion of unhealthy food choices, 74
revised elementary school lunch menus, 138*t*
surgeon general's recommendations for, 160
that allow purchase of less nutritious food/beverages, 73*f*

Schreffler, Laura, 59

Schroeder, Robin, 112

Schwartz, Marlene B., 142–143

Screening, 80–81

"Screening and Interventions for Obesity in Adults: Summary of the Evidence for the U.S. Preventive Services Task Force" (McTigue et al.), 127

Sealey, Geraldine, 139

Sears, Barry, 89

Sebelius, Kathleen, 131, 172

Secondary prevention programs, 57

Self-assessment, Americans', 179–180

"Self-Reported Clothing Size as a Proxy Measure for Body Size" (Hughes), 10

Sensa, 157

"Separate and Combined Associations of Body-Mass Index and Abdominal Adiposity with Cardiovascular Disease: Collaborative Analysis of 58 Prospective Studies" (*Lancet*), 9

Serotonin, 57

Sesame Street (television show), 74–75

"Shared and Unique Genetic and Environmental Influences on Binge Eating and Night Eating: A Swedish Twin Study" (Root), 50

"Why Dietary Restriction Substantially Increases Longevity in Animal Models but Won't in Humans" (Phelan & Rose), 158

"Why It's Good That the Food Pyramid Became a Plate" (Nestle), 165

"Why Men Should Be Included in Research on Binge Eating: Results from a Comparison of Psychosocial Impairment in Men and Women" (Striegel et al.), 150–151

Why We Get Fat and What to Do about It (Taubes), 90

Widom, Cathy S., 50

Wii Fit (video game), 75

Willekens, Frans J., 121, 123

Willett, Walter, 115, 166

Wilson, Amy, 128

WIN (Weight-Control Information Network), 38–39, 49

Wing, Rena R., 114

"With 'Healthy' Foods Like These, Who Needs Junk?" (Jacobson), 73

Witters, Dan, 121, 176

Women

    obese, discrimination against, 141

    overweight/obesity among, 4–6, 13–14

    reproductive health, 44–46

    weight trends, 175

    See also Gender

Woodard, Gavitt A., 113

Wootan, Margo G., 137

Work sites

    companies should be allowed discrimination in hiring overweight, opinion, 182(*t*11.9)

    overweight paying higher insurance rates/discriminated against in hiring, public opinion, 183(*t*11.11)

    overweight/obesity, prevention at, 160–167, 169–171

    prevention efforts in, 160

    surgeon general's recommendations for, 160

    weight-based discrimination and, 141

Workers. *See* Employees

World Factbook: United States (Central Intelligence Agency), 27

World Health Organization (WHO), 131–133

Wyoming, costs of obesity in, 118

X

Xenical, 111

Xu, Xiaohui, 6

Xue, Fei, 6

Y

Yach, Derek, 140

Yancy, William S., Jr., 150

Yang, Zhou, 128

Yanovski, Jack A., 33, 81

Yanovski, Susan Z., 150

Yeager, Selene, 171

YMCA, 128

Yoga, 115

Young, Lisa R., 21

Younossi, Zobair M., 43

Your Guide to Medicare Prescription Drug Coverage (CMS), 119

Yourself!Fitness and Kinetic (video game), 75

Youth Risk Behavior Surveillance System (YRBSS), 64

"Youth Risk Behavior Surveillance— United States, 2009" (Eaton et al.), 76

Z

Zagorsky, Jay L., 151

Zeratsky, Katherine, 149

Zinczenko, David, 90

The Zone: A Dietary Road Map (Sears), 89

Zuckerman, Laurie, 22